**Efferent Organization and
the Integration of Behavior**

CONTRIBUTORS

B. H. BLAND

KENNETH A. BROWN

JENNIFER S. BUCHWALD

MALCOLM B. CARPENTER

JERZY KONORSKI

A. S. MARGULES

D. L. MARGULES

JACK D. MASER

ARYEH ROUTTENBERG

KARL U. SMITH

ARNOLD L. TOWE

C. H. VANDERWOLF

I. Q. WHISHAW

EFFERENT ORGANIZATION AND THE INTEGRATION OF BEHAVIOR

Edited by JACK D. MASER

Department of Psychology
Tulane University
New Orleans, Louisiana

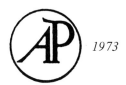 *1973*

ACADEMIC PRESS *New York and London*

ACADEMIC PRESS, INC.
111 Fifth Avenue, New York, New York 10003

United Kingdom Edition published by
ACADEMIC PRESS, INC. (LONDON) LTD.
24/28 Oval Road, London NW1

LIBRARY OF CONGRESS CATALOG CARD NUMBER: 72-77357

PRINTED IN THE UNITED STATES OF AMERICA

Contents

1. Efferent Response Processes: Relationships among Stimuli, Movement, and Reinforcement

Jack D. Maser

2. Physiological and Sensory Feedback of the Motor System: Neural-Metabolic Integration for Energy Regulation in Behavior

Karl U. Smith

3. Motor Cortex and the Pyramidal System

Arnold L. Towe

4. Subcortical Mechanisms of Behavioral Plasticity

Jennifer S. Buchwald and Kenneth A. Brown

5. Comparisons of the Efferent Projections of the Globus Pallidus and Substantia Nigra in the Monkey

Malcolm B. Carpenter

6. The Role of Prefrontal Control in the Programming of Motor Behavior

Jerzy Konorski

7. The Development of Operant Responses by Noradrenergic Activation and Cholinergic Suppression of Movements

D. L. Margules and A. S. Margules

8. Diencephalic, Hippocampal, and Neocortical Mechanisms in Voluntary Movement

C. H. Vanderwolf, B. H. Bland, and I. Q. Whishaw

9. Intracranial Self-Stimulation Pathways as Substrate for Stimulus-Response Integration

Aryeh Routtenberg

List of Contributors

Numbers in parentheses indicate the pages on which the authors' contributions begin.

B. H. BLAND (229), Institute of Neurobiology, University of Oslo, Oslo, Norway

KENNETH A. BROWN (99), Departments of Physiology and Psychiatry, Brain Research Institute and Mental Retardation Center, University of California, Los Angeles Medical Center, Los Angeles, California

JENNIFER S. BUCHWALD (99), Departments of Physiology and Psychiatry, Brain Research Institute, University of California, Los Angeles Medical Center, Los Angeles, California

MALCOLM B. CARPENTER (137), Department of Anatomy, College of Physicians and Surgeons, Columbia University, New York, New York

JERZY KONORSKI (175), Department of Neurophysiology, Nencki Institute of Experimental Biology, Warsaw, Poland

A. S. MARGULES (203), Department of Psychology, Temple University, Philadelphia, Pennsylvania

D. L. MARGULES (203), Department of Psychology, Temple University, Philadelphia, Pennsylvania

JACK D. MASER (1), Department of Psychology, Tulane University, New Orleans, Louisiana

ARYEH ROUTTENBERG (263), Department of Psychology, Northwestern University, Evanston, Illinois

KARL U. SMITH (19), Behavioral Cybernetics Laboratory, University of Wisconsin, Madison, Wisconsin

ARNOLD L. TOWE (67), Department of Physiology, School of Medicine, University of Washington, Seattle, Washington

C. H. VANDERWOLF (229), Department of Psychology, The University of Western Ontario, London, Ontario

I. Q. WHISHAW (229), Institute of Neurobiology, University of Oslo, Oslo, Norway

Preface

The modern, scientific analysis of action began in 1870 with a report by Gustav Fritsch and Eduard Hitzig that movement could be elicited by electrical stimulation of the dog's motor cortex. Neurological research on efferent mechanisms has made dramatic advances related primarily to muscle tone and posture. However, when viewing the richness of complex behavior, even in animals far removed from mammalian forms, one cannot but accept the fact that explanations based on postural mechanisms are grossly inadequate. On February 22, 1971, a conference convened in New Orleans for the purpose of assessing current approaches to the study of efferent organization and to discuss alternative conceptualizations.

During the planning of the meeting it was agreed at an early stage to invite scientists whose research and neuroscientific interests crossed the boundaries of their departmental appointments. The participants were to have a research history which led to the formulation of novel, yet scientifically testable hypotheses of efferent mechanisms. In this way we hoped first to gather from several disciplines recent empirical findings, second, to use this data to reexamine our preconceptions and assumptions regarding the neural basis of patterned movement, and third, to provide one or more theoretical frameworks by which to proceed.

Richard Jessor pointed out in 1958 that it is not always possible or profitable to explain behavioral phenomena in the language of physiology, the major difficulty being a terminology gap—terms which describe phenomena at one level of analysis either do not exist or do not have equivalent meanings at another level. This impediment did not arise at the meeting with the frequency some had predicted. I take this as evidence that the proper time had arrived to compare diverse research strategies and discover commonality of research interests.

Unfortunately, funding limitations placed restraints on the number of participants at the conference. It was decided, therefore, to invite other distinguished scientists to submit papers which would appear in the published proceedings. By design nearly all contributors avoided the spinal cord and peripheral nervous system. These omissions have resulted in a less complete picture than we would have preferred, but they also helped to focus our attention on a limited number of problems.

Acknowledgments

The meeting was held on the Tulane and Loyola University campuses and I wish to express my thanks to the administrations of both institutions for their cooperation. Funds to sponsor the six participants were provided by Tulane University, Loyola University, Louisiana State University in New Orleans, and the National Science Foundation (NSF Grant No. GB-27171). I am particularly indebted to Drs. S. Thomas Elder, Colonel Wallace, and Louis Sutker who served as my organizational contacts at Louisiana State University in New Orleans and at Loyola University. My appreciation and gratitude must also be extended to Nicholas Kierniesky, John Hensley, Debby Leftwich, John Wakeman, and Dr. Davis Chambliss, who generously contributed time and skill in preparation for conference activities. Publication of these proceedings would not have been possible without the support of Dr. and Mrs. Louis R. Maser and the contributors and editor express their gratitude. Finally, my wife, Irma, and daughter, Andrea, must receive a special accolade for their love, understanding, and companionship during a period when I seldom had the time to enjoy their company.

Chapter 1

Efferent Response Processes: Relationships among Stimuli, Movement, and Reinforcement

JACK D. MASER
DEPARTMENT OF PSYCHOLOGY
TULANE UNIVERSITY

I. Purpose

The purposes of this chapter are threefold. The first is to discuss several behavioral categories implicitly used in the papers of this volume. These papers are directed towards an analysis of the neural mediation of movement, and often employ behavior as a quantifiable variable. When the dependent variable is behavior, especially in infrahuman organisms, analysis of the origins of that behavior may be as important as its quantification (Bolles, 1970). Second, although somatomotor responses are a consequence of preceding efferent processes, a distinction should be made between efferent *response* and efferent *motor* processes. It is the contention of this writer that such a distinction would clarify many notions about the organization of the efferent system. Most current neuroscience textbooks present the traditional view that voluntary action is cortically initiated and mediated through the pyramidal system. Extrapyramidal pathways and their structures of origin are said to modulate somatomotor activity following servomechanism principles. Usually discussions of efferent organization omit movements of phylogenetic origin and the incentive properties of environmental stimuli. It will become apparent that the concept of an efferent response process, which includes the present concept of motor process, may result in a more useful model of the efferent system and of integrated behavior. To extend the range of hypotheses and data relevant to a response systems approach, this chapter will attempt to review theoretical points of view not represented by contributors to this book.

II. Behavioral Classification

A. Approach-Withdrawal

Behaviors discussed in this volume may be classified into four categories. approach-withdrawal, respondent, operant, and innate. These categories are by no means inclusive, but they represent a considerable portion of the ongoing activity of animals and man.

The approach-withdrawal dichotomy has the virtue of simplicity. The problem of defining and measuring specific responses, except gross direction of movement, is bypassed. Also, it is tacitly assumed that stimuli eliciting approach behavior are appetitive or positively rewarding, and those eliciting avoidance or withdrawal are punishing or aversive. Grastyan and his co-workers, for example, describe avoidance reactions toward a lever which, when depressed, produced a motoric rebound ipsiversive to the stimulated hemisphere. Motor rebounds contraversive to the site of self-stimulation are related to approach responses (Grastyan, Szabo, Molnar, and Kolta, 1968). In this case, the movements are related to the reinforcing value of the stimulation. Kaada, Rasmussen, and Kveim (1962) use a passive avoidance task in which an approach response must first be elicited toward an appetitive goal, such as food. Following such training, approaches to the goal are punished, resulting in avoidance. A modification of this task has been used by Ursin, Linck, and McCleary (1969). A start box was placed in the center of a straight runway. After meeting approach criterion, rats were shocked upon entering the goal for food. On test trials normal rats actively withdrew to the neutral goal box at the opposite end whereas septally damaged rats either passively remained in the central start box or continued to actively approach the formerly appetitive goal.

In the first of the three studies cited above, the movement effects of intracranial stimulation were correlated with the reward value of the lever press. "Reward value" was judged on the basis of approach to or avoidance of the lever, which had acquired stimulus incentive properties. Limbic structures were lesioned in the latter two studies. The experimental subjects persisted in the previously adaptive response in spite of changed contingencies of reinforcement. Movements involved in approach or avoidance were modified by reward and punishment, and structures not traditionally classified as motor were judged to be somehow involved.

B. OPERANT

The class of operant behaviors may be described as voluntary acts emitted by the organism which may serve to modify his environment. Prior to its use as an instrument of environmental change, the operant is uncorrelated with a reinforcing event. It is, however, emitted at a frequency convenient to the experimenter. Response frequency shifts from some baseline rate when reinforcement is made contingent on its emission. Stimuli which elicit the response are seldom observed or known. If, however, a distinctive cue is associated with the response-reinforcement event, it may come to set the occasion for operant emission. All movements which are equally effective in attaining reinforcement under a given set of conditions are members of the same response class. If the animal emits a behavior in that response class which results in the addition of an appetitive stimulus (positive reinforcement), or in the elimination of an aversive stimulus (negative reinforcement), the frequency of that class of responses will increase in a predictable fashion. (Punishment may be defined as the addition of an aversive stimulus or the subtraction of an appetitive one following a response. Under this condition, response probability decreases.)

This paradigm has been found useful for explaining purposive behaviors (Skinner, 1966). The rat does not press a lever *to obtain* food, but because *in the past* he obtained food when the lever was depressed. We place a telephone receiver to our ear because in the past we have heard voices by doing so. Conceivably, even "aimless" movements eventually affect some environmental change and if this change constitutes a reinforcing event, then in similar situations the probability of that response reoccurring increases. Continued training eliminates excess motion and response topography sharpens, leading an observer to attribute to the organism such constructs as purpose, drive, and "acts of the will." These constructs are of little use to the neurophysiologist working at a lower level of reductionism and who requires a deterministic behavioral mechanism to complement his own observations.

C. RESPONDENT

As a class of behaviors, respondents are distinguished from operants by the operations which produce them (Skinner, 1938). The operations for conditioning an operant involve the arrangement of reinforcement contingent on the emission of a response, but respondent conditioning requires specific eliciting stimuli associated with a previously neutral stimulus. Earlier formulations referred to *pairing* a previously neutral stimulus (conditional stimulus) with a stimulus which reliably evoked some characteristic behavior reflexively (unconditioned response). Following a number of forward pairings in which the conditional and unconditional stimuli do not have simultaneous onsets, the unconditioned response in modified form appears after the presentation of the conditional stimulus alone. When this happens, the conditional stimulus becomes a conditioned stimulus (CS) and the behavior which it evokes is termed the conditioned response (CR).

An important change in behavioral theory has been advanced by Rescorla (1967) which may have implications for neuroscientists. Rescorla argues that behaviors learned through association of conditioned and unconditioned stimuli are better understood if the relevant condition is thought of as a temporal *contingency* between two stimuli, the function of the CS being to signal the probability of US occurrence. The notion of contingency includes what is paired and what is not paired with the US. This conceptual difference with Pavlov's notion of pairing CS and US allows a behavioral analog of neural inhibition. For instance, an animal will learn that the US follows presentation of one conditioned stimulus (CS+) but not the presentation of a second conditioned stimulus (CS−). When a CS− signals the nonoccurrence of shock, its presentation has been demonstrated to actively inhibit expression of the CR, fear (Rescorla and Lolordo, 1965; Hammond, 1966).

Pavlov (1960) originally maintained that the conditioned response represented a mirror of neural alterations. He therefore collected behavioral data as an empirical demonstration of neural excitation and inhibition. Pavlov's behavioral methodology has endured scientific scrutiny, and there is a recent revival of interest in the localization of Pavlovian processes. Theoretical articles by Kimble (1968, 1969) propose that the hippocampus is the locus of Pavlovian internal inhibition. This proposal will be discussed in a later section. Jerzi Konorski, a former student of Pavlov's, will discuss in Chapter 6 various modifications of CS+, CS− conditioning. Konorski describes animals instrumentally manipulating their environment in accordance with the reinforcement contingencies signalled by the CS+ or CS−. When the frontal cortex is experimentally damaged, behaviors "programmed" by CS−, signaling no reinforcement, are dramatically changed.

Except for the operations which produce conditioned responses and modify the frequency of operants, there is no clear distinction between Pavlovian conditioning and operant conditioning. Although initially reflexive, many CRs, such as avoidance behaviors, clearly come under voluntary control. No differentiation has been found in the nervous system for the two forms of learning. Even the autonomic nervous system, long thought to be resistive to operant techniques, has been shown to be susceptible to properly arranged contingencies of reinforcement and therefore voluntary control (Miller, 1969; Pappas, DiCara, and Miller, 1970; Benson, Shapiro, Tursky, and Schwartz, 1971). Miller (1969) contends that demonstrating operant conditioning in visceral structures removes a powerful argument in favor of two fundamentally different learning mechanisms mediated by different neural processes. This does not rule out our distinguishing between operant and respondent conditioning. We will maintain this distinction because of the different operations required at the behavioral level and because of a lack of neurophysiological clarity on how the two assumed processes might be united. Neurophysiologists are reasonably certain of most of the neural pathways mediating the unconditioned stimulus and unconditioned response, but our lack of information is apparent for pathways in which CS-US and CS-CR associations are represented. This absence of sound neurological explanation is even more apparent in the operant situation.

D. INNATE BEHAVIOR PATTERNS

The term "innate" is used here as a behavioral category and not as a behavioral explanation. Nor is this category exclusive. Experiential factors interact with genetic factors early in development, severely restricting the possible usefulness of a dichotomy. Innate behavior patterns have been most useful in the description of action early in ontogony or at low levels of phylogony. Furthermore, careful observation by ethologists has shown that only a fraction of the total movement in most species-typical behaviors is independent of practice (Hinde, 1970).

Behaviors classified as innate include orientating movements (kinesis and taxes) and fixed action patterns. Orientation movements lose their usefulness in phyla exhibiting behavior more complex than that of the Insectivora, but they deserve more attention than they have received as examples of simple efferent organization. Fixed action patterns are more closely related to the movements of interest in this book. The movement patterns are more complex than taxes or kinesis and may be characteristic of a species, higher systematic category, or even of an individual (Hinde, 1970, p. 22). Our attention will focus on species-typical behaviors, the movements of which are initiated or "released" by a given environmental stimulus. Once released, the behavior is, by definition, independent of further external control (Hinde, 1970). There remains, however, the possibility of internal control by proprioceptive feedback.

Species-typical behaviors are preprogrammed through genetic instructions. This conclusion is based on their high degree of behavioral stereotypy, the unique properties of releasing stimuli, and their resistance to major alterations by variables which influence learning processes. These characteristics seem to call for neuronal circuits which are activated by a limited range of environmental stimuli and which produce topographically consistent movements. It has been speculated that a species-typical behavior may be mediated by a group of neurons which, under optimal conditions and in the presence of the proper stimulus complex, has a probability of firing that approaches one. A spinal reflex has a similar probability, although its structural organization would be less complex (Brown, 1969). The functional organization of fixed action patterns would be stabilized by the animal's heredity, and if this were also true of anatomical organization, investigators would be fortunate indeed.

Some of the intriguing questions to be answered by students of the neural basis of responding are: What is the nature of the interaction between preprogrammed innate behaviors and learned operant movements? What is the relationship between stimulation-bound behaviors and positively reinforcing brain stimulation (Glickman and Schiff, 1967; Valenstein, Cox, and Kakolewski, 1969)? What is the neurological basis for a racoon, trained to place a coin in a slot prior to gaining access to food, to begin "scrubbing" the coin as it might a food object in its natural environment (Breland and Breland, 1961)? We hope to provide at least a partial answer to these questions in this volume.

III. Distinctions between Motor and Response Processes

There are six major theoretical inadequacies in the traditional view of efferent organization. Within the efferent motor framework it is difficult to explain:

1. Fixed action patterns.
2. How destruction of frontal granular cortex, septum, or hippocampus produces animals unable to quickly suppress dominant response tendencies or unable to initiate competing responses in the face of changed contingencies of reinforcement.
3. The observation of intracranial self-stimulation in extrapyramidal structures which were not previously considered part of a "reward" system.
4. The complex sequences of behavior which, under appropriate conditions, can be elicited by stimulating the brainstem. This is quite different from the muscle twitches obtained by stimulating area 4 of the cerebral cortex.

5. How stimulation-bound behaviors, once considered "specific" or fixed may be made "plastic" in the sense that a prepotent behavior may, in the presence of appropriate stimuli, be switched to another behavior.

6. The fact that out of a large response repertoire we select and initiate a limited number of movements appropriate to a given set of stimuli. How much of our behavior is the result of an interaction between stimuli with inborn incentive value and stimuli whose incentive is learned?

The efferent motor system is characterized by its participation in reflexive movements, postural mechanisms, and skilled, manipulative acts. These three activities represent a widespread conceptualization of efferent functioning (Granit, 1970; Monnier, 1970; Mettler, 1968; Roberts, 1967; Paillard, 1960). In each of the above activities the concept of volition and reference to modification of movement by changing external events is minimized. Furthermore, limbic structures known to be critical in response initiation, modulation, and suppression are rarely, if ever, mentioned in discussions of efferent organization. The efferent motor system aids movement coordination, but its role in evaluating external incentives is believed to be quite limited.

A response is defined as any change in muscle tension expressed by the organism in its interaction with the environment. The efferent response system functions as the neural basis of movements which are emitted in the presence of a behavioral choice. Sometimes that choice is restricted, as in the stereotyped movements evoked by releasing stimuli (fixed action patterns) or during early stages of Pavlovian conditioning.

The efferent response system provides a conceptual aid when attempting to account for volition and the effects on behavior by stimuli possessing cue or incentive value. Its usefulness lies in relating stimulus incentives to voluntary movement through neural structures not traditionally said to be involved in motor functions. The reflexive, postural mechanisms of the efferent motor system are not oriented to problems raised by stimuli interacting with behavior. The term volition is not used here in the sense of a homunculus "willing" the body to move, but rather is akin to the notion that operant conditioning provides a deterministic framework for apparent voluntary action. That is, an investigation of the organism's history of reinforcement will, in many cases, provide a means of explaining present actions. The neuroscientist, however, believes that behavior is an ephemeral event and the biasing effects of reinforcement must act upon the neural elements mediating behavior (Olds, 1963). In this sense, an explanation of volition must be in terms of the neural substrate mediating operant behavior.

The importance of external events for modulating efferent activity has only recently been appreciated. The fact that behavior is modified by fluctuations in the incentive value of stimuli seems to require that the efferent system interact with neuronal systems subserving learning and emotional processes. Evidence is mounting that efferent neural pathways mediating species-typical behaviors may be modified by environmental influences. This fact requires that the efferent system interact with neuronal systems with specific response functions dictated by the genotype of the species. The traditional efferent motor system is not denied; rather it is viewed as inadequate for describing the rich behavior of a normal organism. Muscular action in the absence of meaningful external stimuli is more appropriately categorized as a motor process than as a response process.

Innate behaviors, because of their topographic constancy, may not appear to be subject to choice or acquired modifications. Experimental evidence exists to argue that point. In a series of studies on the development of color preferences in chicks, Kovach (1971) reported that preferences could be considered neither purely innate nor acquired. Color preferences should be viewed "as constitutionally influenced perceptual and response tendencies which may channel the development of behavior in unique directions from the very earliest states of behavioural ontogeny [p. 397]." Another example is that primary punishment suppresses the apparently innate tendency of some rats to attack and kill mice (Myer and Baenninger, 1966), and secondary punishment of gerbils produces a long-lasting suppression of sand-digging behavior (Walters and Glazer, 1971). Moreover, Walters and Glazer report that secondary punishment enhances the alert-posturing response, also considered an innate response pattern in the gerbil.

The notion which these studies support is that innate behaviors are influenced or dominated by environmental manipulations, and that the efferent system subserving species-typical behaviors must interact with the efferent system subserving acquired behaviors. The fact that some innate behaviors are enhanced and others suppressed relates to a point raised by Bolles (1970) in a discussion of environmental limitations on innate behaviors. Bolles suggests the possibility that studies involving avoidance behavior in the rat may be confounded by species-specific defense reactions to aversive stimuli. Few feral animals survive by *learning* to avoid a predator, but rather initiate immediately innate defensive reactions. Domesticated laboratory animals revert to a restricted class of innate defensive behaviors when placed in aversive surroundings. When an animal is required to learn a response defined by an experimenter and not "dictated" by his heredity, that response will be learned slowly or not at all. Bolles proposes that avoidance responses are rapidly acquired only if they are species-specific defense reactions. The efferent motor system or traditional explanation of movement has simply ignored this problem.

The distinction between response systems and motor systems may be clarified by a comparison of experiments involving the same efferent neural structure. Thus, in a study of motor processes Rinvik and Walberg (1963) demonstrated that the corticorubral and rubrospinal tracts constituted a somatotopically arranged motor pathway functioning to facilitate flexor muscle tone. Distinct from this rubral influence on muscle tone is its possible influence on the response system. Smith (1970) observed a deficit in the ability of rubrally lesioned hooded rats to acquire a one-way avoidance, but found superior performance on a step-down passive avoidance test. Since behavioral testing was not initiated until the operated subjects showed no signs of motor dysfunction, Smith concluded that rubral hooded rats failed to initiate movements in response to appropriate stimuli as quickly as control subjects. The problem of response rapidity has also appeared in septal lesion studies (Maser, 1970; Liss, 1965), where interest centered on response rather than motor control. The Rinvik and Walberg study did not involve learned behavior, innate behavior, or incentive stimuli. The information it provided concerned muscle tone. Smith studied a major nucleus of the same pathway but observed changes in behavior based on reinforcement contingencies.

Supraspinal structures influence spinal cord efferent elements, allowing the response/motor distinction at this level also. In 1962 Lundberg and Voorheeve stimulated the motor cortex while recording intracellular responses from spinal motoneurons to stimulation of afferent reflex systems. When the motor cortex was activated, both excitatory and inhibitory spinal reflexes were enhanced, but this effect was eliminated following section of the pyramidal tract. This often-cited study used an acute preparation, not a behaving organism. In contrast, stimulation of the lateral hypothalamus, a structure rarely thought of as part of the classical motor system has resulted in enhanced lumbar ventral root discharges in response to dorsal root stimulation (Miles and Gladfelter, 1969). Since earlier work by Gladfelter and Brobeck (1962) had shown a permanent decrease in spontaneous locomotor activity, caused by ablation of the lateral hypothalamic region, the Miles and Gladfelter finding suggests that the intact hypothalamus participates in the modulation of spinal motoneuron activity. These authors believe that the decreased locomotor activity observed by Gladfelter and Brobeck (1962) was produced by a lesion-induced decrease in spinal motoneuron background excitability.

The numerous examples of behavior evoked by intracranial stimulation, especially to the hypothalamus, are related to the efferent response system, rather than to the efferent motor system. In this regard we have known since 1870 that movement occurs when the brain is electrically stimulated. However, there is a qualitative difference between stimulating "motor cortex" and observing muscle twitches in a restrained animal (Fritsch and Hitzig, 1870, in Pribram, 1969) and stimulating limbic nuclei and observing biologically significant behaviors.

A. RESPONSE ORGANIZATION IN THE BRAIN

Traditional theory and research on efferent organization focuses on the pyramidal system and on nonlimbic, extrapyramidal structures. The general notion is that movements are initiated by cortical cells originating in the pyramidal tract. Extrapyramidal structures then act to modulate the pyramidal command, largely through influence on gamma efferents in the spinal cord. Granit (1970) and Monnier (1970) are excellent recent sources on the traditional reflex-oriented approach to brain and spinal cord organization. Monnier (1970, Chapter 26), in particular, denotes the pyramidal system as the basis of voluntary skilled motor activity. Noticeably absent from each of the above discussions as well as Roberts (1967) and Paillard (1960) is a substantive discussion of any role for limbic structures in the organization of movement or of possible interactions between innate behavior patterns and the pyramidal-extrapyramidal systems. In this volume, the reader will find a pointed disregard of the pyramidal system's presumed importance for movement and a change in emphasis concerning the role of extrapyramidal structures.

Although the traditional approach to the neurology of movement regards pyramidal and extrapyramidal organization as the most salient feature, the efferent response view stresses the role of limbic nuclei such as the septal region, cingulate gyrus, frontal granular cortex, hippocampus, and hypothalamus. Furthermore, it is suggested that extrapyramidal structures not only influence the role of gamma motoneurons in regulating muscle tone, but also participate in fixed action patterns and interact with limbic response mechanisms (Glickman and Schiff, 1967; Routtenberg, 1971).

The present discussion will be limited to the hypothalamus as an efferent response structure. In later chapters Konorski discusses research on frontal cortex; Vanderwolf, Bland, and Whishaw elaborate on their studies on the hippocampus; Buchwald and Brown discuss behavioral plasticity in decorticate preparations; Carpenter presents anatomical findings important for much of the work on response processes; and Routtenberg sets forth a methodological and empirical discussion relating reward and movement.

B. The Hypothalamus

The small, compact structure called the hypothalamus is already burdened with responsibility for participation in sexual behavior, temperature control, hormone production and release, identification as the "head ganglion" for the autonomic nervous system, eating and drinking, and emotional expression. It is now emerging as an important participant in the mediation of appropriate responding. As the integrative center of the autonomic nervous system and the nodal point in the Papez-MacLean circuit, it is ideally situated to participate in somatic-autonomic integrations.

Involvement in response processes has been observed in diverse experimental situations. For instance, Komisaruk and Olds (1968) correlated firing patterns of single cells in the lateral hypothalamus and preoptic area with the behavior of the freely moving rat. During exploration or locomotion and especially during "voluntary" movement of the vibrissae, these neurons were active. Passive movement of the vibrissae (induced by the experimenter) or spontaneous facial grooming failed to fire the cell. Furthermore, the preoptic area was the site of stimulation-bound feeding and yielded high rates on a test of intracranial self-stimulation.

The lesion studies which demonstrate involvement of the hypothalamus in response modulation have used escape or avoidance tasks in order to rule out confounding due to hypothalamic control over alimentary and temperature regulation. Lesions to the anterior hypothalamus disrupt passive avoidance behavior in a manner very similar to that of septal lesions (Kaada *et al.*, 1962). In fact, the behavioral data of the 18 rats sustaining subcallosal, septal, preoptic, and anterior hypothalamic lesions were so similar that these authors treated all animals as a single group. The group took an average of 43.4 shocks compared with an average of 2.4 for the 24 normal control rats.

Active avoidance and escape behaviors are severely impaired by destruction of the far lateral hypothalamus (Runnels and Thompson, 1969), and Grossman (1970) observed that transection of the lateral connections to the medial hypothalamus produced reliably inferior performance on a signalized two-way avoidance task compared to that of a normal control group or animals suffering parasagittal knife cuts to the lateral hypothalamus. Those rats in the Grossman (1970) study which had received parasagittal cuts lateral to the hypothalamus displayed superior shuttlebox performance compared to normal control animals.

Undoubtedly related to hypothalamic involvement in response processes are consummatory acts and emotional expressions elicited by intracranial stimulation and self-stimulation phenomena. Eating, drinking, and sexual behaviors are highly stereotyped activities, the components of which are recognized by ethologists to be fixed action patterns. These movement patterns are reliably elicited from hypothalamic sites. The prevalent explanation that intracranial stimulation activates fixed or specific pathways has recently been challenged by Valenstein and his co-workers (Valenstein, Cox, and Kakolewski, 1969, 1970; Valenstein, 1969, 1970).

The efferent response process view is highly receptive to the notion that stimulation-bound behaviors are motivated motor acts rather than evoked preprogrammed, stereotyped movements. The role of appropriate goal objects necessary for the elicitation of a given stimulus-bound act emphasizes the importance of stimulus incentives directing movement. It was earlier pointed out that one distinction between response processes and motor processes is the role of stimulus incentives.

Valenstein's (1970) conviction is "that no specific relationship exists between a given hypothalamic site and a particular response [p. 209]." Rather, "the specific response that is elicited will depend on the relative prepotency of the different responses." Figure 1 is an empirical summary of hypothalamic influence on fixed action patterns. Notice that acquired responses are also functionally related to preprogrammed movements, and the resulting behavior may represent a compromise based on reinforcement contingencies. Pathway 1 in Fig. 1 represents a functional pathway from the hypothalamus to any of several fixed action patterns located in the brainstem. According to Glickman

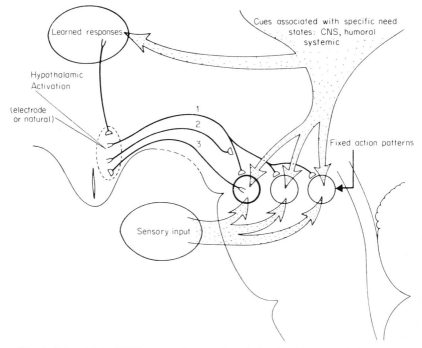

Fig. 1. Valenstein's (1970) conception of the relationship between reinforcement and response systems as suggested by experimental findings. See text for explanation. Reprinted by permission of the author and The Rockefeller University Press, New York.

and Schiff (1967), these fixed action patterns are mediated by extrapyramidal structures and their mere activation is reinforcing. Valenstein's conception of hypothalamic capacity to activate the "reinforcing brain system" is functional connection number 2. When a response is executed and reinforcement follows, the frequency of that response tends to increase, and connection 3 depicts the strengthening of that association.

IV. Current Theoretical Developments

A. VOLITION AND FEEDBACK

The problem of response control discussed here is really the age-old problem of volition. Kimble and Perlmuter (1970) have approached the acquisition of voluntary behavior as a sensory feedback phenomenon. Their conclusion that "voluntary behavior seems never to be prevented by the elimination of feedback" is based on observations in which manipulation of the peripheral nervous system failed to grossly disturb behavior. Since a positive conclusion was not to be found at the periphery, these investigators retreated centrally where feedback loops may be located. Why should central feedback loops not exist between portions of the mechanism concerned with response generation, just as there are feedback loops from muscle to the central nervous system? There is considerable logical demand for feedback between elements of the neural chain which participate in response execution. Note only the often-cited example of the pianist whose fingers race across the keyboard faster than muscular feedback could act to influence successive movements. Oscarson's work suggests to him (in Evarts *et al.*, 1971) that "the organization of many ascending paths suggests that they monitor activity in lower motor centers rather than peripheral events [p. 98]."

Although internal feedback would remove much of the explanatory pressure from a purely peripheral feedback view, the precise extent to which the periphery does regulate the expression of successive action remains an important question. In Chapter 2, Karl Smith discusses the strategy of measuring acts of motor skill to identify specific conditions by which metabolic change or a particular afferent feedback influences successive movements. Action-induced change in muscle metabolism is thought to be a source of feedback data for the nervous system.

Extensive respiratory and autonomic involvement has been demonstrated for the frontal lobe (Livingston, 1967; Livingston *et al.*, 1948) and for the limbic system (Kaada, 1951; Holdstock, 1969). Stimulation of area 4 has even produced blood pressure and respiratory changes at lower thresholds than required for production of somatic motor responses (Sachs and Brendler, 1948). The monitoring of metabolic states by the same structures which regulate somatic events constitutes an important source of feedback. For the nervous system to embark on a course of action without taking into account the current metabolic state is analogous to continuous operation of an automobile without reference to brake fluid, oil, or gasoline.

B. RESPONSE MODULATION

An empirical basis for an alternative hypothesis to replace reflexive, postural mechanisms as neural mediators of movement began to emerge during the 1960s. A suggestion by Stanley and Jaynes (1949) that "act-inhibition" was a major function of the frontal lobe was an early statement of efferent response processes. Performance, not learning, was impaired following frontal injury. The motor control of isolated muscles appeared intact, but response sequences to inappropriate stimuli were not inhibited. On the basis of a more extensive literature, Brutkowski (1965) further identified prefrontal cortex with behavioral inhibition and emphasized its neuroanatomical relationship with limbic-subcortical structures via (1) the caudate-subthalamus-hippocampal complex, and (2) the hypothalamic-amygdaloid complex. A response perseveration deficit resulting from lesions to the first was explained as a loss of inhibition of competing response tendencies, while "drive disinhibition" was induced by lesions to the prefrontal-hypothalamic-amygdaloid circuit.

Amygdaloid functions were reviewed in 1964 by Graham Goddard. He suggested that the amygdala played a role in actively suppressing motivated approach behaviors. This may explain why, when the incentive value of a stimulus shifts from positive to negative, amygdalectomized subjects fail to stop approaching. Emphases on motivational factors were derived in part from the fact that the amygdala participates in autonomic and endocrine responses to stress, and, in part on aversive components of amygdaloid stimulation. At high intensities, piloerection, hissing, urination, sudden flight, and other aversive-associated behaviors are observed. An intact amygdala is necessary for the normal acquisition of avoidance tasks, but not appetitive ones. This further supports the notion that the amygdala is involved in the regulation of fear. The outstanding approach deficit seen in amygdaloid animals is failure to withhold and modify a learned approach response in an aversive situation.

The most significant impact on conceptualizing an efferent response system is found in a classic review by McCleary (1966) entitled, "Response-modulating functions of the limbic system: Initiation and suppression." McCleary succeeded in bringing together a diverse literature, primarily demonstrating response dysfunction following experimental damage to the septal region, cingulate gyrus, frontal lobe, and hippocampus.[1] The dysfunction was characterized by facilitated performance on two-way active avoidance following cingulate damage (King, 1958; McCleary, 1961) or as deficient performance on one-way active avoidance (Lubar and Perachio, 1965) and passive avoidance tasks (McCleary, 1961). Furthermore, the dysfunction was evidenced on appetitive operant tasks: overresponding on fixed interval—1 min (Ellen and Wilson, 1963) and DRL—20 sec (Ellen, Wilson, and Powell, 1964); failure to suppress bar pressing behavior during S— presentation (Maser, 1970; Schwartzbaum, Kellicut, Spieth, and Thompson, 1964); and a deficit in position habit reversal (Zucker and McCleary, 1964).

McCleary's (1966) conclusions were: (1) "it now seems that what is disinhibited by the septal lesion is a response which, first of all, has a high probability of occurrence (or high habit strength) in the particular test situation,

---

[1] Gerbrandt (1964, 1965) had earlier reached similar conclusions. He spoke of mechanisms for response release and control. In the lesioned animal "stabilized" responses could not be suppressed in order for competing "unstable" responses to emerge and allow the animal to adapt to changed environmental contingencies.

if such a response exists under a given set of experimental circumstances." (2) The above conclusion applies to any currently ongoing behavior "even when it was the 'passive' response of withholding an active response." (3) We should not expect to find a unitary deficit. A syndrome which includes response perseveration, hyperreactivity, rage, increased thirst, and increased consumption of sucrose and saccharine may exist in the same septally damaged rat. The difficulty of subsuming these seemingly divergent actions under one mechanism is obvious. Clearly, response perseveration is not a motor deficit. It may be, however, that the response dysfunctions and the affective changes toward environmental stimuli are related through an efferent response process.

McCleary's response modulation hypothesis has been most useful as a heuristic model. The major empirical evidence for a response modulating *mechanism* is that of response perseveration. The danger is a tendency to view response modulation as an explanation of nonperseverative, "normal" movements. Just as instinct fails to explain stereotyped, species-typical behaviors, response modulation fails to explain volitional movement.

C. REACTIVITY

Explanations emphasizing changes in reactivity toward stimuli with incentive properties generally take the form of arousal hypotheses (Kenyon, 1962), or hypotheses relating limbic function to behavioral dispositions (Thomas, Hostetter, and Barker, 1968; Pribram, 1960). Data fitting the arousal hypothesis are provided by Novick and Phil (1969), who show that amphetamine administration to septal rats produces different reactions on tests of reactivity, activity, active avoidance, and passive avoidance. Related to the arousal hypothesis is the notion that limbic damage results in an increase in incentive motivation for positive reinforcement (Beatty and Schwartzbaum, 1967, 1968). When the incentive value of reinforcement shifts, lesioned animals increase responding due to heightened frustration or aversion. Kelsey and Grossman (1971) and Caplan (1970) have used DRL schedules of reinforcement to further support the Beatty and Schwartzbaum (1968) hypothesis. Caplan produced overresponding by withholding reinforcement for a previously rewarded response and also by making reward contingent on response suppression for 1.2 sec or longer. Since both conditions were seen as aversive, the differences between the septal and control animals may be due to a lesion-induced change in reactivity to stimulus reinforcing properties. Kelsey and Grossman (1971) also found that septal rats were unable to perform efficiently on DRL even when prior training did not include CRF. Therefore the observed perseveration was not due to an increased tendency to respond at some previously reinforced level. Since the experimental rats responded more frequently in situations where reinforcement was potentially available, an explanation in terms of response control modulated by motivational variables may be more appropriate than one describing an inability to suppress responding.

D. RESPONSE DECREMENT AND PAVLOVIAN INHIBITION

D. P. Kimble has published several articles proposing the hippocampus as the locus of Pavlovian internal inhibition (Kimble, 1968, 1969). Any of several operations can produce internal inhibition (Pavlov, 1927), including omitting the US; reinforcing the one CS (the CS+) and omitting reinforcement to another (the CS−); reinforcing the CS, but never reinforcing a stimulus compound composed of the CS and an additional stimulus; lengthening the interstimulus interval, which over many trials, will shift the response along a temporal baseline closer to US onset. (See Konorski's chapter in this volume for further explication of these operations and their relation to response inhibition.) Pavlov applied internal inhibition to explain experimental extinction, sleep, stimulus differentiation, and inhibition of delay, and Kimble's proposition is that this same construct be used to explain functions of the hippocampus.[2]

Damage to the hippocampus disrupts this "behavioral braking" mechanism in a manner similar to that of the septum for response inhibition (McCleary, 1966). The behavioral evidence supportive of Kimble's theory is largely taken from response perseveration data following hippocampal injury. More recent and direct support is provided by Micco and Schwartz (1971). CS+ and CS− were established by Pavlovian contingencies as signals of the occurrence of inescapable shock and the occurrence of no shock, respectively. CS+ presentation was then superimposed on a separately established operant for shock avoidance, wheel turning. The result was to facilitate the operant response in normal and hippocampectomized rats. However, only the normal subjects attenuated wheel turning during CS− presentation. As mentioned earlier, CS− may be viewed as an active inhibiter of the respondent evoked by the CS+, fear. Hippocampal destruction interfered with the expression of internal inhibitory properties attributed to the CS−.

Hippocampal rats display a response perseveration deficit remarkably similar to that of septal rats (Douglas, 1967). A strong case might be made that the septum is the neural locus of Pavlovian internal inhibition, and an even stronger case for a septo-hippocampal system mediating that function. Support for functional collaboration of hippocampus and septum is provided by Dafny and Feldman (1969). The reticular formation, hippocampus, and septum were

---

[2] Douglas (1967) has reviewed the hippocampal literature dealing with response perseveration. Although mentioning the Pavlovian model among four alternative hypotheses, Douglas prefers a model in which the hippocampus mediates attention through inhibitory efferent control of sensory reception. Gating-out of the CS implies that the CR would be omitted. Pavlov (1927), Rescorla and LoLordo (1965), and Hammond (1966) demonstrated active suppressant properties, reducing the CR.

stimulated and responsivity of hypothalamic neurons was observed. Reticular formation stimulation produced variable effects among hypothalamic neurons, but stimulation of hippocampus or septum predominantly led to inhibition of both spontaneous and evoked activity.

It is also very probable that the medial septal nucleus paces hippocampal theta activity. Intravenous application of hexobarbital and scopolamine eliminated medial septal cell impulses simultaneously with the cessation of hippocampal theta (Petsche, Stumpf, and Gogolak, 1962). Since the septal units continued to rhythmically discharge in the absence of theta, it is likely that the septal units are driving the hippocampal cells rather than vice versa (Stumpf, Petsche, and Gogolak, 1962). While pyramidal cells of the hippocampus produce theta, septal-hippocampal synchronization is initiated in the septum.

Komisaruk (1970) recently recorded activity in the hippocampus and septum, observing a high, stable correlation with rhythmic (7 Hz) vibrissae movements and cardiac function. The data suggest that motor neurons producing vibrissae movements are driven or modified by septal-hippocampal theta activity. These studies and similarities in response dysfunction previously mentioned indicate that a septo-hippocampal model may be more appropriate than either model alone.

E. ACTION AND REINFORCEMENT

Drawing heavily upon ethological and brain stimulation literature, Glickman and Schiff (1967) hypothesize that, at the neural level, reinforcement involves selective facilitation of motor patterns organized in the brainstem. The mere activation of extrapyramidal pathways subserving innate behavior patterns constitutes a reinforcing event. This may explain high rates of self-stimulation in several extrapyramidal areas. It may have a bearing on species-typical, stimulation-bound behaviors elicited from hypothalamic sites through which either descending extrapyramidal pathways course or diencephalic-midbrain connections originate.

The Glickman and Schiff model has been well received, although some data exist which may call for modification. Baenninger (1970) reports that Siamese fighting fish who "lost" and fled from fights with dominant conspecifics acquired an operant which terminated their view of a mirror. Since male Bettas typically release a complex aggressive display when presented with their mirror image, Baenninger holds a reinforcement explanation in terms of simply facilitating motor pathways to be insufficient. The model should include temporal changes in response strength and variations in stimulus control acquired through prior experience.

Milner (1970) hypothesized that motor activity is modulated by the intensity of goal stimuli and what Morgan (1957) has called the "central motive state." A mechanism for spontaneously generating response patterns is modified by the "response-hold," "response-switch" and "motor arousal" mechanisms. The response-hold process is activated by approach stimuli when the central motive state corresponding to those stimuli has opened the "gate" which permits relevant stimuli to be filtered through. Thus, to a hungry animal, food stimuli would be passed through its own gate to the response-hold system. As long as the current central motive state is active and the external stimulus maintains its incentive value, the response-hold mechanism will sustain the pattern in the response generator. There are no gates between receptors and the motor system in the case of aversive stimuli. Appetitive and aversive stimuli are biologically defined by the nervous system of the species since organisms which approach appetitive and aversive stimuli alike did not survive to reproduce. Noxious stimuli control the response-switch mechanism, whose dominance appears in the absence of positive or negative stimulus incentives. This dominance is evidenced through periodic shifts in response mode. There is no provision in this model for fixed action patterns and learning ability, but one might add only genetically coded memory and a memory potential compatible with learning.

V. Summary

This chapter attempts to provide a framework through which other chapters in this volume may be read. Briefly, this view states that efferent motor processes are not adequate to explain goal-directed behaviors, whether they be simple approach-avoidance movements, complex chains of operants, or innate response patterns. Voluntary behaviors are movements defined by a history of reinforcement and, in this sense, are equivalent to operants. The major inadequacy of the traditional motor approach is failure to take into account the role of stimuli which, through prior history of Pavlovian conditioning or genetic transmission, have acquired incentive properties. The pyramidal tract is deemphasized and the limbic system is viewed as participating in the modulation of movements related to stimulus incentives. The papers which follow are directed toward a neurology of movement which attempts to account for these variables.

Acknowledgment

Dr. Arnold Gerall read an initial draft of this paper and the author acknowledges with gratitude his critical comments.

Chapter 2

Physiological and Sensory Feedback of the Motor System: Neural Metabolic Integration for Energy Regulation in Behavior

KARL U. SMITH

BEHAVIORAL CYBERNETICS LABORATORY
UNIVERSITY OF WISCONSIN

I. Introduction

This chapter presents a revised theory of the role of the motor system in physiological regulation and neural-metabolic integration in energy production for behavior. The chapter revises classical and traditional views of the role and organization of the nervous system in motivation and energy control for response. In particular, we are questioning the scientific validity of past doctrines of physiological and psychological motivation in accounting for energy regulation in behavior and proposing a new view that the motor system and its manifold physiological feedback mechanisms represent a variable control system for dynamically governing, timing, and integrating neural metabolic interactions at all levels of adaptive organic functioning.

The problem of interplay between behavior, or more particularly the skeletal-motor system, and internal molecular, metabolic, and organic functions—i.e., the so-called problem of psychosomatic interaction or mind-body interaction—still stands after three centuries as the central issue of experimental science. Traditional theories in psychology and physiology have had to bypass this problem as an experimental question because their concepts and related experimental methodologies lack the resources to deal with dynamic interactive events on a real-time basis. Behavioral and physiological cybernetics changes this state of affairs by placing both systems concepts and experimental methods on a dynamic, real-time basis.

Using experimental systems concepts of behavioral cybernetics, we propose to probe the manner in which variable integrated modes of response mechanisms serve as the direct dynamic control factors in physiological regulation and vital interaction at molecular, cellular, organic, and organismic levels. For nearly two centuries, physiologists and psychologists have been trying to understand metabolic regulation and related motivated responses in exercise, fatigue, and adaptation as a linear centrifugal process in which internal homeostatic or drive stimuli were assumed to govern both external response and internal vital exchanges in energy regulation. As a result of this classical theoretical orientation and its related dedication to experimental methods of isolating vital functions, only open-ended understanding was achieved of critical psycho-physiological events, such as energy exchange, respiration, circulation, metabolic integration, fatigue, physiological conditioning, etc. The reason for this open-ended understanding is now recognized from a cybernetic standpoint: it is impossible to comprehend the meaning of cellular and organic metabolism as well as other levels of vital interaction without considering a systems role of behavior as the primary basis of differential physiological regulation and energy production.

The theory that we develop here adds a new control dimension to behavior that has not been recognized before in physiology and psychology. That dimension is the dynamic temporal control of internal physiological regulation and interaction by closed-loop feedback guidance and energization of internal cellular and organic processes. Temporal control is exerted through differential response of the skeletal motor system. Behavior and motor system actions are not simply end products of internal processes; they are the differential control mechanisms which serve reciprocally to determine bioenergetic and temporal control at all levels of cellular and vital interaction. The symphony of behavior is the result of interrelated molecular, metabolic, neurohormonal, organic, neural, and interoceptive interchanges, that, by timed feedback control, self-regulates its own bioenergetics, synchronism, integrative patterning, fatigue, physical conditioning, and learning.

This chapter touches on some of the major unsolved problems of efferent integration and psychophysiological regulation in work, exercise, fatigue, and psychophysiological organization. The first problem is the explanation of how muscles interact as motor units to determine the efficiency of energy production, motor skill, and avoidance of fatigue. The nearest physiologists have gotten to the solution of this problem has been to talk about how two muscles can vary from one another to perform positive and negative work (Elftman, 1940; Fenn, 1924). The second problem resolved in part in the chapter is the manner in which body motor responses can control and guide energetic mechanisms such as respiration on both a feedback and a feedforward control basis. Physiologists have tried to deal with these critical predictive relations between motor mechanisms, respiration, and other organic operations by use of general labels such as *work stimuli* or *work factors* in respiration (Asmussen, 1967). The third problem analyzed is the primary bases of energy production for physiological drive within both single muscle cells and motor systems. This problem is resolved generally by the view that muscle cells and integrated motor mechanisms have differential roles in determining various parameters of energy production and utilization. The fourth issue discussed is the determination of physiological (or physical) conditioning in exercise and its relation to learning and motor-skill factors.

The view of motor skill and exercise that we propose is that the motor system and the brain are controlled and organized in terms of physiological feedback from internal processes by muscular contraction and integrated motor responses. These feedbacks constitute the basis of energy production and synchronized neural integration of both cellular and organic metabolism. As indicated in Fig. 1, physiological feedback is defined as the direct molecular, neurohormonal, physiological, organic, and interoceptive effects of dynamic response. These act

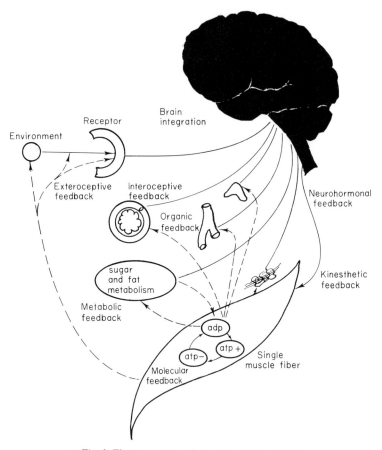

Fig. 1. The parameters of physiological feedback.

reciprocally on a continuous, closed-loop basis to regulate guidance, timing, and energy production in internal physiological regulation and integration. The individual is a unified self-controlled adaptive system organized primarily on the basis of the integration of physiological feedback from dynamic muscle contractions and complex movements of the motor system. Simultaneously, this feedback is used to control environmental effects on sensory systems related to both guidance of behavior and organic metabolism.

As the first explicitly stated control theory of behavior and physiological regulation, cybernetic psychology aims at specifying in detail how specific adaptive response patterns, sensory processes, and physiological mechanisms are regulated in continuous dynamic patterns; how these reactions are guided and timed; how the energy needed to maintain and motivate them is supplied; and organized in functional operations. The central concepts are those of sensory and physiological feedback control. The organism self-regulates its immediate ongoing reactions, its sensory input, and its own vital functions and operations on an integrated closed-loop basis. The primary assumption is that the mechanisms of response organization involve four main parameters of feedback control by dynamic movement. These are (1) sensory feedback from self-generated stimuli or control by the external environment, (2) intramuscular molecular feedback for energy production, (3) organic metabolic feedback for supply of metabolites for energy production, and (4) neural feedback from organic mechanisms that is integrated with external motorsensory as well as other components of physiological feedback. Thus, the concept of dynamic motor-system feedback stated above is not simply a statement of the closed-loop principle; it is a true control and systems theory that specifies how particular behavioral operations reciprocally self-govern behavioral-physiological adaptations.

The concept of feedback has been applied incidentally by several theorists to discussions of the neural mechanisms of posture, respiration, and kinesthetic mechanisms. There have been, however, only the most tentative efforts to reformulate classical thinking about the brain and energy regulation in relation to known facts of feedback control of tracking behavior, continuously regulated activities, feedback processes of receptor and sensory function, and bioenergy regulation. Thus far, the really great promise of feedback doctrine in giving an account of dynamic parameters of interaction between behavior and internal physiological processes hardly has been recognized either in physiology or psychology. It is that promise that we intend to exploit in this chapter with special reference to developing a theory of the way in which muscular energy processes are controlled and integrated with temporal and guidance feedback factors to define behavioral-physiological interaction. The goal is to explain theoretically and to give experimental evidence concerning the way that energy production in single muscle processes and their organic metabolic feedback relationships can be effected by and integrated with compound motor actions or motor skill factors which regulate guidance and feedback timing of both environmental adaptation and internal vital operations. The comprehension of feedback interplay between single muscle processes of molecular energy production and motion factors in dynamically regulating and integrating environmental adaptation and internal physiological processes is the most fundamental problem of efferent organization. We summarize the experimental facts of this field under the principles of psychoenergetic theory.

II. The Brain as a Multidimensional Feedback Control System

Dealing with efferent organization in terms of the integration of single muscle fiber bioenergetic processes and motor-skill (compound motion) feedback effects on physological regulation leads first of all to the role of the brain in energy regulation for behavior. The historical fact is that past theories of conscious and unconscious motivation (Freud, 1920), homeostasis (Cannon, 1929, 1934), and interoceptive physiological drives (Hull, 1943) have attributed to the brain the primary role of determining energy production for response. The basic view was that the strength of internal drive states was supposed to be correlated with the number of motor nerve fibers activated by interoceptive or exteroceptive stimuli. This theory has to be changed not only because it falsely displaces the locus of energy production for response but because it misinterprets the mechanisms of energy production and regulation. As we show below, the primary locus of energy production for behavior is not in the brain or in the viscera, but in the muscle cell itself. The basic mechanism of energy production is not interoceptive drive stimulation of the gut or afferent interoceptive excitation of the brain synapses: rather, it is a feedback control mechanism within the contracting muscle cell which has the capability of also regulating all other metabolic and neural mechanisms related to metabolism and to integrating these energy production mechanisms with variable parameters of motor skill.

As of now, a crucial issue of efferent organization and brain function is how the nervous system is organized structurally and functionally to mediate and integrate the different parameters of sensory and metabolic feedback that are yoked to muscle fiber energy production and to parameters of physiological feedback from compound motion. We attempt to show how muscular demands for energy (adenosine triphosphate) are feedback integrated with neural mechanisms underlying guidance and timing operations of compound muscular response and their effects on internal vital regulation. An attempt is made also to explain how physical conditioning in exercise, learning, and work is related to energy production and its metabolic and neural feedback processes.

The outline of the theory of behavioral-physiological feedback and interaction that we propose is given in some detail in Fig. 2. The main parameters of feedback indicated in Fig. 2 are (1) intramuscular feedback for energy (adenosine triphosphate) production, (2) metabolic feedback of adenosine triphosphate production on aerobic and anaerobic metabolism, (3) organic feedback of motor response on circulation and respiration, (4) neurohormonal feedback of ATP production on organic metabolic regulation, (5) kinesthetic feedback of the gamma efferent system in muscle contraction, (6) interoceptive feedback from motor activity and material and gas input produced by motor activity, and (7) external motorsensory feedback.

The theory diagrammed in Fig. 2 is a homeokinetic feedback doctrine of behavioral-physiological integration. It states that the brain functions as a central timing and synchronizing mechanism for the integration of organic-metabolic (including neurohormonal), exteroceptive, interoceptive, and kinesthetic feedback from muscle energy production and compound motion. The timing

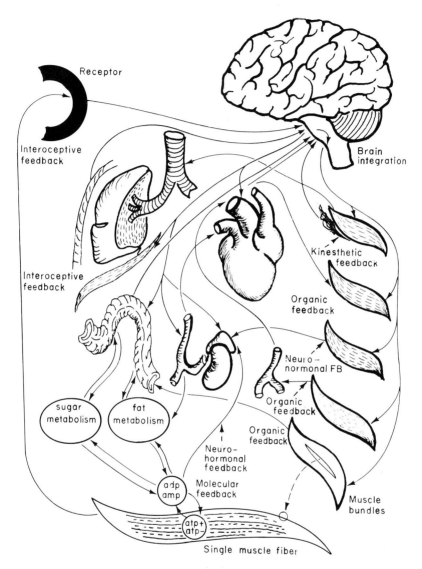

Fig. 2. The motor-system feedback theory of behavioral-physiological integration in energy regulation and motivation.

operations are feedback governed as delay circuits whose frequency characteristics are determined primarily by length of the nerve circuits and response characteristics of particular motor, sensory, and biochemical mechanisms. Three main motor operations are integrated by the brain through such timed integration. The first is the guidance of articulated components of the skeletal motor system through exteroceptive feedback and space-organized, feature detection neurons of the cerebral cortex. The second is the timed control of receptor-efferent mechanisms, including the gamma efferent system of muscles, that operate through space-structured and time-synchronized feature detection neurons of the cerebellum, pons, and basal ganglia of the nervous system. The third consists of the limbic and autonomic systems that are differentiated for control of both generalized (sympathetic) and organ-specific (parasympathetic) neural activation. This primitive organic motor system is related to the sensory input channels of both the receptor-efferent and skeletal motor mechanisms at all levels of brain function. It can thus be integrated neurally with both guidance of receptors and motor response as well as with feedback timing of sensory operations by receptor-efferent energy-regulating processes. In this view, the receptor-efferent nervous system, and especially the gamma efferent kinesthetic system is closely allied with energy production and utilization in muscle contraction. It serves as the basis of self-governed neuronic detection and control of metabolic and muscular demands in regulating the force and velocity of movement. Our theory is that the extrapyramidal motor system operates as a coordinate efferent outflow, controlling energy regulation in conjunction with action of receptor-efferent mechanisms. The pyramidal motor system acts primarily in relation to articulated motor mechanisms (the hands, feet, limbs, head, tongue, eyes, lips, jaw) for environmental guidance of specific movements.

Our view is that the central circuits of the extrapyramidal motor system provide a neural bridge of postural and travel movements for checking and controlling dynamic compliance between the metabolic state and the level of energy production in movement guided by single muscle cells. The cerebellar circuits of this system sense both exteroceptive and proprioceptive time and force functions of postural travel components in guided movement, while the cortical sensory projections of this system detect oxygen demands of local muscular sites and can adjust postural and travel movements relative to oxygen depletion of special neural circuits involved in focal guided movements. The receptor-efferent legs of this system generate motor signals that can produce sensory effects that comply or fail to comply with the existing patterns of movement-controlled sensory input. The receptor-efferent branch produces afferent effects that signal time and force compliances between kinesthetic and interoceptive feedback from larger muscles and specific exteroceptive feedback from articulated movements. These differential sensory signals, detected by the brain, result in central adjustments of all three motor systems.

III. The Locus and Mechanisms of Energy Production for Behavior

In this section, evidence is presented relative to the validity of the theory that the motor system and its single contracting muscle cells are the primary locus of energy production for behavior and hence the mechanism of motivation. This evidence does not come from our own research, but consists of extrapolation of results of molecular, biological, and physiological research on the processes of energy production in muscle and the effects of exercise on organic metabolism.

Quite clearly, one of the primary demands for both immediate and sustained motor response is that of energy supply. As noted earlier, past psychologists and physiologists tried to explain the source and distribution of energy supply for response by creating the various doctrines of unconscious motivation and physiological drives based on interoceptive stimulation and physiological homeostasis. Hull (1943), for example, spoke of the drive stimulus as any internal interoceptive effect which, when reduced, could serve as a reinforcing effect in learning. Although forming two of the most cherished scientific dogmas of the twentieth century, the doctrines of unconscious motivation and homeostatic drives have turned out to be most incorrect for explaining motivation, inasmuch as both misplace the locus and misidentify the mechanisms of energy production by muscular contraction. As current evidence indicates, these mechanisms are feedback processes located in muscles themselves which act to regulate by secondary feedback circuits all other levels of energy exchange in the body.

The nature of the feedback coupling of dynamic activity of muscle and cellular and supracellular energy metabolism has been known in a general way for three decades. This coupling was first suggested by the remarkable facility of higher organisms, including man, for varying the intensity of their metabolic activity according to the level of their physical behavior. Asmussen, Christensen, and Neilsen (1939) determined the extent of this variation by measuring oxygen consumption of human leg muscle and of the entire body as a function of work load. There was an increase in oxygen consumption by the muscle tissue of about twentyfold in lightly working over resting muscle, and a further threefold increase in muscle oxygen consumption when work load was again increased by a factor of three. Over this same work load range, oxygen comsumption in the whole body increased by ten times. It was estimated that with a work load variation between relaxation and maximum exercise, oxygen consumption in the muscle would increase one hundredfold. These increases in oxygen consumption are accompanied by, and integrated with, temperature variations in muscle tissue and by dilation of capillary vessels supplying the tissue.

A. Energy Production by Muscular Feedback Control

The two primary questions posed by a motor-system feedback theory of energy production by muscle activity are: (1) how does the metabolism of single muscle fibers proceed only rapidly enough to supply the energy required at any given time; and (2) how are the different bioenergetic control mechanisms dynamically integrated during exercise and motor skill at the metabolic and neural levels? Before going into these questions, we will review the main features of molecular energy metabolism in contracting muscle fibers, which encompasses the mechanisms of adenosine triphosphate production, carbohydrate metabolism, and oxidative versus anaerobic metabolism (Fruton and Simmonds, 1960; White *et al.,* 1964). Evidence indicates that energy metabolism is yoked to muscle action by both positive and negative feedback mechanisms, thus allowing the coupling of energy production to energy expenditure.

Chemical energy production in cellular metabolism depends upon two major processes: the breakdown of carbohydrates and the consumption of oxygen. When we speak of chemical energy in the cell, we essentially mean one specific molecule, a compound called adenosine triphosphate (ATP). As shown in Fig. 3, ATP can be considered as the end product of cellular energy production. It is essential for such activities as amino acid synthesis, protein synthesis, carbohydrate breakdown, muscle action, and production of body heat, as well as a host of other processes. Under *aerobic* (oxygen present) conditions, ATP is produced at the expense of sugar and oxygen. Cells also can produce ATP under *anaerobic* (oxygen absent) conditions, albeit in a more inefficient manner. It is the control of these processes that is our main concern here.

The primary site of ATP formation in cells of higher organisms is in the mitochondria, which are specialized organelles located in the cell cytoplasm. In muscles, carbohydrate (primarily glucose) and oxygen permeate into individual cells from capillary blood vessels supplying the tissue. Within the cells, carbohydrate catabolism (breakdown), oxygen consumption, and ATP production proceed in the mitochondria by processes described below. Muscle fiber contraction during work, exercise, and other physical exertion utilizes the ATP so produced.

There are five main physiological components of energy regulation involving: (1) glucose phosphorylation, (2) glycolysis, (3) citric acid cycle, (4) fat production, (5) ATP production. All of these components are dynamically regulated and integrated by muscular contraction through variously synchronized feedback controls. The immediate low-energy sources of ATP are two closely related molecules, adenosine diphosphate (ADP) and adenosine monophosphate (AMP), by which low-energy feedback mechanisms replace ATP as it is expended under conditions of motor work in which the muscle fiber is not stretched. Conversion of ADP or AMP to ATP by oxidative phosphorylation requires oxygen (respiration) and reducing power. Reducing power is supplied in the form of a molecule called reduced nicotinamide adenine dinucleotide (NADH), which is produced primarily by citric acid cycle reactions but also by glycolysis.

Much more ATP is produced from carbohydrate metabolism if sugar is broken all the way down to CO_2 under aerobic conditions, when the citric acid cycle and oxidative phosphorylation can proceed. In fact, the process of

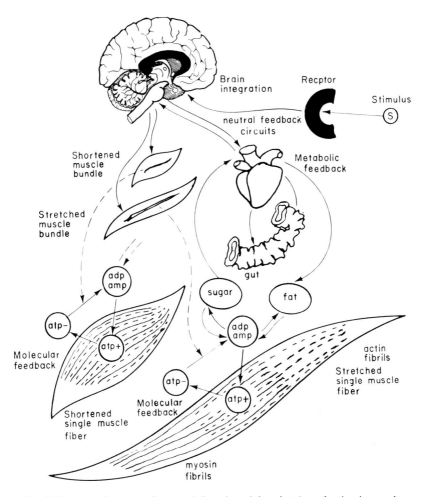

Fig. 3. The muscular locus of energy (adenosine triphosphate) production in muscle.

anaerobic glycolysis, when carbohydrate catabolism stops at lactate, releases only about 7% of the energy obtained when glucose is broken down completely to CO_2. Therefore, the energy needs of the cell can be met with considerably less glucose under aerobic conditions. A further consideration is that fat can be mobilized for energy only if oxygen is available.

B. Selective Feedback Control of Aerobic and Anaerobic Metabolism by Muscle

One of the most critical processes that links single-muscle fiber energy production with motor-system regulation of internal vital function is related to respiration. The functional relationship between respiration and carbohydrate metabolism was discovered over 100 years ago, when Louis Pasteur noted that yeast consumed a much greater quantity of sugar under anaerobic conditions than when oxygen was present (White *et al.,* 1964; Fruton and Simmonds, 1960). This phenomenon, later termed the Pasteur effect, has subsequently been observed in a wide variety of animal tissue preparations and in microorganisms. The basic observation is that oxygen somehow decreases the rate of carbohydrate breakdown to pyruvate in glycolysis, so that glycolysis is much more rapid under anaerobic than under aerobic conditions. In trying to interpret the Pasteur effect, one is immediately struck by the fact, discussed above, that energy production is much more efficient under aerobic conditions. With oxygen present, glucose catabolism in glycolysis can proceed at a moderate pace and still produce a substantial amount of energy. The important inference of the Pasteur effect, however, is that cellular energy feedback controls the rate of its own production and simultaneously can influence organic respiration and other levels of bioenergy regulation under motor system control.

Evidence indicates that ATP, and its precursors ADP and AMP, can exert multifaceted feedback control over the rate of carbohydrate catabolism, thereby regulating the rate of ATP production. This control seems to be achieved primarily through positive or negative modulation, by ATP, ADP, and AMP, of the activities of specific enzymes along the glycolytic pathway and in the citric acid cycle. Regulatory features of the system have been incorporated into a model termed the adenylate control hypothesis, recently reviewed by Atkinson (1965, 1966) and depicted generally in Fig. 3.

Adenosine triphosphate (ATP) controls its own production directly by inhibiting the enzyme which catalyzes the entry of pyruvate into the citric acid cycle, thereby restricting the operation of the cycle and the concomitant production of reducing power which is needed for energy production. ATP complements this process by also inhibiting one of the enzymes in the cycle. The action of ATP is reversed by that of AMP and ADP, which enhances the activity of another of the enzymes in the cycle to increase the production of energy. The general result is a coordinate control of the citric acid cycle: if the ATP concentration is high, the cycle is inhibited, but if it is low due to excessive energy expenditure, the resultant high concentrations of AMP and ADP tend to enhance NADH production.

The feedback relationship of ATP pictured in Fig. 1 allows multifaceted control of energy metabolism. If the amount of energy in a cell or tissue drops owing to any extraordinary exertion, the flow of carbohydrates and the production of NADH is augmented in a ramified manner. Glycogen breakdown increases, the production of ADP is enhanced, and operations within the citric acid cycle are boosted. On the other hand, if the cell begins to accumulate excess energy in the form of ATP, this enhancement of carbohydrate flow is reversed owing to ATP inhibition of AMP, ADP, and NADH production and the flow of pyruvate into the citric acid cycle.

C. The Feedback Bridge Between Muscular Work and Energy Production

The view that the muscle acts as a dynamic regulator and integrator of vital interactions in both cellular and organic bioenergetic regulation has been validated by experimental studies of the mechanisms of contraction. This research has given rise to the sliding filament theory of striated muscle contraction, which Huxley (1969) reviewed recently. Muscle fibers are made up of a large number of individual filaments, bundled together along their longitudinal axes to form the fiber. Muscle filaments may contain one of two types of protein molecules, actin or myosin, and the actin and myosin filaments overlap each other in a highly precise manner within the fiber to form a characteristic lattice or array appearance when viewed in cross section. When the muscle changes length, during either contraction or stretch, the sliding filament model proposes that the length of the filaments themselves remains the same, but that the overlapping arrays of myosin and actin filaments slide past each other. Actin is drawn further into the array of myosin filaments as the muscle shortens, and withdrawn again as the muscle is stretched. During contraction, the traverse difference between the filaments increases considerably, accounting for the familiar muscle bulge caused by contraction.

It is now fairly certain that the sliding of actin and myosin filaments represents the energy-consuming stage of muscle action, and the ATP is directly required in the interfilament interactions which allow sliding to occur. Moreover, this interaction is the base control mechanism whereby single-fiber molecular events in energy utilization and production are yoked to blood distribution and the mechanisms of organic metabolism. That is to say, we can correlate the molecular control features of single-fiber muscle metabolism and the energy demands and output of muscle contraction with the more outward psychophysiological manifestations of work, exercise, and motor skill for different cases of muscle exertion. At rest, energy demands on muscle tissue are slight and the rate of oxygen consumption is low (Asmussen et al., 1939). Blood circulation is minimal—only one capillary of every hundred supplying the tissue may be open and carrying blood (Krogh, 1922). It is probable that the decreased blood supply is a feedback response to decreased demand of the tissue for oxygen (Lardy, 1956). As the muscle begins to contract in work or exercise there is an immediate and dramatic increase in capillary blood flow along with concomitant increases in tissue temperature and heat production. Although the control mechanism is still unknown, there is little doubt that this rapid response of capillary circulation in muscle tissue to contraction is a direct feedback mechanism of muscle bundle activity. The action of contraction releases neurohormones that act immediately on the arterioles and capillary muscles, while the mechanical events of contraction influence the baroreceptors in a rapid way to cause positive response of the arterial system to the increased demands for blood flow. These feedback control processes can act with high speed on the heart through mechanical pressure responses of the arterial system or on the nervous system by stimulation of temperature and peripheral pressure receptors closely associated with the arterial system.

The mechanism of blood circulation controlling oxygen supply to acting muscle thus may be said to be composed of two phases—(1) a fast phase that is regulated rapidly and directly by local muscle contraction and which is directly yoked by closed-loop mechanoreceptors and neurohormonal feedback control to energy production within a given number of contracting fibers within a muscle bundle; and (2) a slow phase that is governed by the baroreceptive and neural feedback circuits of the heart itself, which may be varied especially in rate of response by the more articulated and rapid muscle control circuits.

It is this two-dimensional control of oxygen supply by peripheral muscle and circulatory feedback control which makes possible a third fundamental bridge between single fiber energy production and the compound activity of the motor system. This bridging integrative feedback yoke is represented by the capability of the organic system to change systemic control of energy resources and oxygen supply at different levels of exertion. In resting muscle, energy is derived primarily from fat oxidation, not carbohydrate oxidation (White *et al.,* 1964). Although other factors may be involved, the two major reasons for this mode of metabolism are probably that the low concentrations of inorganic phosphate and ATP limit the rate of liver glycolysis, and the epinephrine-induced factors necessary for muscle glycogen breakdown to glucose are not available.

Every athlete knows that sudden, violent exertion from a resting condition may cause adverse muscle effects, reflecting the inability of the tissue to convert instantaneously from a passive state to one of accelerated energy metabolism. The common "warmup" program circumvents this problem. Enhanced secretion of epinephrine caused by the activity and also by anticipation of the pending contest induces vasodilation of capillaries feeding the muscle tissue, and oxygen supply to the tissue increases. Epinephrine also initiates a series of biochemical changes which ultimately stimulate glycogen breakdown, thereby raising glucose levels in the muscle. At the same time, the rate of oxygen consumption rises markedly, reflecting a higher energy demand due to muscle contraction. Inorganic phosphate and ATP levels increase and the rates of glycolysis and oxidative phosphorylation become appreciably higher than their values in resting muscle.

Sudden, violent bursts of muscle activity, such as occur in athletic sprints or similar intense, short-term exertions, introduce still another profound systemic shift in muscle metabolism. At near maximal work levels, ATP reservoirs in mammalian skeletal muscle become exhausted within a few seconds (White *et al.,* 1964). Furthermore, the maximal increase in ATP utilization for contraction is manyfold greater than the maximal increase in cellular oxygen consumption. Thus, neither the energy reservoir nor respiratory metabolism is adequate to meet the energy demands of muscle for intense activity, and the tissue switches to anaerobic glycolysis for ATP production. When the ATP level is high because of energy expenditure, glycolysis is enhanced at a number of points. By catabolizing glucose at a high rate, the muscle is therefore able to keep pace with intense energy demands for an appreciable period of time by primarily anaerobic metabolism. This is why intense physical activity is always accompanied by the appearance of large quantities of lactic acid in the blood.

Although anaerobic metabolism can meet the needs of short-term muscle exertion, sustained muscle use over a longer period must be fueled by oxidative metabolism. This is because the carbohydrate reserves of muscle, in the form of glycogen, are limited, and are rapidly depleted by anaerobic glycolysis. Over the long term, oxidative phosphorylation, which entails oxygen consumption and ATP production, must be able to keep pace with the expenditure of energy. A further feature of long-term muscle use even at moderate levels is that the primary energy source is fat, not carbohydrate. Equating these effects with athletic performance, the 100-yard dash man relies almost entirely on his glycogen reserviors, while the marathon runner consumes mainly fat for energy production. Moreover, there is little reason to question the view that peripheral muscle activity levels exert feedback control over liver glycogen manufacturing in relation to these varied states of rest and exercise. It can achieve this control by both biochemical and neural feedback effects of muscle activity on the liver.

A very direct feedback relationship between cellular metabolism and body respiration is demonstrated by the well-known "oxygen debt" incurred after a period of intense activity or exertion. The respiratory manifestations of this phenomenon are simply that oxygen consumption after intense physical activity continues to exceed the basal rate and is of greater magnitude than oxygen consumption during the activity. The metabolic and physiological basis of this oxygen debt is the necessity for the body to restore the energy balance of the muscle tissue by oxidative phosphorylation of ADP to ATP, catabolizing in the process some of the excess lactic acid provided by anaerobic glycolysis during the intense work. However, most of the excess lactic acid is used to restore the depleted glycogen reserves of the tissue, a synthetic process which requires energy and thus further prolongs enhanced oxygen consumption. The oxygen debt, therefore, is a direct manifestation of feedback relationships between external and internal respiration, energy production by single muscle cells, and biosynthetic metabolism at organic levels.

D. COORDINATE DIMENSIONS OF PHYSIOLOGICAL FEEDBACK

The feedback control of ATP within the single muscle cell and of its precursors ADP and AMP in supracellular metabolism constitutes the base of the primary dynamic circuits of energy production. For these primary controls in muscular contraction to be sustained, other levels of organic energy supply, conversion, uptake, distribution, and mobilization must occur. These derivative levels of energy exchange are determined by the several dimensions of ATP and muscle controlled feedback pictured in Fig. 2. Besides the molecular and metabolic levels of physiological feedback already discussed, the other phases of energy exchange are reciprocal modes of neurohormonal, organic, interoceptive, and kinesthetic feedback tied to ATP production.

Superimposed on the feedback control properties of ATP, ADP, and AMP in energy metabolism summarized by the adenylate control hypothesis, are the influences of the body's endocrine system on carbohydrate metabolism, respiration, and energy production. In muscle, the most prominent such influence is that of epinephrine, the hormonal product of the adrenal glands (White et al., 1964). Epinephrine secretion by the adrenal medulla is enhanced by behavioral conditions of exercise, excitement, anxiety, exertion, or stress, apparently by direct stimulation of the adrenals by the nervous system. Epinephrine promotes glucose production from glycogen (a process called glycogenolysis). Under aerobic conditions it also enhances energy production from fat by promoting fat breakdown. In addition to these effects, epinephrine also causes marked dilation of capillary blood vessels feeding skeletal muscle. Therefore, epinephrine has a threefold positive effect on energy metabolism at times of tension or stress when the organism needs energy: (1) it enhances carbohydrate supply through glycogenolysis; (2) it provides an additional energy source through fat mobilization; and (3) it increases oxygen supply to muscle tissue by means of vasodilation and is responsible apparently for the immediate vasodilatory response to compound muscle activity.

E. ORGANIC DIMENSIONS OF PHYSIOLOGICAL FEEDBACK

According to the present view, all major internal organic mechanisms of the body have reciprocal, dynamic, isomorphic, feedback links with the action of the skeletal-motor system. Aside from motor control of capillary circulation, the most noteworthy of these circuits is that of the motor regulation of venous circulation. The skeletal muscles are the outer sector of the circulatory system. Contraction of muscles is needed to pump blood back to the heart and if tonic control of the muscles is lost, as it may be when lying on an inclined surface at about 65 degrees, venous blood pools in the lower limbs cause fainting. Venous pressure is specifically regulated by the level of muscle contraction in the larger muscle groups. The same muscles also regulate blood and energy distribution by their marked capability for storing blood. That is, they have a capacity not shared by any other tissues and organs of the body in being able to increase and decrease the volume of blood contained by 15 to 20 times.

External respiration is specifically yoked metabolically and neurally with dynamic movements of other movement systems. Asmussen (1967) has discussed this yoked relationship as the work factor in respiration. As the arms, legs, and head are moved, the muscle systems of the chest and abdomen are caused to move both by mechanical and neural effects of the related motions. As will be shown later, the external respiratory system is one of the most refined and articulated tracking systems of the body, and can quickly adapt to and follow other movements with high precision. Such precision body tracking is observed in both speech and athletic skills in which the chest and abdomen not only generate specialized movements, but simultaneously alter and maintain breath pressure as related movements are in progress. A fast phase of respiration that is time compliant with the fast phase of circulation in exercise is thus achieved by direct feedback integration of respiratory and body movements.

The most direct organic effect of motor activity on respiration and the gut is in controlling ingestion of food, water, and gas. Besides causing stimulation of the interoceptors of these organ systems, the gas intake and ingested food and water induce mechanical changes in the organs concerned and alter their integrative relations with body movements. All of the processes of eating, drinking, and respiration are productive, self-regulated, feedback-controlled adaptations and in no sense follow the specifications of stimulus-response or homeostatic theories of behavior and motivation.

F. KINESTHETIC-NEURAL FEEDBACK OF MOTION

When viewed from a cybernetic standpoint, the motor system is also designed and organized to reciprocally control sensorimotor factors in energy production. Inasmuch as the alpha fibers are specialized for active work and energy production for contraction, the same cells lack specialization for signaling the sensory effects of their own action. However, the muscle spindles and their gamma efferent neurons located adjacent to the alpha fibers can correlate their activity with both the degree of stretch and rate of contraction of surrounding alpha fibers (Granit, 1970). These kinesthetic receptors also may be partly specialized as chemoreceptors to sense oxygen level and lactic acid level resulting from their own activity and from surrounding alpha fibers.

The main effect of kinesthetic feedback from motor activity, of course, is the sensory input from the muscle spindles which may be integrated with proprioceptive guidance mediated by joint and tendon receptors. The primary central projection regions of this system are on the cerebellum and not the cortex, which apparently receives kinesthetic connections from only a few muscle regions, such as the eye and tongue musculature. The thought of the past has been that the cerebellar mechanisms of kinesthetic projection are concerned primarily with timing of movement and posture. Another possible effect of such kinesthetic feedback on the cerebellar system is that of a feature detection of energy demands in the larger muscle systems. The cerebellar cells not only sense muscle-spindle differences in regard to the stretch of the spindle and the rate of contraction, they also detect changes in sensitivity of the spindle as regulated by state of energy production in the spindle and in surrounding alpha fibers.

G. Motivational Manifestations of Energy Regulation

The short-term and long-term motivational aspects of energy regulation are well known to everyone in the form of rest, active relaxation, fatigue, boredom, exhaustion, depression, hyperactive states, and endurance in exertion. It is of note that these states, which can be given a direct explanation in terms of a biomotor control hypothesis, have never been described in any complete way in traditional thinking. One is reminded of the controversy carried out over nearly three decades by Hill (1922) and Fenn (1930) regarding the efficiency of energy utilization by muscles in work. Inasmuch as these two eminent investigators used different methods of assessing efficiency of energy expenditure (Fenn studied walking in man and Hill investigated performance in nerve muscle preparations and of human subjects in a bicycle ergograph), they came up with very different estimates of energy utilization by muscle. We now know why such estimates can vary: the mode of contraction determines almost completely the efficiency of energy production and utilization. With unstretched fibers, muscles can replace almost completely by their own feedback resources the energy expended for contraction. Under other conditions of work, they can reconstitute almost none of the ATP used for contraction.

A demonstration by Hill (1960) illustrates the general meaning of feedback processes in bioenergetics of muscle activity. In studies of nerve muscle preparations, Hill found a marked difference in susceptibility of such preparations to fatigue when the muscle was required to do work while being shortened, considered negative work, and while being stretched, considered positive work. The finding was that there was rapid fatigue in positive work and little or no fatigue in negative work. As indicated in Fig. 4, these recovery effects of positive and negative work were explained in terms of the differences in biochemical recovery of muscle under the two conditions. Positive work or contraction requires the accelerated expenditure of chemical energy in the muscle at a rate which far exceeds the capacity of the muscle to replenish energy supplies. On the other hand, the muscle performing work while in a shortened state may act with nearly 100% efficiency, because energy demands are far smaller and energy production is able to keep pace with expenditure.

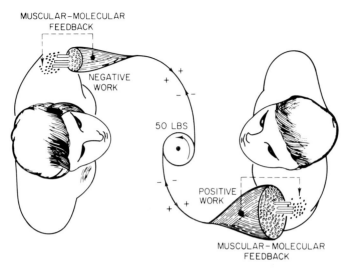

MUSCULAR–MOLECULAR
FEEDBACK

NEGATIVE
WORK

50 LBS

POSITIVE
WORK

MUSCULAR–MOLECULAR
FEEDBACK

Fig. 4. Hill's demonstration of the principle of variable physiological feedback in energy regulation. (Based on Hill, 1960.)

The connection between so-called positive and negative work and its relation to motor coordination and motor skill has gone all but unrecognized in muscle physiology. Elftman (1940) discussed this relationship in terms of the advantage of two-joint muscles over one-joint muscles. This advantage was thought to ensue from the fact that one of the muscles in two-joint muscle mechanisms can perform negative work while the other is engaged in positive work—i.e., work in the process of being stretched. The recent clarification of the molecular energy production mechanisms in muscle make the notions of positive, zero, and negative work as originally defined by Fenn (1924) somewhat dubious. All work in single muscle fibers, whether stretched or nonstretched, is positive. The critical point is that in the fiber not undergoing stretch, energy consumed can be replaced almost completely by self-governed feedback control within the individual fiber whereas this is not true for the contracting muscle undergoing stretch. In the intact organism, the processes of motor coordination and motor skill in compound muscle systems can adjust the relative duration of contraction of muscles undergoing stretch (or imposed work) and increase the duration of contraction of muscles performing self-governed (i.e., nonimposed work) and thereby increase the efficiency of energy utilization and production to very high levels. Thus, the meaning of positive and negative work in muscle physiology can be comprehended only by knowledge of the details of energy production in single muscle fibers and its relation to motor coordination in regulating the conditions of imposed work on contracting muscles in compound motor systems. Or more specifically, one of the primary dynamic factors in efferent organization deals with the way that compound muscles can be made to interact to regulate the efficiency and conditions of energy utilization and production within single-contracting cells. Muscle coordination, and hence motor skill, is a fundamental aspect of energy regulation at molecular, cellular and organic levels.

IV. Systems Feedback Research on Behavioral-Physiological Interaction

In the preceding section, we have attempted to deal with one of the primary problems of physiology and psychology—i.e., the mechanisms of integration of the bioenergetics of the single contracting muscle cell with the metabolic activity of the total muscle, compound muscle mechanisms, and the processes of organic metabolism concerned with energy uptake, conversion, mobilization, and distribution. Although the story was often skimpy, we have shown that this bioenergetic integration, which probably underlies every other parameter of psychophysiological regulation and organization in the body, depends fundamentally on several special modes of reciprocal feedback interaction. The reciprocity occurs between muscle cell activity and compound muscle interaction. It operates primarily to vary the efficiency of ATP production in the single muscle cell and the parameters of organic metabolism that serve to supply the precursors of different patterns of energy production within the single cell.

The most important conclusion from these facts of intramuscular bio-energetic integration for psychology is that this dynamic efferent organization is the most significant basis of time synchronism in all aspects of behavioral-physiological interaction related to respiration, circulation, liver function, and motivation. It represents not simply an expression of exercise, but the roles of motor coordination and skill in governing most of the critical dimensions of vital interaction. In this section, the attempt is made to expand the story of the physiological feedback effects of motor coordination and efferent integration. We will show that efferent integration and organization of muscle activity for physiological regulation at the organismic level is also based on feedback coordination of motorsensory activities and on feedback linking of body movements and physiologically related behaviors of respiration and circulation.

A. PSYCHOENERGETIC THEORY OF ORGANISMIC ENERGY REGULATION AND EFFERENT INTEGRATION

For nearly two decades it has been apparent to us that feedback theory in psychology offers much more than a recasting of traditional stimulus-response and homeostatic dogmas in the form of informational engineering doctrines, sampled data theories, and other anomalous statistical reiterations of the reflex concept. The theory brings to psychology and physiology the first concrete concepts and methods for studying and measuring systems interactions between behavior and physiological functions on a continuous operating basis. Eventually these methods, as applied especially in the form of real time, computerized techniques of analyzing biofeedback phenomena, will displace the artificial and circumscribed statistical techniques that psychologists in particular depend upon to give some experimental clues regarding nonreal time interactions.

We believe that a systems theory in physiology—i.e., systems concepts of respiration, circulation, liver function, digestion, brain function, reproduction, development, genetic expression, and evolutionary selection—is impossible without a detailed inclusion of behavioral factors in formulas for vital regulation. Specifically, experimental knowledge of behavioral feedback effects on vital function can now be shown to be essential for specifying both the detailed and articulated control mechanisms for metabolic processes and to be needed especially to give the first real clues as to how the bioenergetic, timing, and guidance operations of molecular, cellular, organic, and organismic mechanisms are integrated on a dynamic basis.

B. Application of Systems Tracking Techniques to Study of Behavioral-Physiological Interaction

One of the first experimental challenges presented by the feedback theory of physiological integration was met by initiating studies of the behavioral aspects of respiration as a continuous tracking process. From the very first steps in this field, the effort seemed highly promising because the notions of respiratory tracking and behavioral feedback control touched on many of the problems of continuous control and guidance of respiration. Respiration is modulated by both external skeletal-motor and internal organic mechanisms. Moreover, physiological investigators in the fields of circulation and respiration have been either uninterested in trying to deal with the events of breathing behavior or have failed to account for several very critical phenomena of external respiration. (1) The rate and volume of voluntary respiration exceeds by a large percentage value the variance in exercise-induced or CO_2-induced rate and volume changes. (2) Exercise-induced rate and volume changes exceed by a large percentage value the variance in rate and volume changes induced by changes in pulmonary CO_2. (3) The fast phases of exercise induced changes in respiration are not dependent on the slower chemically induced changes in internal or pulmonary respiration. (4) The fast phases of respiration, as observed in speech, singing, musical production, and prior to exercise have anticipatory, predictive, and feedforward control properties that are neurally or neurohormonally regulated and can control respiration within a single cycle of slower chemically governed internal respiration. (5) The fast phases of respiratory behavior do not depend simply on the mechanics of breathing; rather they are closely allied with other body movements such as those of speech, head movements, arm movements, and lower limb movements. (6) The interactions between body movements and the fast phases of respiration are exemplary forms of motor coordination and motor skill and are not simple effects of exercise. We know this because the movements of respiration are distinctly specialized in relation to their coordination with other body movements. For every distinctive motion pattern of the body there is an accompanying distinctive breathing pattern.

The application of behavioral tracking methods to study of respiration and other self-governed vital interactions demonstrates the essential features of experimental systems research on behavioral-physiological feedback. In the first applications of these methods to study of respiratory tracking, we wished to determine to what extent the properties of respiratory activity follow the specifications of a motorsensory feedback concept of control and organization of movement. Studies were done on the systems capabilities of respiratory activity to control exteroceptive signals or targets, such as the way that respiratory movements are used to control speech sounds. In subsequent studies, the dynamic systems interactions between respiratory movements and limb movements were investigated in order to determine to what extent natural or built-in feedback integrations occur between such movements. Evidence regarding marked differences in respiration during tracking periods and rest periods between such periods provided information on the interaction between respiration and skeletal-motor adaptation and its energy production processes.

The measurement of continuous, real time dynamic interactions between movement and sensory input and between different movement controlled feedback mechanisms also involves the capability for using error measures as the basis of generated real time movement produced feedback to a subject. The subject can then operate, not simply in terms of perception of his movements or of some extraneous knowledge or results, but in terms of a continuous indication of his system's error or accuracy in relating his movements with one another or with some stimulus display. Although psychologists and physiologists have approximated such methods in the study of error in manual visual tracking, they have not been able to manipulate sensory feedback factors in a controlled way. The real time, or analog-digital-analog computer system, however, has made detailed and highly controlled systems experimentation possible in both psychology and physiology.

In experimental systems research, as on respiratory interactions, we do not attempt to dissect out particular component reactions and isolate them experimentally as discrete events. Rather, the effort is to maintain the subject as far as possible in a normal state and then use controlled dynamic feedback procedures to separate modes of response for measurement. Thus the individual is investigated, not in some artificial way, but as he normally operates as a control system to govern particular stimulus conditions and physiological processes.

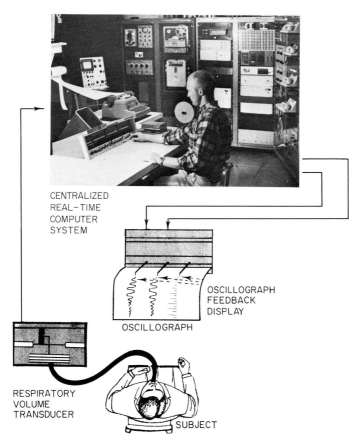

CENTRALIZED
REAL-TIME
COMPUTER
SYSTEM

OSCILLOGRAPH
FEEDBACK
DISPLAY

OSCILLOGRAPH

RESPIRATORY
VOLUME
TRANSDUCER

SUBJECT

Fig. 5. Components of a real time computerized laboratory system for study of respiratory tracking.

Figure 5 illustrates the arrangement of the components of the hybrid computer laboratory setup for conducting systems studies on respiratory tracking. The laboratory consists of an experimental transducing station coupled with a central analog-digital-analog computer facility. The latter contains a main digital computer coupled with analog-digital and digital-analog converters, as well as oscilloscope, oscillograph, frequency generating, stimulating, timing, tape-recording and electronic switching equipment. The subject's task is to use a mouth tube to actuate a respiratory bellows, which records the breathing movements. Electrical signals from these movements actuate the computer system which measures them and outputs an electrical signal that actuates a sensory feedback display which the subject sees or hears to guide his movements.

The detailed components of the real-time computer system are shown in Fig. 6. This diagram illustrates how the respiratory transducing station is tied into the signal converting and signal conditioning equipment of the laboratory. The column to the left of the central computer system indicates the analog signal-conditioning equipment which may be coupled with the respiratory

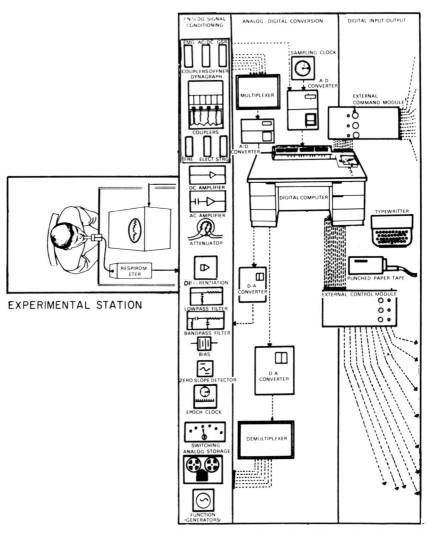

Fig. 6. Detailed components of the real time computerized laboratory for systems studies of respiratory tracking.

transducer and used to control visual, auditory, and tactual feedback displays that the subject observes. The central part of the block diagram describes the signal converting and multiplexing equipment of the laboratory. The column to the right illustrates digital input and output apparatus that may be operated by the computer system to summarize measurements of respiratory responses or to control digital displays related to respiratory movements of the subject.

Figure 7 illustrates the steps in data conversion and experimental computer programming involved in an experiment on respiratory tracking with a visual feedback display of breathing movements. The subject operates a breath volume transducer, as described earlier, and observes a visual indication of his movements on an oscillograph display. The breathing movements of the subject are transduced to continuous electrical form by a linear potentiometer located in

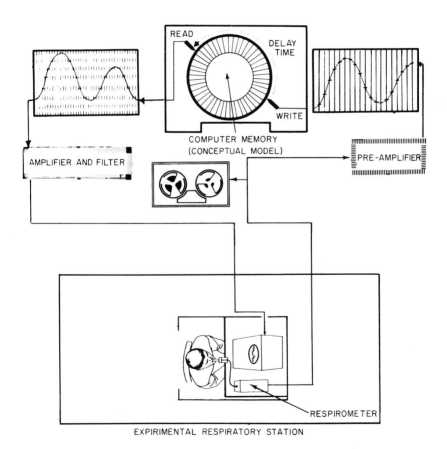

Fig. 7. Steps in data conversion and computer programming used in experimental automation and real time feedback control in studies of respiratory tracking.

the respirometer. The transduced respiratory signal is amplified, converted to digital form at 128 samples per second, and transmitted to the digital computer. The digital computer is programmed to perform a number of different experimental operations on the signal, including (1) measurement of response magnitude, (2) time interval between breath peaks, (3) error magnitude in following the pattern of a target wave that the computer generates which is displayed on the oscillograph, (4) scheduling the order of trials and observations in which the respiratory tracking is measured, (5) giving warning to the subject of the beginning and ending of trials, (6) making experimental calibrations of the respiratory transducer before each trial is begun, (7) differentiating the movement signal and measuring response velocity, (8) storing and summarizing all of the experimental measurements in memory, (9) varying the feedback parameters of the respiratory movements such as their magnitude, velocity, time delay, intermittency, etc., (10) comparing the measured magnitude, time, and velocity characteristics with similar measurements of other responses, such as arm movements, which may be transduced along with the breathing movements, and (11) outputting a digital signal of some measured characteristic of the respiratory movements or of some systems characteristic of these movements in interacting with other body movements. This digital output signal is converted to continuous or analog form to operate the oscillograph feedback display which the subject observes.

Initial studies were done on oral breath pressure control and breath volume tracking to ascertain the interrelations between breathing, heart action, and other body movements. The subject's task in these experiments was to maintain steady pressure by watching a visual feedback display. The subject's breath control movements were transduced, and the electrical signal of the movements amplified, converted, and programmed as described above. The digital computer was programmed to produce a variable sine wave movement in the feedback signal of breath control movements, which the subject had to compensate. The computer measured the accuracy of the subject in this continuous compensatory tracking. In these studies, the computer was programmed to receive signals from a zero setting of the transducer and a feedback indicator, and to establish the voltage corresponding to these readings as zero. The computer then measured the magnitude of variations from this zero calibration.

Oscillograph records of oral breath pressure and breath volume tracking in these studies showed that tracking movements have all the characteristics of self-generated, continuously regulated, closed loop reactions. They consist of uninterrupted oscillatory movements which display a dominant frequency pattern. As the subject continued to practice, the error of the tracking movements was reduced and the irregular movements tended to drop out. However, the subject never achieved a perfect performance. During initial learning, a number of very high velocity movements occurred. Also, variation in the records occurred which corresponded to the heartbeat. As the trials progressed, this ballistocardiographic effect on the movements decreased. During learning the velocity of the movements did not decrease with practice in an orderly way.

Besides the effects of the cardiac rhythm, the breath control reaction showed variations related to postural shifts, the breathing cycle, and articulated movements of the lips, tongue, and jaw. Thus, movement control of breath pressure was a compound activity made up of a number of components which had variable relations with heart action, posture, and articulated activities of mouth and head. These reciprocal interactions were neither accidental nor unimportant for respiratory control. They reflected the fact that the external respiratory mechanism is an ultraprecise tracking system of the body and interacts continuously with other organic and movement mechanisms.

Results of several special experiments on delay of the visual feedback on ventilation rate and breath pressure tracking showed that these mechanisms are not simple stimulus released reflex mechanisms, but depend continuously on reciprocal sensory feedback derived from actual movements. To produce delay of the feedback of respiratory tracking, the computer setup was programmed to store the incoming signals of respiratory motion for a predetermined period of time and then to transmit these stored signals to the subject as a delayed feedback of the breath motions. The overall perceptual effect of such delay was to cause the subject to sense a discoordination between his breath movements and the sensory effects of these movements as observed on the oscillograph feedback display. The more refined oral breath pressure tracking was affected most by feedback delay, the breath volume movements were affected less, and the ventilation rate tracking was affected least.

Overall, the findings indicated that the process of external respiration, a skeletal-motor activity on which almost all levels of internal respiration and energy exchange depend, is regulated and learned in precise ways in relation to movement controlled, sensory feedback factors. The effects of feedback delays on breath control movements suggested in addition that the rhythmic timing and learning of external respiration can be altered by changing the temporal factors linking skeletal-motor activity and sensory inputs.

With visual feedback delay, the subject showed no consistent evidence of improvement with learning, and was just about as irregular in controlling his movements at the end of practice as he was in the first trial. The effect of the feedback delay was to cause gross irregularities in motion, decrease in the frequency and marked increase in the magnitude of movement, and distortion in control of velocity of breath control motions. The results of the effects of feedback delay on learning breath control movements were extended by observations on the characteristics of performance with delays of different magnitude. The results of these observations confirmed the results on learning with feedback delay in showing that the motorsensory lags altered the regularity, accuracy, and velocity of different parameters of breath control. In addition, these studies brought out that the frequency characteristics of self-controlled breath tracking varied systematically with different magnitudes of delay. The conclusion is that integration of different body movements with motions of the respiratory system depends on precise modes of feedback timing of movements and sensory stimulation of the respiratory system.

Experiments similar to these initial learning and feedback delay studies with respiratory tracking were carried out on emphysema patients. The studies were done by remote real time computer feedback control with the patients located in a hospital some 150 miles from the computer laboratory. An analog dataphone connection was used to transmit the electrical signals of the subject's tracking movements to the computer laboratory and a second line was used to send the computer programmed feedback signal back to the feedback display of the patient subject in the remote hospital observation room (Smith and Henry, 1967). The results of breath pressure tracking were that the patients were significantly poorer in breath pressure tracking than a normal control group. However, the patients' behavior was not affected as much by feedback delay of the respiratory tracking as was that of the normal group. This finding agrees generally with results of other feedback delay studies in indicating that, with less precise movement control, the effects of feedback delay are somewhat less than they are with exact movement guidance.

C. Manual Tracking of Respiration Produced Target Stimuli

In order to study the behavioral feedback mechanisms of physical conditioning, two studies (Smith and Putz, 1970; Smith and Sussman, 1970) were conducted to determine to what extent manual-visual tracking movements may be learned in relation to target stimulus patterns and to compare the efficiency of such learning with similar environmentally produced target variations. For purposes of the experiment, processes of interrelating respiratory activity and visual-manual activity shall be referred to as body tracking or steering, while the comparable task of following an environmental target will be called stimulus tracking. The experiment consisted of comparing respiration related body tracking and stimulus tracking under conditions in which the visual targets in the two modes of tracking were very nearly identical. In body tracking, a subject's breathing movements were transduced by means of a pneumograph, and the electrical signal from these movements used to vary a visual target. The subject's task was to negate these respiration produced target variations by moving a hand control device. If the subject performed perfectly, his hand movements were identical to his respiratory movements except that they moved the target indicator in an opposite direction. The accuracy in performing this task was compared with tracking a computer generated variation in the visual target which was approximately equal in frequency to the respiration produced target variations. The study determined the relative rate at which the respiration related and stimulus tracking were learned, the degree of transfer of learning between the two tasks, and the effects of feedback delay upon them.

The subject's main task consisted of using a small spring-wand hand control to position a light target on a projection screen. By moving the hand control, the subject could compensate any movement of this light spot from the center or zero point on the screen. In one experimental condition, the target light was caused to vary in position in relation to the subject's respiration, and the task was to correct for this respiration perturbed variation in the target position. In a second condition, a hybrid computer system was used to produce variations in movement of the target spot in a sine wave pattern approximately equal to the rate and magnitude of the normal respiration rate. In this case also, the subject's task was to correct for the externally controlled variation in the position of the target by using his hand control to keep the target on center. The two conditions of performance were compared in regard to error level in tracking, the course and rate of learning the two tasks, the effects of feedback delays of several magnitudes on error level, and the extent of transfer from one task to another.

The design of the experiment involved 24 female college students who were divided into two groups of 12 subjects each. The first was designated the respiratory group, and the second the stimulus-tracking group. The respiratory group practiced for 25 trials with the respiratory controlled target and then were tested in 15 transfer trials with the stimulus tracking. The stimulus tracking group practiced for 25 trials with the computer generated target wave, and then were shifted to 15 trials with the respiratory related tracking. In both series of trials feedback delay test trials were interspersed every five trials in the practice series and every three trials in the transfer series. Six feedback delay magnitudes between hand motion and action of the visual cursor were used, 0.0, 0.2, 0.4, 0.6, 0.8, and 1.5 sec. The entire design of the experiment was based on the fact that the two modes of tracking—i.e., respiratory controlled and stimulus controlled tracking—were exactly comparable in terms of the calibration of the hand motion feedback display relationship and in terms of the relative degree that the computer and the respiratory waves perturbed the feedback display.

This experiment utilized the real time computer system to control and equate the two modes of tracking performance and to regulate the magnitude of the feedback delays. The computer system and real time dynamic programming were used to interrelate hand action, as recorded by the hand motion transducer, and the hand-yoked light spot on the feedback display. The feedback display consisted of a vertical cylindrical white screen extending for some 90 degrees over the subject's visual field. A spot of light 1 inch in diameter was continuously projected from a light galvanometer on the screen and moved horizontally across it at the subject's eye level when she was seated in a dental chair facing the feedback display. The screen also had a marker at its center, and the subject was required to keep her hand-yoked light spot aligned with this marker.

The subject controlled the projected light spot on the screen by operating a hand motion transducer. This transducer consisted of a bronze spring wand about 12 inches long that was anchored to a support and fitted with strain gauges. Lateral movement of the wand produced proportional movement of the light spot. The polarity of movement of the system was adjusted so that the movements of the hand motion transducer and that of the light spot were in the same direction. The ratio of hand motion to movement of the light spot was approximately 1 to 13. The strain gauge wand served to transduce hand movements linearly to their electrical analog and these electrical signals were processed by the computer system.

To transduce the respiratory movements and to use these signals to control the feedback display of the breath related tracking, a pneumographic strain gauge transducer was used. This consisted of a rubber tube which was fitted around the subject's chest and, when stretched by breathing motions, actuated a small spring wand fitted with strain gauges. These transduced breathing movements were amplified and admixed electrically with the feedback signal of the hand motions. During calibration of the movement of the light spot with respect to hand movement, a switch was automatically activated to block the effect of the breathing on the feedback display and thus to calibrate the manual-visual part of the tracking system independently of the breathing movements.

The computer system was used to control all aspects of the experiment. To accomplish the main function of controlling the interaction between hand motion and feedback display, the transduced electrical signals of hand motion were processed in the manner described earlier for respiratory movement signals.

The task in the stimulus tracking was produced by programming the computer to generate a sine wave variation in the movement of the light spot on the screen. The frequency of these induced variations in the indicator light was approximately that of resting respiration in the individual. The subject had to compensate for these computer generated stimulus changes to keep the indicator on center on the screen. An oscillograph readout system, which recorded both the computer generated target wave and the respiratory generated wave, was used to calibrate these two systems so that the wave amplitudes resulting from them were equal.

The digital computer was programmed to control feedback delays of the visual signal of the hand motion in the stimulus and respiratory perturbed tracking. Besides a normal condition, five magnitudes of delay were used—i.e.,

0.2, 0.4, 0.6, 0.8, and 1.5 sec. The order of presentation of these delay trials in the training and transfer conditions of the experiment was varied by subjects. The principle of storing the input hand motion signals for control of delay magnitude is illustrated by the circular diagram of the digital computer memory in Fig. 7. Following computer program instructions, the input signal was written into memory, stored for the specified magnitude, and then outputted after this delay interval to govern the movement of the light indicator.

The procedure of the observations on particular subjects was controlled in large part by computer automation. Once an individual subject was seated in a dental chair in front of the screen, the computer system took over to govern all the main experimental operations. Besides governing the magnitudes of feedback delay, the computer system generated warning signals of the beginning of calibration procedures before each trial, carried out the calibrations of feedback display with respect to movement of the hand motion transducer, generated the target wave for the stimulus tracking, admixed the transduced signals of breath control with the feedback signals of hand motion, computed the tracking error, timed trials, regulated the sequence of trials and of test trials with given magnitudes of feedback delay, reduced the error values of each sample measurement to mean values for each 5 sec of performance, and coded and tabulated these means according to a predetermined format for later statistical analysis. At the end of the observations on a particular subject, the tabulated means were punched out on paper tape. Later the taped data for all subjects were assembled, transferred to IBM cards, and analyzed by statistical methods.

The main results of the experiment consist of: (1) learning functions for the initial training of the respiratory related and stimulus tracking groups, (2) transfer data for the two groups in shifting from the training tasks to stimulus tracking and respiratory perturbed tracking respectively, (3) delay functions for the two training groups and the two transfer groups, and (4) a complete set of oscillograph records for the different conditions of learning and performance.

It will be remembered that the first aspect of the observations consisted of 25 practice trials by the two experimental groups—the respiratory perturbed and the stimulus tracking groups. The learning curves for the two groups are described in Fig. 8. These curves indicated that the respiratory group was superior in tracking to the stimulus tracking group throughout the 25 trials. The general form of the two curves is much the same, with that for the respiratory mode being somewhat more irregular.

Effects of delay of the visual feedback of hand motion were determined by delay trials interspersed in both the practice and transfer series. The delay functions for the two modes of tracking in the two trial series are given in Fig. 9. In this graph, the steering (body tracking) curves represent the respiratory guided tracking, while the stimulus tracking curves represent the environmentally controlled tracking. The two training series of delay trials are marked

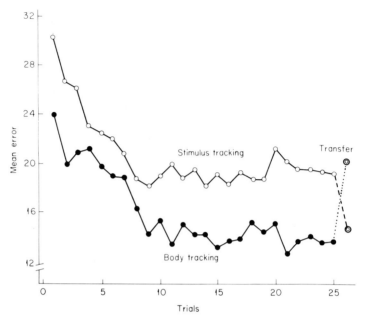

Fig. 8. Learning curves for manual-visual tracking with respiratory produced and environmentally produced stimulus patterns. (From Smith and Sussman, 1969.)

separately from the transfer series and indicated by five dotted lines. The performances affected most by delay were the respiratory transfer series and the stimulus learning series. The effect of the delay on the stimulus tracking training series and the respiratory transfer series was very similar, with the latter being consistently the least affected. The results indicate that only the target delay values of 0.8 and 1.5 sec produced differentiative effects on performance, and that these effects were not consistent with regard to the conditions.

Oscillograph records of the performances also showed that both the respiratory related and the stimulus tracking were markedly perturbed by increasing magnitudes of delay, and error was increased. In the case of the respiratory mode, breathing became quite irregular with delays of 0.4 sec and above. The frequency pattern of hand motion was reduced with delay values above 0.6 sec, and along with this change in rhythm, the velocity of movement was reduced. With one exception, similar variations in performance with increasing delay intervals also can be observed in the records for the stimulus tracking. In this case, the regularity of respiration did not change with the level of feedback delay.

A three-way analysis of variance was carried out on the data of the experiment which encompassed the variables of order of presentation of the training and transfer conditions (0), delay magnitude (DM), and tracking modes

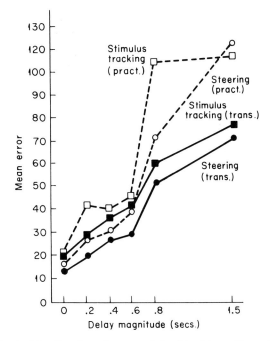

Fig. 9. Feedback delay functions for manual-visual tracking with respiratory produced and environmentally produced targets. (From Smith and Sussman, 1969.)

(TM). Both delay $(P < .01)$ and tracking modes $(P < .05)$ were statistically significant. Proceeding from these findings, Neuman-Keuls range tests (Winer, 1962) were carried out on the learning and delay means. The tests made included only the first four and last three trials of the training series. The results indicate that the means of the first four trials were significantly different from those of the last three trials for both the stimulus tracking and the respiratory perturbed tracking.

The results of the range tests related to delay magnitude showed that the differences in performance related to delay magnitudes were not significant below the value of 0.6 sec. Above that value, error increased significantly with each magnitude of delay.

Results of this experiment suggest that in rehabilitation and exercise training, body tracking in accurately integrating external motorsensory and respiratory related movements and functions is more rapid than, and therefore precedes, stimulus or environmental tracking tests. This superiority of body tracking of self-generated, organically related stimulus variations was found to persist in transfer tests. The results show that feedback delay affected processes of integration of movement and organic mechanisms of body tracking in much the same way that it affects accuracy in stimulus tracking.

The findings give some definite ideas of how external motorsensory and autonomic mechanisms are coordinated in physical conditioning. In keeping with assumptions stated earlier, these two sectors of function were shown to be feedback yoked and to depend on precise conditions of closed loop timing for coordination. Results also showed that feedback delay in an external motorsensory circuit may impair respiration. One main conclusion is that physical conditioning can be achieved in part by regulating external motorsensory operations, not only to improve smoothness and accuracy in performance but to reduce fatigue and to create more efficient organic function and behavior. A second conclusion is that a relatively high level of accuracy for the integration of motorsensory and autonomic function precedes learning of tracking environmental stimuli. The patterns of such integration differ markedly in stimulus tracking and in body tracking essential for stimulus conditioning.

The experiment just described was repeated and the effects of practice and visual feedback delay on body tracking and stimulus tracking compared in somewhat more detail. Results showed that learning functions over trials as well as over days of practice differed for the two types of tasks. Again, it was found that the pattern of respiration became specialized and differed markedly in the body tracking and in the stimulus tracking. The results of this study, as well as those of the previous experiment, suggested that specific training in coordinating breathing with specific external movement processes could contribute materially to physical conditioning of skilled movements.

D. Integration of Respiration with Arm Movements in Physical Conditioning

In collaboration with Luetke (Smith and Luetke, 1969), several studies were conducted regarding the way respiratory movements and visually guided arm movements are coordinated in tasks such as swimming. An initial investigation indicated that tracking of visual targets by control of breath volume was significantly more precise than manual tracking of comparable visual targets. Then, in subsequent studies, feedback control of arm and respiration integration was compared in two tracking modes, namely: (1) when changes in breathing served as a target indicator which tracked nonvisually by hand motions; and (2) when hand and arm movements served as an indicator which was tracked nonvisually by control of breath volume. The experiment was designed to simulate to some degree the arm movements used in swimming and the coordination required in this skill between arm movements and breathing. The question of physical conditioning posed was: is it better to train the swimmer to make his breathing track his arm movements or the reverse?

The apparatus used in the experiment consisted of a breath volume transducer which was constructed from the parts of a commercially sold metabulator. An arm transducer was devised and mounted 6 inches above the top of the breath volume transducer. The subject's task consisted of breathing into the mouth tube of the breath volume transducer either to track arm movements or to generate respiration movements that were tracked by the arm. In this situation, the term tracking refers to the fact that the respiration had to follow the pattern of hand motion or vice versa. The hand transducer consisted of a near frictionless linear potentiometer. In doing the task, the subject's nose was closed by a nose clamp and vision was occluded by a pair of opaque goggles. The respiratory and hand-arm movements were recorded on an oscillograph and also on a magnetic tape recorder. These records were later measured in terms of timing errors between the respiratory and hand-arm motions. The error measures also were classified in terms of whether a given hand or breath movement led or lagged behind the indicator movement.

The study involved comparison between eight experimental conditions divided into two groups of four main conditions. In the first main condition the rate of the target generating movement (either respiration or hand movement) and the timing of tracking motion had to be adjusted to every peak change in the target movement. In the second main condition the timing of the tracking motion had to be adjusted to every other peak change in the movement generated target variations. There were eight conditions in which the two modes of tracking were varied in terms of the rate at which the target movement was generated and the timing of tracking motion with the wave peaks of the movement generated target. The tracking targets in the two conditions were intrinsic and not visual or auditory—i.e., they were tactual, kinesthetic, and interoceptive inputs, as produced by the movement system that generated the intrinsic target patterns to be tracked by the other movement system.

The subjects used in this study were eight expert swimmers. An experimental design was used in which each subject performed under all eight conditions in a given order. Four subjects performed the first trial with arm tracking of respiration generated targets and the other four began with the hand tracking of the breath generated targets. The trial length was kept at 20 sec to prevent carbon dioxide buildup in the breath-volume transducer from affecting the results.

The results of the experiment indicated that four conditions of breath tracking of hand generated targets gave error values below those of hand tracking of breath generated targets. The mean relative error for breath tracking was 6.56, while that for hand tracking was 11.99. Tracking was more precise when tracking movements were coordinated with every other peak of target motion.

The timing between the two movement systems was assessed by measuring the interval at which the tracking movements led or lagged behind the target generating motions. The time measures expressed the percent of the times that the target movements led or lagged behind target motion. For breath tracking, the percentage of target lag values greatly exceeded the lead values. For the four conditions of hand tracking, however, the hand led the breath generated target a greater percentage of time. In other words, the respiratory movements tended to follow the hand movements even when they were supposed to serve as a target source. These time data mean that in both modes of tracking the breath movements were coordinated with and tracked the arm movements. The time data conform to the error data in showing that in physical conditioning in such activities as swimming, respiratory operations, and body movements governing energy production are coordinated externally as well as internally, and that the mechanism of this coordination is based primarily on high precision respiratory tracking.

The results of this respiratory behavioral research confirm that in all aspects of breath control tracking, respiratory behavior displays various high speed characteristics that are integrated with and may influence the slower general activities of inspiration and expiration. The results indicate that the control characteristics of inspiration in tracking may differ from expiration in the form and pattern of movement and be affected differently by conditions that require adjustment of breath control to coordinate with other movements. Inspiration is the leading control process in the fast phase of respiration. Both fast inspiration and expiration are affected by feedback delay, and in a manner which indicates that both involve predictive, anticipatory control features which are degraded under conditions of delay. The results show that the frequency of the rhythmic oscillatory rate of fast respiration is decreased as the magnitude of respiratory feedback delay is increased. The results prove that fast respiratory behavior is feedback timed in terms of its closed loop delay functions.

The results add to physiological data on exercise (Asmussen, 1967) in showing that the fast phases of respiration are cross-linked with body movements and that this interaction can influence the slower phases of the respiratory rhythm. The findings of this study, however, go beyond the exercise data in indicating that respiratory tracking is one of the most articulated and exquisite tracking systems of the body in interacting with arm and hand movements. Respiratory movements not only can adjust to other body movements with a speed and accuracy that equals that of the eye but perform this body tracking in a predictive feedforward way that anticipates or projects the pattern of body movement. This predictive interactive relationship between respiratory behavior and body movements influences both the accuracy of motor skills involved and the basic pattern of respiratory control.

Exercise physiologists (Asmussen, 1967; Dejours, 1964) have recognized that respiration has a body movement-related fast component that has projected anticipatory effects on the general pattern of respiration in exercise. Asmussen refers to these interactions as the work stimuli or work factors in respiration, which he supposes are regulated by neural processes. We think these terms, work stimuli or work factors, represent overgeneralized ideas and fail to convey the fact that the dominant features of respiration are these predictive motor coordinate interactions. The present findings, along with similar data from speech research, suggest that the fast phase of respiration is a dominant aspect of breathing, which serves to link it in a coordinate way as a rapid, energy regulatory process with every movement pattern of the body. In some movements such as speech, singing, and musical instrumentation, respiration is the base control mechanism for all the articulated detailed movements to be performed. In other movements, such as general body movement skills, the fast component of respiration operates as a rhythmic graded control process which serves to regulate the timing and force gradations of body movements. The findings confirm our theory that every movement pattern of the body has a highly distinctive respiratory pattern accompanying it, which acts in the dual feedback role of projecting the energy demands of the movement or skill and simultaneously governs many of the feedback timing and gradations of force of the motor skill.

The findings of respiratory tracking research agree in detail with many of the fundamental facts regarding the rate of respiratory movements in speech, as clarified especially by Stetsen (1951) in studies on the motorphonetic control of speech movements. Stetsen was the first to demonstrate that respiratory movements function at several different levels in controlling speech sounds. The primary movement is that of the intercostals in producing syllable pulses. As this articulated syllable pulse production proceeds, abdominal and diaphragm movements maintain breath pressure at a relative constant level while one or more syllable pulses are produced in breath groups to give expressive and grammatical phrasing to speech. Not only that, but the system also can adjust the force of intercostal movements within breath groups to vary speech power and expression and to dynamically interact with tongue, jaw, and lip movements, and thereby aid in articulation of syllables. As in the case of respiratory tracking movements, all of these variable control features of speech respiration have precise feedforward control characteristics that are essential for the guidance of sustained speech. The facts of both speech respiration and respiratory tracking confirm the theory that breathing behavior is a multi-dimensional motor coordination in itself that operates along with various feedback control parameters to interact with and govern in part energy and guidance factors of other body movements.

These studies on respiratory tracking also clarify a number of features of physical or physiological conditioning in exercise. As we showed earlier, a critical aspect of interaction of body movements with respiration in practice and exercise is that learning proceeds more consistently and rapidly with interactive body movements, including respiration, than it does with environmentally related stimuli. Since respiration is feedback linked to every phase of metabolism and energy production, the implication of this finding is that a most significant feature of motor-skill learning is the varied physiological feedbacks which respiration related learning imposes in a reciprocal way on the internal physiological system. We believe that such physiological learning is not only the key to physical conditioning in exercise but to the physiological bases of motor skill learning itself. That is to say, the various modes of physiological feedback are themselves primary determinants of learning and operate during practices to alter the efficiency of dynamic efferent integration for the feedback control of the parameters of energy regulation, including external and internal respiration. Our results give a number of substantial evidences that physical or physiological conditioning is far more than sports specialists and exercise physiologists have thought it to be—i.e., as either skeletal muscle or heart muscle building. Our view, which is confirmed in a limited way here, is that physical toning or conditioning in exercise and skill is a type of coordinated behavioral and physiological learning in which various parameters of physiological feedback are progressively more efficiently integrated and guided as learning proceeds. Externally, the results suggest that physical conditioning depends critically on feedback-controlled respiratory tracking of body movements that serve as a bridging mechanism between skeletal motor demands for guided movement and energy production for motor skill and internal oxygen metabolism.

V. Central-Neural versus Motor-System Feedback Control of Organic Rhythms

A. RATIONALE

As we have mentioned a number of times earlier, the fact is widely recognized that behavioral processes and motor factors have a marked influence on all of the main organic systems of the body and that these influences encompass external motor determination of the fast components of some rhythms along with dominant voluntary control over respiratory regulation. However, exercise physiologists have offered no methods to explore these behavioral systems processes which more often than not possess characteristic features of articulated, feedforward control that dominate the determination of the different organic rhythms, and especially those of respiration and circulation. The theory and experiments on biofeedback tracking, as carried out in an introductory way in the respiratory tracking studies, open the investigation of behavioral and neural components of organic rhythms as a field of experimental systems research.

In psychology and medicine, the problem of the interplay between behavioral and physiological factors in control of internal processes related to organic rhythms has been stated in the generalized ideas of psychosomatic influences on organic disease, theories of unconscious motivation (Alexander, 1950), and visceral conditioning (Pavlov, 1927; Miller, 1969). These views hold that psychological factors can influence organic rhythms through the neural or mental effects of reinforcement or associative learning.

The behavioral feedback view of physiological regulation presented earlier is a biofeedback concept that shifts the theoretical focus on behavioral-physiological integration from speculation about assumed learning and physiological-drive mechanisms to direct study of self-regulated, motor control mechanisms that can be shown to influence organic rhythms and other internal bioenergetic processes. The main theoretical issue raised by this feedback view is whether behavioral control of internal organic rhythms is based on direct stimulus and reinforcement conditioning of neural systems or whether action of peripheral skeletal motor mechanisms governs all critical modes of self-regulated and/or learned control of organic rhythms. An original series of experiments, using computerized laboratory feedback methods, initiated this systems biofeedback research on self-control of heart rhythms and brain rhythms. The view used to plan these studies holds that open-loop stimulus conditioning and reward factors can influence organic mechanisms only by altering external skeletal motor control of these processes. The view was that reactive motor processes can influence organic processes and their rhythms in any one of three ways—i.e., by metabolic feedback from energy production during response, by organic feedback effects of response on circulation and respiration, and by neuro-hormonal and kinesthetic feedback which regulates limbic and autonomic output.

To evaluate the validity of the views just stated, experimental systems studies were made of self-regulation and feedback entraining of organic rhythms. The term, feedback entraining of organic rhythms, refers to a procedure of yoking exteroceptive stimuli to peak responses of organic reactions, such as heart rate or the alpha rhythm of the electroencephalogram, and then changing slightly the frequency of occurrence of the feedback-yoked stimuli to see if this change will alter the frequency of the organic response. The technique is a refinement of direct associative conditioning of external stimuli with organic response to provide a type of pure sensory or neural feedback conditioning that has not been studied heretofore in either physiology or psychology.

B. Self-Regulated Feedback Control and Stimulus Feedback Entraining of Heart Rate

Figure 10 illustrates the real-time computerized, experimental systems methods for study of self-regulation of the heart rhythm. Subjects were fitted with electrocardiogram electrodes and seated in front of an oscillograph display. The transduced EKG signal was amplified, converted to digital form, and subjected to programming by the digital computer for measurement of the time intervals between successive heart-pulse peaks. The computer was programmed

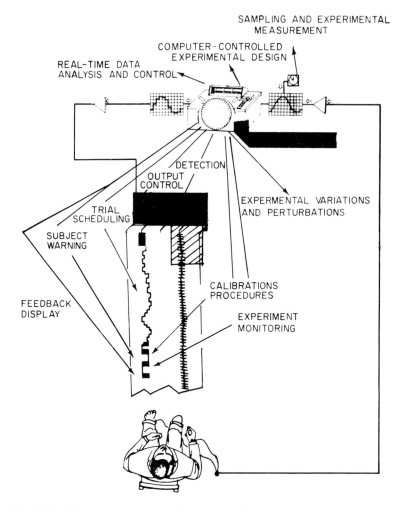

Fig. 10. Real time computer methods used to study self-governed feedback control and feedback entraining of the heart rate. (From Ansell *et al.,* 1967.)

to measure the time differences between successive heart pulse intervals and to output this difference measure as a visual feedback display to the subject. As the subject sat relaxed, he saw the oscillograph cursor move in small millimeter steps to the right or left of a zero line. Steps to the right indicated increases in heart rate (decrease in the heart-pulse interval) and those to the left, decreases in heart rate (increase in the heart-pulse interval). The subject observed this differential feedback display of his heart rate and attempted to negate variations in it, or in additional studies, to produce variations in it.

Several experiments on computerized study of self-regulation of heart rate showed that subjects can vary this rate in two and possibly three patterns (Ansell, Waisbrot, and Smith, 1967). Rapid self-produced compensation of intrinsic variations in heart rate are typically limited to one to five beats per minute. At somewhat longer intervals of 15–30 sec, subjects can self-generate increases in rate. At longer intervals, slowing of induced increases in heart rate can be accomplished. Observation and questioning of the subjects in these studies suggested that one or more of several methods were seized upon to reduce or increase heart rate. These included tensing up the neck, working the abdominal and chest muscles, generally tensing or relaxing, thinking of dull or exciting events, and changing breathing rate. The general conclusion was that these methods involved direct or indirect techniques of affecting venous circulation by movement, stimulating the carotid arteries of the neck, altering breathing rate or the general state of attention and the musculature through thought.

To test whether similar changes in heart rate could be produced by stimulus feedback entraining, the heart signal was transduced and subjected to computer programming as described above. However, in this case, the computer was programmed to detect the real time occurrence of each heart-pulse peak in milliseconds, and to output a digital voltage corresponding to this time point. This digital voltage was then used to activate a discrete light or sound click so that at each heartbeat the subject saw a light flash or heard a sound. Thereafter, in controlled observations, the computer was programmed to produce artificial changes in frequency of the heart produced external stimuli. The computer detected the actual heart rate over a period of a 2-min trial and increased or decreased the detected moving average rate by adding or subtracting one, two, three, or five stimulus occurrences each 10 sec. Changes in heart rate during these feedback entraining trials were automatically measured. Results of many different atempts to entrain the heart rate by these methods indicated that no systematic increases or decreases in the measured rate occurred with the direction of the entraining procedures, even with hours of exposure to the entraining stimuli. Typically, the only heart changes observed were a slowing of rate as the experimental observations proceeded. These changes were attributed to relaxation and accommodation to the experimental situation. The results thus suggest that external stimuli cannot be conditioned to drive the heart rate in a manner like that which can be achieved by self-regulation procedures.

The observations on self-regulation and feedback stimulus entraining of the heart rate were preceded by similar efforts to analyze self-regulation and feedback entraining of the alpha rhythm (Smith and Ansell, 1965). These studies of self-regulation and entraining of the electroencephalogram were carried out exactly as the heart-rate studies were programmed except that, in the brain wave entraining research, the peaks of the electroencephalogram above a predetermined voltage value acted automatically to induce feedback-yoked stroboscope flashes, sound clicks, or electrical tactual stimuli. A beginning series of observations were carried out to determine if these feedback-yoked stimuli stabilized the brain wave pattern in any consistent way. In later observations, the effect of varying the frequency of the feedback-yoked stimuli on the amount of alpha frequency was observed.

The results of the brain wave feedback research were like those later found in the heart rate studies. By relaxing and controlling visual attention, subjects breathing, and level of muscular tension in the experimental situation, subjects could produce variations in the amount of alpha rhythm in the electroencephalogram, sometimes amounting to as much as 15 or 20% of the duration of such waves. However, no such systematic variations occurred with yoking of external stimuli to the heart wave or as a result of directional entraining of the rhythm by changing the frequency of the feedback entraining stimuli. Since the feedback entraining procedure represents a specific mode of differential conditioning, it was judged that the claims of others for stimulus conditioning of the heart and brain rhythm cannot be substantiated by accurately controlled feedback research.

The general evidence from our studies of self-regulation and entraining of organic rhythms is that significant directional changes in organic rhythms by self-regulation or by learning procedures typically involve motor feedback factors and effects. The evidence is that if a rhythm can be changed by learning, it can be altered as well by self-governed control with adequate feedback displays. In contrast, attempts to bring the same rhythms under control by simulus entraining methods did not work.

The conclusion just stated has been strengthened in relation to stimulus-induced changes in brain rhythms by findings of Keesey and Nichols (1966). Their results show that intrinsic rhythmic variations in the pattern of the electroencephalogram under stabilized vision antecede by 400–700 msec appearances or disappearances of vision. In other words, the brain wave pattern is not modified or conditioned by afferent input under stabilized vision; rather, these changes in the electroencephalogram, which are known to be affected by motor produced neural activation, precede the changes in vision.

The main outcome of these initial computerized biofeedback studies on organic rhythms was to crystallize methods and theory of research on voluntary and motor control factors related to organic rhythms as a sector of experimental systems research. The results suggest that self-governed organismic processes which can influence internal physiological and organic mechanisms are not necessarily psychosomatic neural states but rather may represent reciprocal interaction between various modes of skilled motor activity in self-regulating different parameters of physiological and organic response. Voluntary self-control of organic processes in man seems to have a potential of influencing internal vital rhythms which is as great or greater than that which can be achieved by any procedure of conditioning and learning. However, such control is obviously limited and appears to be defined in general by different ways in which the skeletal motor system can be made to alter respiratory and circulatory processes and to influence the neural state. Our evidence would suggest that the phenomena of voluntary self-control of organic rhythms generally are much the same as the events of motor systems regulation of the different parameters of physiological feedback, as discussed in the first experimental section of this paper.

A first specific outcome of our computerized, biofeedback research was to point up the fine distinction between what may be called pure sensory feedback conditioning and learning as opposed to associative Pavlovian and operant conditioning. This distinction is important because an entire school of classical and operant conditioning investigators are now busily engaged in trying to identify feedback learning, such as we have studied in the biofeedback sensory entraining research with the crude associative stimulus conditioning of Pavlov (1927) and Thorndike (1932) respectively. As we showed in the work on stimulus entraining of organic rhythms, the direct association of repetitive sensory input signals with the frequency of the heart or brain rhythm has no noticeable effects on these rhythms. Accordingly, any effects which stimulus or operant conditioning have on organic rhythms in man is due to factors other than direct sensory feedback effects of the organic processes involved. We believe that the effectiveness of operant and associative stimulus conditioning in producing changes in organic rhythms is related to the mediation of motor control processes which are improved as a result of practice and suggestion in biofeedback conditioning observations.

The broadest practical issue opened up by the studies of stimulus feedback entraining of organic rhythms is that of effectiveness of various types of feedback learning or conditioning in altering disturbed physiological states, such as cardiac and neural disorders. The evidence we have obtained is that specific stimulus conditioning effects may have only limited potential in altering internal states and that any of the therapeutic and rehabilitative training effects which ensue from these discrete methods are in fact the result of motor systems-controlled feedback learning.

The methods and results of this research thus conform to the earlier summarized experimental data regarding motor system factors involved in regulation of physiological integration in physical conditioning. Physical conditioning cannot be achieved by the momentary effects of discrete stimulus or reward conditioning of the brain and organic system. Changes in the efficiency of physiological integration in skill and in instances of organic or behavioral disorders are dependent on either improved voluntary or learned control of the motor system and its influence on various parameters of vital energy regulation and production.

VI. Dynamic Efferent Organization in Physiological Feedback Regulation and Learning: Theoretical Summary

This chapter was set up to define a new behavioral cybernetic approach to analysis of the motor system and its dynamic efferent organization for control of different parameters of physiological feedback, metabolic integration, and energy production for behavior. The challenges faced in the chapter were fivefold, i.e., (1) to demonstrate that the motor system functions in significant dynamic ways to control many parameters of physiological feedback and energy production and operates not simply as an end product of reflex control and physiological drives; (2) to provide evidence that the primary psychophysiological foundation of learning and motivation is based on efferent integration of single muscle cell activity in controlling energy production with compound muscle functions and motor system operations, which can regulate the physical state of single muscle cells as well as the organic metabolic precursors of muscle energy production; (3) to determine whether basic forms of vital regulation involve a behavioral component which operates to determine the fast phases of oscillatory organic rhythms and therefore influence the internally governed aspects of the organic rhythms; (4) to show that biofeedback regulation of organic rhythms may be related to efferent organization of physiological feedback and motor system control of organic processes; (5) to present evidence that dynamic efferent organization, physiological regulation, energy regulation for motivation, and learning involve a process of physical conditioning.

The main conclusion from the facts assembled in this chapter is that the efficiency, synchronism, and accuracy of motor system and physiological integration are changed as a result of the neural feedback effects of the response. This serves to regulate parameters of energy uptake, conversion, distribution, mobilization, utilization, and production.

The different sections of the chapter dealt with the first four critical issues. A wide spectrum of facts was presented to show that the essential features of the mechanism of energy production for movement and its precursors in energy uptake, conversion, mobilization, and distribution consist of compound muscle control. This, in turn, determines the efficiency and mode of energy production within the cell as well as organic metabolism at more complex levels. Another series of experimental facts was presented to show that the modes of motor system exertion act to regulate differentially the mode of organic metabolism, the pattern of liver function, the rhythms of respiration and circulation, and the neurobehavioral and neural states of metabolism. The motor system is organized not simply to determine the pattern of skill and to control the external environment, but to systematically govern and integrate all levels of physiological regulation and vital organization for energy production.

The impact of the motor system on metabolism, energy production in muscle cells, and cellular physiological integration is not limited to molecular, organic-metabolic, and neurohormonal feedback, but can affect organic functions and their systems control components directly. In keeping with our central assumption, experimental results indicated that the skeletal behavioral component of respiration represents an articulated fast phase of the breath control system, which acts as an exquisite, bridging, feedback controlled tracking mechanism for integrating all primary patterns of body movement with both internal energy regulation and circulation. Not only that, but this bridge is of a highly variable nature so that every specialized body movement involves a distinctive pattern of respiration. Evidence was presented that this integrative linkage between body movements and respiration is the base of the predictive, feedforward control influences of body movements and exercise on respiration. Additional findings showed that a similar feedback linkage between muscle activity and capillary circulation constitutes a fast phase of circulatory and heart operations that can govern the predictive and exercise control of various parameters of circulation and heart action. These various series of facts add up to the conclusion that metabolic integration also depends on efferent integration and its neural and metabolic feedbacks.

Evidence regarding the biofeedback effects of behavior on organic rhythms was assembled from initial computerized studies of self-regulation of brain and heart rhythms under conditions in which closed loop feedback effects were yoked to oscillatory peaks of the rhythms. Results indicated that voluntary control of brain and heart rhythms with external sensory feedback depends materially if not entirely on motor-systems adjustments that can influence various aspects of neural activation, circulation, and respiration. Findings on feedback stimulus entraining of brain and heart rhythms, in which external stimuli were yoked to the oscillatory peaks of these rhythms and then varied to create a process of direct sensory conditioning of the organic rhythms, had no discernible effects on either type of rhythm. These results suggest that the current efforts of learning investigators to interpret biofeedback processes in learning, training, and behavioral therapy in terms of operant or classical conditioning processes are misconceived. Rather, the critical learning events of self-governed biofeedback are mediated by dynamic motor-system factors. Our conclusion is that the evidence for reinforcement learning in visceral control is no better than the evidence being supplied by clinical psychologists in confusing the issues and facts of training individuals in self-regulated control of brain rhythms and heart functions by use of discrete episodic sensory feedbacks which are conceived as reinforcements for learning.

We believe that the upshot of present facts regarding the role of physiological feedback in determining learning is that a cybernetic systems approach to behavior rather than a general reinforcement doctrine hereafter will represent the primary control theory of learning and performance. This possibility can be judged to be likely also because S-R reinforcement and conditioning concepts cannot explain how continuous interacting feedback effects from different movements can be sensed as dynamic systems effects of movement and thus used to guide movement learning and projected feedforward control of physiological regulation and motivation. Our own view is that the processes of continuous and dynamic control of neural and metabolic events underlying physical conditioning and motor learning cannot be specified in any accurate way by modified stimulus-response and reinforcement doctrines of behavior because these views are essentially a denial of the possibility of continuous self-governed control of behavior and its related vital operations.

The implications of the results are not limited to the specific theoretical sectors used to assemble the experimental data and to design our own studies. Several general concepts of a behavioral cybernetic interpretation were given some support by the combinations of experimental data summarized in the different sections of this chapter.

The present studies add to the behavioral feedback concept of physical conditioning. This concept is that physical conditioning is a type of physiological learning based directly on the metabolic, neurohormonal, kinesthetic, interoceptive, and organic feedback effects of motor systems action. This physiological learning is coupled with exteroceptive feedback effects of motorsensory response which induce learning change. There is an integration of energy production in specialized muscle groups with movement and receptor guidance as well as the various parameters of visceral behavior and metabolism. In this learning, the brain detects the patterns of receptor inputs from the various organic systems as well as from kinesthetic, interoceptive, and exteroceptive inputs resulting from the same motor patterns. The brain converts these feedback feature detections to coordinated efferent control of the limbic, extrapyramidal-postural, extrapyramidal receptor-efferent, and pyramidal motor systems. The outcome of such dynamic efferent coordination and neural feature detection is to integrate both the parameters of physiological feedback resulting from movement and behavioral physiological interactions for control of energy production. Physical conditioning consists of feedback induced physiological effects that lead to improved integration of the parameters of energy regulation as well as guidance and synchronism in motor skill behavior.

The present studies revise our understanding of the relationships of work, exercise, and motor skill. For over a century physiologists and psychologists have kept themselves at arm's length from one another in discussing these processes with the aim of preserving their traditional understanding of these events as separate processes supposedly determined by quite different neural and biochemical events. As a result of these dissective approaches, physiologists have protected the field of exercise as a preserve for studying biochemical homeostasis, while psychologists have isolated their concerns by talking about motor skill and the motor system as learned psychomotor behavior. The feedback concept of motor-system physiological regulation and efferent organization dissolves this divorce of motor skill psychology and exercise physiology by asserting that everything which physiologists have said about work and exercise is overgeneralized and serves mainly to bypass the most crucial roles of the motor system in reciprocally influencing all limits and parameters of physiological regulation. However, to know really how efferent organization and motor skill affect vital functions and operations, it is necessary to alter also the limited and superficial psychological views of psychomotor skill as an end product of conditioned neural integration, stimulus control, and physiological drive, which supposedly has no known impact on internal functions. A needed extension of the behavioral concept is that motor skill phenomena represent all of the detailed variable control factors and dynamic integrative functions of exercise and work in influencing physiological regulation in exercise. Motor skill, efferent organization, motor systems feedback on vital regulation, and exercise are all one and the same thing, and their most significant property in reciprocal behavioral-physiological interaction is in controlling and integrating energy production, guidance of behavior, learning, and synchronism of parameters of organic function in metabolism. Motor skill psychophysiology is the key to some of the deepest mysteries of respiration, circulation, physical conditioning, sugar metabolism, and all of the predictive features of organic regulation.

Overall, this chapter achieves in a limited way a needed minor revolution in psychology—the so-called handmaiden of physiology—in suggesting that the two terms of psychophysiology are on an equal scale in dealing with problems of learning, vital regulation, and adaptation. The central problem of vital organization in adaptation is the mechanism of interaction between single cell metabolism in energy regulation and motor system operations in feedback regulation of both single cell metabolism and organic functions. Motor skill and physical conditioning based on motor skill are the critical control aspects of efferent organization, both of which bridge dynamically the needs and potentials of energy production and the regulation of organic precursors of such production. The proper view is that the motor system is simply not a dependent variable of physiological drive and regulation; rather, the skeletal motor system is the dominant, dynamic center of all vital regulation which has variable control over more primitive operations. The time has come for psychophysiologists to recognize that the development of the skeletal motor system represents the dynamic forefront of vertebrate evolution and that the patterns of efferent organization for regulation of motor skill have determined the selective development of both the brain and the capacities of the visceral system in energy regulation.

Acknowledgment

The work described in this report has been supported by research grants from the National Science Foundation, and by a training grant from the Biological Sciences Section of the National Institute of Mental Health.

This paper was prepared with the assistance of Thomas J. Smith, Physiology Department, University of Wisconsin.

Chapter 3

Motor Cortex and the Pyramidal System

ARNOLD L. TOWE

SCHOOL OF MEDICINE
UNIVERSITY OF WASHINGTON

I. Introduction

Consult any textbook of physiology and you will learn, by implication if not by direct statement, that movements are conceived in a limited region of the cerebral cortex, either *de novo* or in response to information received from other regions of the brain, and that each movement is coded by the cortex as a unique pattern of nerve impulses which is transmitted by the corticospinal tract[1] to

---

[1] The corticospinal tract is that portion of the pyramidal system that projects into the spinal cord; it generally amounts to about half of the total pyramidal system.

appropriate alpha motoneurons. The rest of the brain is left in a supportive role, the primary task being performed by this simple, "two-neuron" system.[2] In this paper we will briefly examine some of the experimental data that bear on this simple model. It will first be necessary to settle on some working definition of motor cortex, and then to examine the general anatomical properties of the postulated "hot line" from the cerebrum to the outside world. The popular concept under examination is caricatured in Fig. 1.

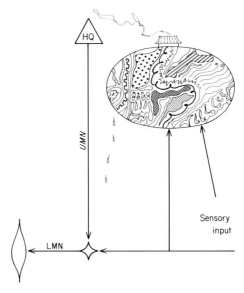

Fig. 1. Caricature of the "hot line" view of the mammalian nervous system. HQ, headquarters; UMN, upper motoneuron; LMN, lower motoneuron. "Mod egg" is the rest of the central nervous system. Headquarters is seen sniffing incense when the breeze is right and it is so inclined; it must occasionally compromise its output with minor effects from elsewhere in the nervous system. An alternative caricature would move headquarters to the "mod egg" and subordinate the "hot line" entirely to the role of messenger—too modest a role for such an important set of neurons in the view of many scientists.

A. MOTOR CORTEX

A precise definition of the term motor cortex is as elusive as the concept itself, and can only be approached through the various experimental maneuvers that reveal some cerebral involvement in the regulation of movement. In a sense, the entire nervous system is motor, for it exists primarily to develop output, be it muscular contraction or glandular secretion. Yet, alpha motoneurons are

[2] Neurologists often refer to corticospinal fibers as upper motoneurons, and to alpha motoneurons as lower motoneurons.

clearly more motor than are the group IA afferent fibers that excite them. In the case of the cerebral cortex, we wish to sort out degree of involvement, in the sense of immediacy and specificity. The experimental maneuvers that allow such sorting seem limited to stimulation, ablation, and recording, though an histological criterion for the identification of motor cortex has also been promoted. Unfortunately, the results of these different approaches to definition do not always converge onto the same tissue.

Our fundamental belief in the existence of motor cortex as a discrete and definable entity derives primarily from the oft-repeated observation that electrical stimulation at the surface of the cerebral cortex causes muscles to contract. These contractions, which occur mainly contralateral to the side of cerebral stimulation, are usually recognized and described as movements, ranging in magnitude from the barely detectable flick of a single digit to massive, convulsive contractions involving many muscles. The region of cerebral cortex which, when weakly stimulated, causes relatively isolated muscle contractions, or simple movements, is properly designated as electrically excitable motor cortex.[3] Within this region, a high degree of topographical organization can be recognized in many mammals (Woolsey, 1958).

The electrically excitable motor cortex is generally regarded as occupying the precentral gyrus,[4] a belief due largely to the efforts of Leyton and Sherrington (1917). However, apparently in no mammal, not even in man (Foerster, 1936; Penfield and Rasmussen, 1952), is this tissue so neatly restricted. A supplementary motor area, defined by the criterion of electrical excitability, is present in the frontal lobe of many species (Penfield and Welch, 1951; Woolsey, Settlage, Meyer, Spencer, Pinto Hamuy, and Travis, 1951). The rostral part of the parietal lobe, traditionally called somatosensory area I, and even tissue caudal to this, qualifies as electrically excitable motor cortex (Kennard and McCulloch, 1943; Sugar, Chusid, and French, 1948; Vogt and Vogt, 1919; Welker, Benjamin, Miles, and Woolsey, 1957; Woolsey, 1958; Woolsey, Travis, Barnard, and Ostenso, 1953). No problem is immediately posed for the pyramidal tract "hot line" belief, however, for about half of the pyramidal tract fibers originate in this postcentral cortex. Following surface stimulation of the postcentral gyrus, I waves can be recorded from the medullary pyramids (Patton and Amassian, 1954, 1960), and even D waves can be obtained if the stimulating electrodes are thrust a millimeter deep into the tissue (Towe and Kennedy, unpublished observations on *M. mulatta*).

A similar definition of motor cortex would be difficult, if not impossible, to obtain through lesion studies. Most mammals get along adequately in the

---

[3] This designation is often shortened to motor cortex, with a consequent loss of clarity.

[4] Not all primates and none of the nonprimate mammals possess a precentral gyrus; however, all mammals possess some agranular neopallium, generally located rostrally in the cerebrum.

laboratory following recovery from large cerebral ablations, especially if the lesions are bilaterally symmetrical (Travis and Woolsey, 1956). On the other hand, such lesioned animals could not compete successfully with normal mammals, for they lack the required speed, agility, and adaptability. The "higher" primates (including man) show marked motor deficiencies following pericentral ablations, but Travis and Woolsey (1956) have demonstrated that with care, locomotor functions can be retained, even through heroic cerebral ablations. In the case of humans, the deficit is more profound and persistent following parietal than following precentral gyrus lesions; a marked paresis[5] develops.

Recordings from cerebral cortex yield an even more puzzling picture with respect to the idea of motor cortex. Both Evarts (1968, 1969) and Fetz (1969) find increased activity on some precentral gyrus neurons prior to muscle contraction, when that contraction is trained in an operant situation. However, it is not clear what is being trained, the muscle contraction or the precentral neuron activity, among other possibilities. Furthermore, the muscle contraction and neuron activity can readily be dissociated (Fetz and Finocchio, 1971). According to Fetz (personal communication), at most recording sites the neuron activity is predominantly related to contraction of proximal limb muscles, whereas threshold stimulation at these sites causes contraction of distal limb muscles. In the case of the frontal eye fields, defined by the criterion of electrical excitability, Bizzi (1968) was unable to find neuron activity clearly preceding spontaneous eye movements; activity increased during and after the saccads, eliminating such neurons from a "hot line" role. Again, in an area just caudal to the arcuate sulcus of *M. mulatta,* where neuron activity is clearly related to jaw movements, Luschei (personal communication) reports that stimulation yields contraction of buccal muscles rather than contraction of jaw muscles. Further, Luschei finds that a neuron in this tissue may fire in close relation to, and preceding, a single jaw bite but fail to fire when a closely following second bite of the same "topography" occurs. Finally, Ward, Ojeman, and Calvin (personal communication) find in humans that neuron activity in precentral cortex only infrequently relates to "voluntary" contraction of facial muscles, whereas surface stimulation at that location regularly causes contraction of those very facial muscles.

Such disjointed findings leave our intuitive idea of motor cortex in a shambles. We would do well to retreat to the firmer ground of electrically

---

[5] The term paresis is often transmuted to paralysis, and the expression "paralysis of voluntary movement" is used in connection with cerebral lesions. In the stimulus-response frame of reference that still dominates our thinking, voluntary movement is a category obtained by exclusion of certain movements from the stimulus-response core. Unfortunately, movements seem to move in and out of that category with a will all their own, depriving the expression of clear meaning.

excitable motor cortex, and sort out these ablation and recording studies later. Some studies seem to tie the precentral gyrus activity to output[6] that generates immediate payoff; others seem to reinforce the idea that precentral gyrus can create output *de novo*. Cerebral cortex neurons, and especially pyramidal tract neurons, are only loosely coupled to afferent input in the American opossum (Towe and Biedenbach, 1969), yet this lowly creature is so highly successful that it has survived almost unchanged for some 60 million years. If its "motor cortex" plays an important role in initiating or regulating behavior, or movement, it would seem to do so quite independently, for no tight coupling with other neurons has been found.

B. Pyramidal System

An unequivocal definition of the pyramidal system is no less difficult to attain than one of motor cortex, for presumed function has become thoroughly entangled with ideas about anatomical organization. The development of thinking about the prominent corticofugal pathway that characterizes this system has left a fascinating trail across nearly two centuries of time and has touched all those who know the term nervous system. The story is much too involved to recount here; let a few highlights suffice. The existence of a corticospinal system in man was first clearly realized by the phrenologists Gall and Spurzheim (1810), and the idea that this system "mediated" volitional movements quickly appeared. Magendie (1834) was first to test the notion by transecting the pyramids in the rabbit, obtaining only minor motor disturbances. Over the past century, variations on that experiment have been performed on a host of different species by a host of different investigators, always with the same result: minor motor disturbance. Yet, the idea that "paralysis of voluntary movement" invariably results from pyramidal tract lesion persists to this day. The reader should consult the classic paper of Schäfer (1910) and the recent paper of Bucy, Ladpli, and Ehrlich (1966) to obtain some flavor of that controversy. In textbooks, the effects of pyramidal tract section have been exaggerated out of all proportion to their magnitude, and the associated changes in cutaneous sensitivity have been ignored.

For anatomical analysis, the pyramidal tract has been defined in different ways, leading to quite different ideas about the pyramidal system. Three major approaches may be recognized, the first of which is no longer followed. Early on, the pyramidal tract was identified through an abundance of very small fibers. Since it was thought to be exclusively a corticospinal pathway and to be the *sine*

---

[6] In thinking of output, we must distinguish among muscle contraction, movement, and behavior. Any behavior may be composed in a number of different ways, through different movements. Less obviously but equally important, any movement may be produced through different degrees of muscle contraction and is characterized by reciprocal action.

qua non of voluntary activity,[7] description began at the pyramidal decussation and proceeded caudally. The extent of the pyramidal tract within the spinal cord was thus somewhat exaggerated. With the development of methods for staining degenerating fibers, and with the idea that the muscle contractions caused by cerebral stimulation depend upon conduction via the pyramidal tract, a new, refined, and powerful approach was in hand. One could simply identify the electrically excitable motor cortex in his animal of choice, ablate that tissue, close the exposure, and await degeneration. During the interim, one had the additional advantage of being able to observe the motor consequences of cerebral ablation—the consequences routinely being ascribed solely to pyramidal tract deprivation. At the appropriate time, the brain was perfused, and all tissue caudal to the pyramidal decussation carefully removed for histological study. This procedure, as we now understand it, underestimates the pyramidal tract, for most investigators adjust their criteria for electrically excitable motor cortex so that a single, circumscribed region confined to the frontal lobe is obtained. They thus miss about half of the corticospinal fibers and, by ignoring the brainstem, fail to recognize the extraordinarily diffuse character of the pyramidal system. Interpretation is further confounded by the fact that the rate of axon degeneration varies with fiber size (Russell and DeMyer, 1961; van Crevel and Verhaart, 1963a).

The third major approach, to define the pyramidal system through the compact collection of fibers on the ventral surface of the medulla oblongata—the medullary pyramids—has led to an ever-expanding view of the system that has yet to come to full flower. The approach has forced recognition of the massive contribution of this system of fibers to the brainstem nuclei, through collaterals, *en passage* synapses, and terminal connections. It has led to a clearer recognition of "aberrant" pyramidal bundles and to agreement that probably all pyramidal tract fibers emanate from cell bodies in the cerebral cortex. The pyramidal system comprises corticobulbar as well as corticospinal fibers; collaterals terminate in pons and midbrain tegmentum and even the dorsal thalamus (Clare, Landau, and Bishop, 1964). The distinction between pyramidal and extra-pyramidal "motor pathways" has become clouded, for the former directly interacts with the latter at the red nucleus (Tsukahara and Fuller, 1969, Tsukahara, Fuller, and Brooks, 1968) and at midbrain and bulbar tegmental sites (Kuypers, 1958a,b,c, 1960; Niimi, Kishi, Miki, and Fujita, 1963) as well as at the level of spinal interneurons. For the moment, then, we will think of the pyramidal tract as those fibers originating in the cerebral cortex that emerge caudal to the pons as a compact bundle on the ventral surface of the medulla oblongata. We will think of the pyramidal system as comprising the pyramidal tract, its cells of origin, and all its diverse and far-flung terminations. As will

---

[7] This knowledge was held at a level of confidence scarcely justified by the data existing in the latter half of the nineteenth century.

become evident later, it is through the characteristic pattern of terminations of the pyramidal tract, as seen in both cat and monkey, that the definition of the pyramidal system may be broadened to include a more obscure tract known as the corticotegmental tract, or bundle of Bagley (1922; Haartsen and Verhaart, 1967).

II. Organization of the Pyramidal System

The outstanding feature of the pyramidal system is its high degree of variation, not only between species, but also among individuals of the same species. In the brief review that follows, emphasis will be placed on generality, at the expense of most species variation. The discussion will be carried on as far as possible at the level of mammalian order. Literature citations will be restricted mainly to classical papers, to those that illustrate conflict of interpretation, and to those from which the reader may conveniently "work backward" into the bulk of this immense literature.

The pyramidal tract runs a similar course from the cerebral cortex to the caudal brainstem in nearly all mammals thus far studied. From the cerebral cortex, fibers pass through the rostral or middle region of the internal capsule, to take up a medial or middle position within the pes pedunculi.[8] They then scatter into numerous fascicles as they pass through the pons, and thereafter regroup into a compact bundle medially along the ventral surface of the medulla oblongata. After crossing just caudally to the decussation of the medial lemniscus, the fibers take up any of a number of positions in the spinal cord, according to the species. They course primarily through the dorsal half of the spinal cord and terminate around neurons in the dorsal horn and intermediate zone, a few making direct contact with the dendrites of alpha motoneurons. Many fibers leave the pyramidal tract to terminate in the lower brainstem. In the bats, a prominent pyramidal decussation can be recognized just caudal to the pons (Dräseke, 1903; Fuse, 1926a; Merzabacher and Spielmeyer, 1903; van der Vloet, 1906). Fuse (1926d) thought he could identify a similar decussation in the giant anteater, but Verhaart (1967) was unable to verify this in the two specimens that he examined. From the findings of Bergman (1915), one might expect that the elephant would show a similar pattern. Other unusual "levels" of pyramidal decussation have been identified (Addens and Kurotsu, 1936; Chang, 1944, Goldby, 1939), though their precise interpretation is uncertain. Those corticospinal fibers that follow an uncrossed route through the spinal cord have occasionally been shown to cross at the level of termination. The reader should consult Valverde (1966) to gain an appreciation of the diverse zones of influence of any single pyramidal tract fiber.

[8] Frontopontine fibers occupy the most medial part of the pes pedunculi, but are numerous only in those mammals that possess large prefrontal lobes.

A. CEREBRAL ORIGIN

The cell bodies that give rise to the pyramidal tract are concentrated along the border between the frontal and parietal lobes, although they are also scattered sparsely through other regions of the cerebral cortex. In man and the "higher" primates, about 60% of the pyramidal tract fibers arise from Brodman's areas 4 and 6 of the frontal lobe, and about 40% arise from Brodman's areas 3, 1, 2, 5, and 7 of the parietal lobe (Barnard and Woolsey, 1956; Jane, Yashon, DeMyer, and Bucy, 1967; Lassek, 1952; Levin and Bradford, 1938; Liu and Chambers, 1964; Mettler, 1944; Minckler, Klemme, and Minckler, 1944; Peele, 1944; Russell and DeMyer, 1961; Uesugi, 1937). Other cerebral areas supply a small number of fibers to the pyramidal tract. A similar situation exists in the slow loris (Campbell, Yashon, and Jane, 1966) and the tree shrew (Jane, Campbell, and Yashon, 1969), the latter being of disputed primate affinities. In the domestic cat, this tract arises from cells mainly in the anterior and posterior sigmoid gyri and in the depths of the cruciate sulcus (Gobbel and Liles, 1945; Jabbur and Towe, 1961; Kennedy and Towe, 1962; Nyberg-Hansen and Brodal, 1963; van Crevel and Verhaart, 1963b; Walberg and Brodal, 1953), though again, fibers arise from other regions. In the sheep and the goat, this tract seems to arise from the superior frontal gyrus and adjacent tissue (Bagley, 1922; Haartsen and Verhaart, 1967; Verhaart and Noorduyn, 1961). In the American opossum, the pyramidal tract originates almost exclusively from the granular tissue of the postorbital and parietal areas of Gray (1924), although a few fibers arise from the agranular tissue rostral to the orbital sulcus (Bautista and Matzke, 1965; Biedenbach and Towe, 1970; Martin and Fisher, 1968; Towe and Biedenbach, 1969). Regarding other mammalian forms, too little is known. What studies have been done have primarily followed the second approach to definition outlined above—to ablate electrically excitable motor cortex and then to trace the resultant degeneration—leaving much of the cerebral origin of the pyramidal tract in doubt.

B. CORTICOSPINAL PATTERN

The greatest variation in anatomical organization of the pyramidal system occurs in its corticospinal component. Even within the single species, *Homo sapiens,* the variation is almost unbounded. The primary bundle forms in the dorsal portion of the lateral funiculus, after decussating just caudally to the crossing of the medial lemniscus. It comprises anywhere from 60% to nearly 100% of the corticospinal tract, and usually can be traced to sacral levels of the spinal cord. An uncrossed bundle is frequently present in the ventral funiculus. This bundle may comprise as much as 30% of the corticospinal tract, though it disappears by midthoracic levels of the spinal cord (Bumke, 1907; Minckler *et al.,* 1944; Nicolesco and Hornet, 1933; Nyberg-Hansen and Rinvik, 1963; Obersteiner, 1896; Probst, 1899; Rothmann, 1900; van Lenhossék, 1889;

Verhaart, 1970; Weil and Lassek, 1929). In addition, uncrossed fibers in the dorsolateral funiculus, and crossed fibers in the dorsal and ventral funiculi, may often be seen (Bumke, 1907; Obersteiner, 1896; Rothmann, 1900; van Lenhossék, 1889). Not content with such a variable pattern, one or both of the corticospinal tracts may fail to decussate, following instead an uncrossed route in the ventral or dorsolateral funiculi (Verhaart, 1970; Verhaart and Kramer, 1952). The lesser primates show less variation from one specimen to the next, though they generally show the pattern described for man (Barnard and Woolsey, 1956; Campbell *et al.,* 1966; Fulton and Sheehan, 1935; Glees, Cole, Liddel, and Phillips, 1950; Kuypers, 1958c; Liu and Chambers, 1964; Schoen, 1966; Shriver and Matzke, 1965; Tilney, 1927; Verhaart, 1954, 1966, 1970). On the other hand, the taxonomically uncertain tree shrew shows a crossed pathway confined to the dorsal funiculus (Jane *et al.,* 1969; Verhaart, 1966). The generalized primate pattern is illustrated in Fig. 2(A); *Tupaia* follows the pattern shown in Fig. 2(C).

The carnivores show a pattern of corticospinal pathways almost identical to that of the primates, though the ventral funicular components are much reduced or even absent, depending on the species (Buxton and Goodman, 1967; Kuypers, 1958a; Niimi *et al.,* 1963; Nyberg-Hansen and Brodal, 1963; Simpson, 1912; van Lenhossék, 1889). The crossed lateral funicular bundle accounts for nearly the entire corticospinal pathway of lagomorphs (Munzer and Wiener, 1902; van der Vloet, 1906; van Lenhossék, 1889). Oddly, the pattern in monotremes is much

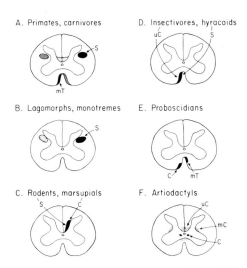

Fig. 2. Generalized patterns showing spinal pathways followed by corticospinal fibers in several mammalian orders. Symbols show caudal extent of the different pathways. uC, upper cervical; mC, midcervical; C, throughout cervical cord; mT, midthoracic; S, through sacral segments.

like that of lagomorphs, the crossed lateral bundle being evident beyond midlumbar levels (Goldby, 1939). Both Ziehen (1908) and Abbie (1934) thought they could resolve a small, ventrally disposed medullary pyramid that crossed in the ventral funiculus, to disappear into the ventral horn in the first cervical segment. However, Kölliker (1901) had earlier traced a pathway that decussates in the pons and runs a lateral course through the bulb, to enter the dorsal part of the lateral funiculus; several more recent studies agree with Kölliker (Addens and Kurotsu, 1936; Fuse, 1926b; Goldby, 1939). The pattern for lagomorphs and monotremes is shown in Fig. 2(B).

Both marsupials and rodents specialize in a crossed dorsal funicular pathway [Fig. 2(C)], but this is about all they have in common. The corticospinal fibers of marsupials rarely can be traced beyond upper thoracic levels (Bautista and Matzke, 1965; Biedenbach and Towe, 1970; Goldby, 1939; Martin and Fisher, 1968; Towe and Biedenbach, 1969; Ziehen, 1897, 1908), whereas they extend throughout the length of the spinal cord in most of the rodents thus far examined (Barnard and Woolsey, 1956; Douglas and Barr, 1950; Goldby and Kacker, 1963; Goldstein, 1904; King, 1910; Ranson, 1913; Reveley, 1915; Simpson, 1914, 1915a,b; Valverde, 1966; van Lenhossék, 1889). There are many minor variations, but the Canadian porcupine is markedly deviant. It not only displays a large, crossed dorsal pathway, but also a significant uncrossed ventral bundle that likewise extends to sacral levels, an uncrossed dorsal funicular bundle that extends through the thoracic cord, and a minor crossed lateral bundle that disappears in the cervical cord (Simpson, 1915a).

The insectivores, modern forms of the stem mammalian line, show yet another pattern: the medullary pyramids plunge directly into the spinal cord without crossing and disappear in the upper cervical cord (Bischoff, 1900; Dräseke, 1904; Kozenberg, 1899; Linowiecki, 1914; van der Vloet, 1906). Verhaart (1967) has recently found a similar condition in the rock hyrax, though the pathway in that species evidently extends to the sacral cord. This condition is illustrated in Fig. 2(D). The closest living relatives of the hyracoids, the proboscidians, possess an uncrossed ventral funicular bundle, which terminates within the cervical cord, but in addition possess a somewhat larger, crossed bundle that occupies the dorsal part of the ventral funiculus and descends to the midthoracic cord (Verhaart, 1963; Verhaart and Kramer, 1959). This condition is shown in Fig. 2(E).

Most but not all of the pyramidal tract fibers in chiropterans decussate shortly after they emerge from the pons; however, a standard caudal bulbar decussation is also present, the fibers forming a small bundle in the dorsal funiculus and disappearing in the cervical cord (Dräseke, 1903; Fuse, 1926a; Merzabacher and Spielmeyer, 1903; van der Vloet, 1906). In the flying fox, Hatschek (1903) found the pyramidal fibers grouped laterally to the inferior olive rather than along the ventral surface of the bulb—reminiscent of the ipsilateral accessory pyramidal bundle found in man (Probst, 1899). Its position is intermediate between that of the "normal" bulbar pyramidal tract and the bundle of Bagley found in artiodactyls (Bagley, 1922; Haartsen and Verhaart, 1967; Verhaart and Noorduyn, 1961).

In artiodactyls, an almost symmetrical pattern of degeneration occurs in the cervical cord following unilateral cerebral lesions (Haartsen and Verhaart, 1967). Most fibers enter the intracommissural bundles and extend through the cervical cord. Sparse lateral bundles pierce the reticular substance to midcervical levels, and dorsal funicular fibers extend only through the upper cervical segments (Bagley, 1922; Bischoff, 1900; Dexler and Marguiles, 1906; Haartsen and Verhaart, 1967; King, 1911). In addition, the corticotegmental tract described by Bagley (1922) for the sheep and recently by Haartsen and Verhaart (1967) for the goat descends to caudal bulbar and even upper cervical levels. Its terminations, however, seem to be confined to brainstem cell clusters. The tract originates in the superior frontal gyrus, along with other fibers of the pyramidal system. It can be seen as a distinct bundle, dorsal to the substantia nigra in rostral midbrain, that moves dorsally in the tegmentum, lateral to the red nucleus, to assume a somewhat dorsolateral position through pontine and bulbar levels. Its distinctive pattern of terminations will be outlined in a later section. The spinal pattern of corticospinal fibers in artiodactyls is shown in Fig. 2(F).

The edentates present yet a different condition, with lateral and ventral funicular bundles occupying both sides of the spinal cord, the crossed bundles being the larger (Fisher, Harting, Martin, and Stuber, 1969; Fuse, 1926c, d; Strominger, 1969). In the armadillo, the crossed ventral bundle is dominant. It occupies the dorsal part of the ventral funiculus and has some fibers disposed after the manner of the ventral intracommissural bundle of the ungulates (Fisher et al., 1969; Strominger, 1969). Although most of its fibers terminate through the cervical enlargement, a few can be traced into midthoracic levels. In the sloth, on the other hand, the crossed lateral bundle is dominant. It occupies the far lateral margin of the spinal cord and projects only as far as upper thoracic levels (Fuse, 1926c; Strominger, 1969). None of the other components projects farther than the cervical cord.

C. Fiber Composition

The pyramidal tract is similar to most other central pathways in that it consists primarily of small fibers (Haartsen, 1961). About 90% of the pyramidal tract fibers in each of the species thus far studied have been found to be less than 3 μ in diameter, and usually about 70% are of the order of 1 μ or less. Man is no exception. Figure 3 shows an approximation to the recent data for man obtained by Lankamp, as quoted by Verhaart (1970); it does not depart significantly from previous estimates. Included are conduction times for 300-mm

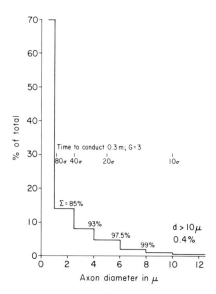

Fig. 3. Fiber spectrum of human medullary pyramid, as measured by Lankamp and quoted by Verhaart (1970). Time marks show conduction time over 0.3 m, calculated by using the linear relation: three times fiber diameter in microns equals conduction velocity in meters/second.

distance, the distance from cerebral cortex to cervical enlargement.[9] The implication is that about two-thirds of the pyramidal tract fibers would require a tenth of a second or more to conduct that distance—a rather long time. Accurate calculation is not yet possible, however, because the constant of proportionality for the human pyramidal tract is not known, and the correction for shrinkage in histological preparation may not be adequate. Further, fewer than one-third of the pyramidal tract fibers that emerge just caudal to the pons actually project that far into the spinal cord, and whether that fraction preferentially contains the larger fibers is still a matter of conjecture (Lassék, 1942b, 1952; Shibasaki, 1968; Shibasaki and Wasano, 1969; Verhaart, 1948).

The total number of fibers comprising the medullary pyramids of different mammalian species has come under considerable study. Even so, it is quite difficult to give an accurate description, for several reasons. Adequate identification of the smallest fibers is often almost impossible without the aid of the electron microscope. Because fibers leave the medullary pyramids in large numbers to enter the brainstem, the level at which the count is made becomes critical; usually, from 40% to 60% of the pyramidal tract fibers that emerge from

[9] A proportionality constant of 3, derived from the study of the cat pyramidal tract (Towe and Harding, 1970), was used.

TABLE 1

MEAN NUMBER OF FIBERS IN PYRAMIDAL TRACTS[a]

A: Mammals with extensive corticospinal tracts	
Man	1,000,000
Chimp	800,000
Seal	748,000
Spider monkey	505,000
Macaque	400,000
Gibbon	300,000
Dog	285,000
Cat	121,000
Rabbit	102,000
Ferret	90,000
Rat	73,000
Mouse	32,000
B: Mammals with scant corticospinal tracts	
Cow	540,000
Deer	490,000
Mule	412,000
Goat	260,000
Sheep	238,000
Hog	210,000
Opossum	40,000

[a] Biedenbach and Towe, 1970; DeMyer, 1959; DeMyer and Russell, 1958; Lassek, 1941, 1942a; Lassek and Karlsberg, 1956; Lassek and Rasmussen, 1939, 1940; Lassek and Wheatley, 1945; van Crevel and Verhaart, 1963b; Verhaart, 1970; Verhaart and Noorduyn, 1961.

the pons disappear into the brainstem. Clear identification of the borders of the tract, and of isolated, aberrant bundles, is often difficult. Nonetheless, a rough picture is emerging; it suggests that the larger the mammal, the greater the number of fibers in its medullary pyramids. This general rule may be seen in Table I to apply to two groups of mammals, those with and those lacking extensive corticospinal tracts. As outlined previously, and illustrated in Fig. 2, only the primates, carnivores, lagomorphs, monotremes, and rodents are known to possess extensive corticospinal tracts. The counts for most of these, shown in Table IA, were taken at a midolivary level, making them reasonably constant. However, the counts for some species differ so widely between different studies that only rough median values are stated. Some of the variation in counts may reflect the extreme variability in the pyramidal system. For example, the range reported for man is about 900,000, the reported counts varying from about 500,000 to nearly 1,400,000. Within the single study by DeMyer (1959) on 21 human specimens, the total count varied from 749,000 to 1,391,000. In studies on the domestic cat, the count has varied from 56,000 to 186,000. Van Crevel and Verhaart (1963b) reported a range of 50,000 but found the count to vary directly with the size of the cat. A similar variation in count with body weight has been reported for the ferret (Verhaart and Noorduyn, 1961). In the case of the animals listed in Table IB, only the pyramids are included; apparently the counts for the ungulates would nearly double if the bundle of Bagley were included (Verhaart and Noorduyn, 1961).

It is often remarked that man is unique among mammals in having an enormous number of pyramidal tract fibers. This statement is misleading, for man has the expected number of pyramidal tract fibers for a mammal of his size in possession of a significant corticospinal component. Both the chimpanzee and the seal overlap the human range, and several other species are close. Relative to body weight, an animal such as a mouse has about 50 times as many pyramidal tract fibers as man. Figure 4 shows the mean number of pyramidal tract fibers per kilogram of body weight for different mammals. Because body weights have not been reported with the fiber counts, the data are plotted in terms of the range of normal body weights for the different species. Thus, a fairly accurate

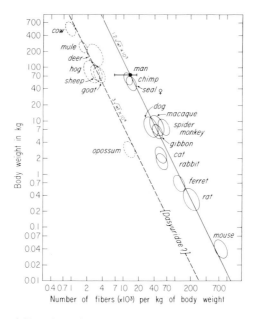

Fig. 4. Number of fibers in medullary pyramid per kilogram of body weight for several mammals, stated as a function of adult body weight. Horizontal bar at 70 kg shows range of fiber counts for man; dot on bar shows the usually quoted number of 1 million fibers per 70 kg. Further explanation in text.

point defining the mean number of fibers for an animal of some average weight for the species is captured within each ellipse. The data for mammals with extensive corticospinal components are distinguished from those for mammals in which the pyramidal tract disappears rapidly within the cervical region, because the latter appear to constitute a distinct set.

Although the data are both scanty and variable, it appears that within each group of mammals the total number of pyramidal tract fibers, as measured at a midolivary level, is directly proportional to the square root of mean body weight, suggesting that the total number of pyramidal tract fibers does not vary directly with gross brain weight (Dubois, 1897; Jerison, 1970; Sacher, 1970).[10] A proportionality constant of 1.2×10^5 fibers/kg$^{1/2}$ applies to mammals with an extensive corticospinal tract, whereas it is one-fourth of that for the less well-endowed forms.[11] It may be significant that inclusion of the Bagley bundle would change the latter constant from one-fourth to one-half that of the well-endowed forms, and that in the well-endowed forms, about half of the pyramidal system consists of corticospinal fibers. Thus, if the corticospinal component is an addition to, and not a simple extension of, the simpler pyramidal system (Bagley bundle included), then addition of this component to the ungulates and marsupials would again double the constant of proportionality, raising it to that for mammals possessing the full pyramidal system. Whether this line of thought holds important implications for our concept of the pyramidal system remains to be determined. The small pouched mammals, such as the dasyurids, may hold the key to whether or not the suggested separation of the mammals into two sets—those with and those without an extensive corticospinal component—is valid. However, from the present perspective on his pyramidal tract, man shows up as just another mammal.[12]

D. PATTERN OF TERMINATIONS

When pyramidal tract terminations are under consideration, the usual focus is upon the ventral horn region of the cervical and lumbar enlargements, with only scant allusion to other sites of termination. Yet, the pyramidal tract fibers in many mammalian forms fail to penetrate even to the cervical enlargement. These mammals possess an electrically excitable motor cortex, though in some cases

[10] The commonly obtained exponent of 2/3 for brain weight-body weight studies does not fit the data; an exponent less than 1/2 would be required to fit the combined data.

[11] The quantitative relationship shown in this discussion was obtained by a "visual" fit to the data expressed in Fig. 4. An accurate fit, obtained by a stepwise multiple regression on 21 carefully estimated pairs of data points, has yielded an exponent of four-ninths rather than one-half (Towe, in press).

[12] One might compound the sacrilege by suggesting that, because of its extreme variability, the pyramidal system of man is not under strong selective pressure; it may be more a gift of his ancestors than the *sine qua non* of man.

the character of the evoked contractions differs from that of other forms (Bagley, 1922). Significantly, these mammals perform many behaviors that inspire the term voluntary—with as much justification as with primate and carnivore behavior. Many, such as the antelopes, are up and about in minutes after birth, and within the hour attain motor control equal to that of the adults. Only speed and stamina are lacking, though these will come with size and conditioning. Frolicking in antelopes, like play in primates and carnivores, may have evolved not only for its effect on the development of the nervous system but also as a physical conditioning device.

In those mammals with extended corticospinal tracts, the rate of loss of corticospinal fibers with distance along the spinal cord remains in some dispute. Many investigators believe that most of the fibers—all of the large ones—synapse exclusively on those alpha motoneurons that innervate the distal limb muscles. Others believe that the large fibers project farther down the spinal cord than do the smaller fibers. Figure 5 shows the approximate decline in the number of corticospinal fibers relative to that fraction of the pyramidal tract fibers that enters the spinal cord. Except for the first four cervical segments, the pattern of loss seems to be about the same in the four species and across the three mammalian orders represented. In calculating the relative innervation density of different body regions, Weil and Lassek (1929) and Lassek, Dowd, and Weil (1930) failed to detect any relative increase within the cervical and lumbar enlargements. To the contrary, in man they found a significant decrease in the number of pyramidal tract fibers terminating per unit of muscle mass in those segments. The four upper cervical segments in man, dog, kitten, and mouse received five times as many pyramidal tract fibers per unit of muscle mass, as the rest of the spinal cord, and the segments T3-T11 received the next greatest density of innervation. The vast majority of corticospinal terminations are onto structures other than alpha motoneurons. A single corticospinal fiber in cat may influence neurons over many segments, for it typically ends through a couple of segments onto interneurons, which themselves terminate through several

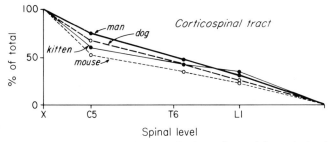

Fig. 5. Percentage of corticospinal fibers projecting as far caudally as the levels indicated for four mammals, as counted by Lassek, Dowd, and Weil (1930).

segments (Scheibel and Scheibel, 1966). Valverde (1966) finds that individual pyramidal tract fibers in several species of rodent terminate over vast areas of the brainstem before apparently descending into the spinal cord.

The precise sites of termination of pyramidal tract fibers evaded definition for many decades; the suggested sites were more reflections of the viewer's expectations than of the body of data itself. Fibers were regularly observed to disappear into brainstem tegmentum, into the reticular substance of the intermediate column of upper cervical levels, and into the dorsal horn. These were usually thought to distribute to the motor nuclei of the brainstem and into the ventral horn of the spinal cord. Yet, some remarkably accurate perceptions came out of that era. For example, in 1903 Probst observed that numerous fibers leave the pyramidal tract to terminate in large numbers along the ventral aspect of the dorsal column nuclei of the cat. Nonetheless, growth in understanding had to await improved histological methods. In 1941, Szentágothai-Schimert asserted that pyramidal tract fibers terminate, not on motor cells, but rather upon interneurons, thus ushering in a new phase in the study of the pyramidal system.

From the third working definition stated in the introduction, the pyramidal tract includes all those fibers that emerge caudal to the pons to form the compact bundle on the ventral surface of the medulla oblongata known as the medullary pyramid. Before reaching this level, however, collaterals are distributed to nucleus ventralis lateralis of the dorsal thalamus (Clare et al., 1964), to the red nucleus (Tsukahara and Fuller, 1969; Tsukahara et al., 1968), to the pontine nuclei (Allen, Korn, and Oshima, 1969; Kitai, Oshima, Provini, and Tsukahara, 1969), and apparently also to medial and dorsolateral midbrain tegmentum (Kuypers, 1958a,b,c; Niimi et al., 1963). These endings are mainly ipsilateral to the cells of origin of the pyramidal tract fibers. Caudal to the pons, fibers leave the pyramidal tract to distribute to the medial and dorsolateral tegmentum, to the inferior olive, to the hilus of the dorsal column nuclei and to the main and spinal nuclei of the trigeminal nerve (Kuypers, 1958a,b,c, 1960; Kuypers and Tuerk, 1964; Niimi et al., 1963; Petras, 1969; Zimmerman, Chambers, and Liu, 1964). These endings are bilateral, but tend to become mainly contralateral toward the caudal part of the bulb. Because about half of the pyramidal tract fibers disappear in the bulb, many are properly termed corticobulbar. From the corticospinal component coursing through, many collaterals and en passage terminations are formed. In the spinal cord, the corticospinal fibers terminate primarily in the dorsal horn and intermediate zone, with a few terminations directly in the ventral horn (Campbell et al., 1966; Fisher et al., 1969; Hoff, 1932; Hoff and Hoff, 1934; Jane et al., 1969; Kuypers, 1960; Kuypers and Brinkman, 1970; Liu and Chambers, 1964; Niimi et al., 1963; Nyberg-Hansen and Brodal, 1963; Petras and Lehman, 1966; Scheibel and

Scheibel, 1966; Valverde, 1966; Zimmerman *et al.*, 1964). These endings are mainly contralateral.[13]

The primates show more ventral horn terminations than do other mammals, and the concentration apparently increases from the prosimians to the apes. However, whether other mammals ever develop equivalent connections is as yet unclear, for alpha motoneurons send their dendrites into the intermediate zone, up into the dorsal horn, and even into the lateral funiculus, where *en passage* connections could be made. Because the spike on mammalian alpha motoneurons originates in the axon hillock region, such distant dendritic connections would have minimal effect.[14] In fact, most pyramidal tract terminations seem to be onto dendrites, except for the axo-axonic relationships that are presumed to yield presynaptic inhibition.

The overall pattern of pyramidal tract terminations in the brainstem and spinal cord is made up of contributions in different amounts from different cerebral regions. The only abstractions that can be made at this stage are that topographic order is in the main preserved and that fibers from frontal cortex mainly innervate "motor" interneurons whereas those from parietal cortex mainly innervate "sensory" interneurons (Kuypers, Fleming, and Farinholt, 1962; Nyberg-Hansen and Brodal, 1963). Physiological observations support these statistical statements which derive from anatomical data (Fetz, 1968). It is perhaps significant that the pyramidal tract, which may have originated as an outgrowth of the corticopontine system, still influences cerebellar tissue, not only via the pontine nuclei, but also via the lateral reticular nucleus and the inferior olive.

E. BAGLEY BUNDLE

In 1922, Bagley announced the existence in the sheep of a corticotegmental bundle that has since proved to be of great potential significance in our understanding of the pyramidal system. He was following the standard technique of ablating electrically excitable motor cortex to produce degeneration in the pyramidal tract, but rather than discarding what was often regarded as irrelevant tissue, he examined both the midbrain and the medulla oblongata. Thus, he happened upon the corticotegmental bundle. Its fibers originated in the electrically excitable motor cortex, but could be traced no farther than the facial nucleus, wherein Bagley thought they terminated. This bundle has since been identified in the horse, pig, camel, llama, fallow deer, cow, blesbok, and goat (Haartsen and Verhaart, 1967), running the same course in all of these animals. Although not an aberrant pyramidal tract bundle, its pattern of terminations identifies it as part of the pyramidal system.

---

[13] The reader is encouraged to consult the literature cited for details about these terminations.

[14] Barrett and Crill (1971) have recently shown that the amount of current drawn from the soma by distant synapses in alpha motoneurons may be larger than previously believed.

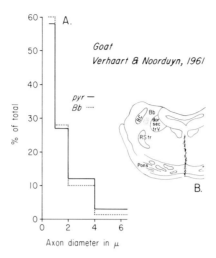

Fig. 6. A. Fiber spectrum of pyramidal tract (solid line) and Bagley bundle (dashed line), as counted by Verhaart and Noorduyn (1961). B. Cross-section of brainstem, showing position of the Bagley bundle (Bb) relative to the brachium conjunctivum (BC), rubrospinal tract (RStr), and the dorsal secondary tract of the trigeminal nucleus (dor sec tr V), as shown by Verhaart and Noorduyn (1961).

As illustrated in Fig. 6(A), Verhaart and Noorduyn (1961) found the fiber spectrum of the corticotegmental bundle of Bagley to resemble that of the medullary pyramid. However, its dorsolateral position in the brainstem [Fig. 6(B)] suggests that its pattern of termination would differ significantly from that of the pyramidal tract. Haartsen and Verhaart (1967) determined that the bundle of Bagley terminates profusely in the ipsilateral spinal trigeminal nucleus and the adjacent dorsolateral tegmentum; it also terminates in the hilus of the dorsal column nuclei and subjacent reticular substance, apparently bilaterally. Unlike the situation in carnivores and primates, the spinal trigeminal nucleus in ungulates apparently receives no crossed input from the cerebrum. The pyramidal tract of the goat sends no fibers to the spinal trigeminal nucleus, and none to the dorsolateral tegmentum. However, it supplies the medial reticular formation, the dorsal column nuclei and the base of the dorsal horn, bilaterally.[15] Thus, the combination of pyramidal tract and Bagley bundle in the goat begins to resemble the pyramidal system of carnivores. Considerably more data are required before that argument can be pushed. However, support for the idea comes from an unexpected quarter.

In 1896, Obersteiner remarked that the parrot possesses a pyramidal tract, and shortly thereafter, Kalischer (1901, 1905) came to the same conclusion. In

---

[15] In the face of contrary evidence Haartsen and Verhaart (1967) state that: "A cortical area for the hindlimb is not evident, because no pyramidal fibers can be traced beyond the seventh cervical segment." This interesting illustration of how a concept shapes the data could be multiplied a hundred times over.

1961, Zecha claimed that not only a pyramidal tract, but also a Bagley bundle could be found in both the parakeet and the parrot. Then, in the summer of 1970, Karten (1971, personal communication) found a pyramidal tract in both the owl and the pigeon, having previously identified the Bagley bundle in the pigeon (Karten, 1969). Thus, the antiquity of the pyramidal system was extended from the Triassic to the Carboniferous period! Apparently, Johnston (1915) thought he could identify a pyramidal tract in a turtle, but no such claim has been made for other extant reptilian forms. The striking similarities between ungulates and birds in the location and pattern of terminations of both the pyramidal tract and the Bagley bundle[16] make convergent evolution highly improbable.

According to Karten (1971), the pyramidal tract originates in the anterior "wulst"–the eupallial tissue–and runs a course similar to that of mammals, terminating in the red nucleus and in medial, magnocellular reticular formation. It also terminates bilaterally in the dorsal column nuclei, and after decussating, enters the dorsal funiculus. The Bagley bundle, on the other hand, terminates in the pontine nuclei, the dorsolateral tegmentum (parvicellular reticular formation), the spinal trigeminal nucleus, and bilaterally in the hilus of the dorsal column nuclei; it does not seem to supply spinal cord neurons. The Bagley fibers originate from cells in the anterior two-thirds of the archistriatum, tissue which has been homologized with amygdala,[17] but which Karten has cogently argued is conjunctive cortex. Thus, if the two tracts are combined, one obtains a system comparable to the mammalian pyramidal system; no terminations have been identified in the inferior olive of the bird.

Figure 7(A) portrays the current conception of the avian visual system and "pyramidal system" as elaborated in conversations with Dr. Karten. The lateral visual fields are mapped topographically via the thalamofugal system onto the posterior "wulst" (Karten, 1969). The neurons in this tissue have small visual fields (Revzin, 1969) and hence will be called visual s (Vs) neurons. These neurons project to the periectostriatal zone of conjunctive cortex (Karten, 1969; Kozenberg, 1899). The tectofugal system projects to ectostriatum via nucleus rotundus (Karten, 1969; Revzin and Karten, 1966), the neurons in that region having wide visual fields (Revzin, 1969, 1970); they will be called visual m (Vm) neurons. Evidently, ectostriatum is a source of corticofugal fibers (Karten, personal communication). The "network" so formed[18] is analogous to that

[16] Zimmerman et al. (1964) describe a scanty collection of corticotegmental fibers in the rat which is, in part, similar to the bundle of Bagley.

[17] The posteromedial third of the archistriatum is probably homologous with amygdaloid tissue.

[18] This condition of the avian visual system recalls that seen in the eye of the males of many dipteran species, in which "large field" facets are added along the rostrodorsal, medial edge of the compound eye, sometimes so many as to cause the eyes to meet in the midline.

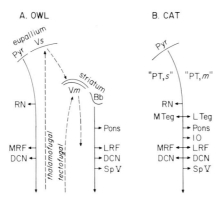

Fig. 7. Conceptualization of the general organization of the pyramidal system in the owl and the cat, with the visual system of the owl included. Explanation in text.

deduced for postcruciate tissue of the cat, in which the small-field (s) neurons primarily modulate the excitability of the wide-field (m), corticofugal neurons (Towe, Whitehorn, and Nyquist, 1968).

Because the avian pyramidal tract develops from tissue which, a little posteriorly, contains Vs neurons, it is suggested that these pyramidal tract fibers are also small-field cells, analogous to the PT,s neurons of the cat. On the other hand, both the Vm neurons of the ectostriatum and the Bagley bundle cells of anterior archistriatum derive from dorsal eminence tissue. It is therefore suggested that the Bagley bundle fibers are wide-field cells, analogous to the PT,m neurons of the cat. If this hypothesis proves to be correct, then the pattern of terminations of wide-field and small-field pyramidal system fibers in mammals may be largely solved. The test resides with the goat, in which both the Bagley bundle and the pyramidal tract originate from the same cerebral tissue, but follow widely separated courses in the brainstem, facilitating discrimination among cells of the two types by antidromic means. Figure 7(B) shows the cat pyramidal system, with the sites of termination divided into those suggested to be PT,s and those suggested to be PT,m (Bagley bundle equivalent). If the two components, pyramidal tract and Bagley bundle, of the owl or of the goat are combined, one arrives at an almost complete cat pyramidal system, with the major exception of the extensive corticospinal component.

III. Physiological Considerations

Much of what is now known about the synaptic action of pyramidal tract fibers that terminate in the brainstem and the spinal cord has been discussed by Wiesendanger (1969) in his comprehensive review, and will not be repeated here. It is evident that the pyramidal system exerts both an excitatory and an inhibitory action, and that the inhibition may be either direct or through a presynaptic mechanism. It is also evident that the pyramidal system is directly affected by cutaneous, auditory, visual, and proprioceptive influences, and that interhemispheric, intrahemispheric, and cerebellar (Casey and Towe, 1961) inputs modulate the activity of this system. It has recently been discovered that the brainstem terminals of PT,m fibers receive a presynaptic inhibitory influence from cutaneous input originating anywhere on the body surface, and that PT,s fibers either do not terminate in the medulla oblongata or are spared this inhibition (Towe and Holt, unpublished observations). Thus, the pyramidal system, with at least 300 million years of antiquity, is thoroughly entangled with much of the brain and exercises all known synaptic options.[19] The degree of its influence at different terminal sites varies with the species of mammal.

A. Fast and Slow PT Neurons

The monotonically decreasing fiber spectrum of the pyramidal tract, because of its rate of curvature relative to the nonlinear transformation from fiber size to conduction time, implies the existence of at least two groups of pyramidal tract cells, distinguishable on the basis of their antidromic response latencies. In 1965, Takahashi published his observations on the membrane properties of cat pyramidal tract cells, dividing them into a fast and a slow group on the basis of the V-I curves, membrane time constants, and spike durations. The antidromic response latency that divides the two groups occurs at the time predicted from knowledge of the cat's fiber spectrum and the antidromic conduction distance involved (Towe and Harding, 1970). This division of pyramidal tract cells into a fast and a slow group has proved to be of fundamental importance; several recent studies have found a differential distribution of cerebral (Naito, Nakamura, Kurosaki, and Tamura, 1970; Takahashi, Kubota, and Uno, 1967) and brainstem (Allen *et al.*, 1969, 1970; Kitai *et al.*, 1969; Tsukahara and Fuller, 1969; Tsukahara *et al.*, 1968) effects ascribable to these two groups. Such an arrangement undoubtedly exists at other brainstem and spinal sites, although this remains to be demonstrated. It is clear that at least the fast pyramidal tract neurons of primates have an excitatory effect on some cuneate nucleus neurons (Harris, Jabbur, Morse, and Towe, 1965) and on some alpha motoneurons (Kernell and Wu, 1967b).

B. Synaptic Action on Alpha Motoneurons

Because of the popularity of the "hot line" notion of corticospinal-motoneuronal relationships, an examination of pyramidal effects on such

[19] Some investigators would insist that its direct inhibitory action is mediated by interneurons, but such an arrangement remains to be determined.

neurons is in order. In no mammal does more than a small fraction of the corticospinal fibers form direct synaptic connections onto ventral horn cells. On the other hand, the oft-repeated idea that such connections occur only in primates is certainly incorrect; direct terminations have been found on several other mammalian forms. Even where direct terminations may be difficult to find, they may be present on the extended dendrites. Yet, no physiologically detectable monosynaptic action of pyramidal fibers onto motoneurons has been demonstrated outside the primate line. Single shocks and even short trains of shocks applied to electrically excitable motor cortex of the cat fail to activate motoneurons when only the pyramidal tract connects the brain with the spinal cord (Lloyd, 1941a,b; Stewart and Preston, 1967). The classical work of David Lloyd (Lloyd, 1941a,b, 1968) has demonstrated unequivocally that the pyramidal action is primarily through interneurons, and that an extended repetitive train of shocks is required to bring an alpha motoneuron to firing level. In the intact cat, on the other hand, discrete muscle contractions are readily produced by single shocks to the cerebral cortex. Thus, these cerebrally evoked muscle contractions do not depend upon the pyramidal tract, caudal to the trapezoid level, for their production. Transection of the medullary pyramid at an olivary or trapezoid level has essentially no effect on the threshold or latency of these cerebrally evoked muscle contractions (Towe and Zimmerman, unpublished observations). These findings do not rest well with the "hot line" notion.

Transection of the pyramidal tract at an olivary or trapezoid level also has little or no effect on the normal behavior and movement of the cat (Laursen, 1966; Laursen and Wiesendanger, 1966; Wiesendanger, 1969; Wiesendanger and Tarnecki, 1966), the contrary assertions of Ranson (1932) and Sarah Tower (1935) notwithstanding. A similar transection has no clear effect on the normal behavior of the monkey, but does affect the character of the movements comprising the behavior (Bucy et al., 1966; Lawrence and Kuypers, 1968a,b; Schäfer, 1910; Travis and Woolsey, 1956). The animal retains full motor control in the sense of initiating and sustaining directed and well-organized output, but the movements are no longer carried out smoothly. The effect is best seen in the finely graded movements of the forelimb digits, and hence has led to speculation that the primary role of the pyramidal system in the life of the animal is to control the digits. The effect may also be seen as a mild decrease in strength—especially of the grip—a circumstance that has often been transmuted to "profound weakness" or even "paralysis." Anyone who has watched a healthy, pyramidotomized monkey bounding off the four walls and the ceiling of its enclosure can only stand in awe before the concepts that attend such an agile creature.

Yet, a direct corticomotoneuronal effect does exist, and is stronger on motoneurons supplying the intrinsic than the extrinsic muscles of the hand

(Clough, Kernell, and Phillips, 1968). Whether cell body size or synaptic locus is responsible for this difference is immaterial to the conclusion. Preston and Whitlock (1961) found both excitatory and inhibitory events on lumbar motoneurons of the monkey following cerebral stimulation after apparently all of the brainstem except the pyramidal tract had been lesioned. Since that time, work has proceeded, primarily in the laboratories of Charles Phillips, on corticospinal effects onto the motoneurons supplying muscles of the forearm and hand of the baboon. Because other motoneurons, for example those at thoracic levels, have not received similar experimental attention, the findings must be evaluated in other ways.

A single shock to the proper cerebral site (Landgren, Phillips, and Porter, 1962b) evokes an excitatory postsynaptic response on some motoneurons after a brief delay (Landgren, Phillips, and Porter, 1962a; Phillips and Porter, 1964). The latency is so short that the fibers mediating the effect are clearly among the largest in the pyramidal system (and hence in the extreme minority). The rate of rise and decay and the duration of these excitatory responses suggest that the synapses are farther out on the dendrites of the motoneurons than are those supplied by the group IA afferent fibers (Porter and Hore, 1969), an interpretation consistent with the histological picture. The corticomotoneuronal EPSP[20] produced by a D wave is of small amplitude, and cannot be increased beyond a few millivolts without involving the I waves as well as the D wave (Phillips and Porter, 1964; Porter and Hore, 1969). Rather than steadily increasing in size with increasing shock strength, as occurs when the group IA volley is increased (Homma, 1966), the corticomotoneuronal EPSP becomes complex by the addition of later components (Phillips and Porter, 1964). These components may result from repetitive firing of corticospinal neurons (D and I waves) and/or input via other pathways. Two important implications accompany these findings. One is that a synchronous barrage on corticospinal fibers, with one action potential per fiber, cannot discharge a motoneuron, unless that motoneuron is already close to its firing level. The other is that cerebrally evoked muscle contractions do not depend solely on the corticospinal tract for their production. Lewis and Brindley (1965) corroborated this latter conclusion by showing that essentially the same pattern of muscle contractions can be obtained after transection of the medullary pyramid as occurs in the intact baboon. Rather than using single shocks, however, they used a 100 cps stimulus. To be sure, both threshold and fatigability of the evoked contractions increased after pyramidotomy, but electrically excitable motor cortex remained, nonetheless. Had the reverse experiment also been performed—transection of the brainstem, leaving only the pyramidal tract intact—then measurement of the

---

[20] EPSP refers to the *excitatory postsynaptic potential* that can be recorded by an intracellular microelectrode.

subsequent pattern, thresholds, and fatigability of the evoked muscle contractions would have revealed the relative importance of the corticospinal input
in the cerebrally evoked muscle contractions.

In the usual study of cerebrally evoked muscle contractions, either strong
single shocks or repetitive trains of shocks are used; in either case, corticofugal
cells fire repetitively. A sufficiently weak, single shock may produce only one
action potential on each fiber, as in the situation described above, but a stronger
shock will produce both D and I waves in the medullary pyramid [Fig. 8(A)]
and spinal cord (Kernell and Wu, 1967a,b; Patton and Amassian, 1954, 1960).

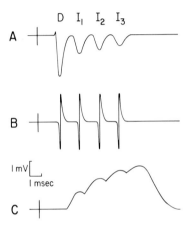

Fig. 8. Schematic representation of D and I waves (A) and fast PT fiber response (B) as
seen at medullary pyramid or in dorsolateral corticospinal pathway, and of intracellular
postsynaptic response of alpha motoneuron (C) following a single, strong shock to the
precentral gyrus. The potentiation of the synaptic response may rise to several millivolts
before plateauing.

As shown in Fig. 8, single corticospinal fibers fire repetitively during these
waves, the intervals between spikes being about 1.5 msec. The corticomotoneuronal EPSP [Fig. 8(C)] grows rapidly in amplitude, reaching a plateau
rather quickly. This "potentiation" is quite unlike the action of group IA
afferent fibers on the same motoneurons when the IA fibers are driven
synchronously at the same frequency (Landgren *et al.,* 1962a; Phillips and Porter,
1964). The potentiation dies away with a time constant of about 10 msec (Porter,
1970). If weak cerebral shocks are repeated at iterative rates higher than about
200/sec, a similar potentiation will occur (Hern, Landgren, Phillips, and Porter,
1962; Kernell and Wu, 1967b; Landgren *et al.,* 1962a; Phillips and Porter,
1964; Porter and Hore, 1969), and the alpha motoneuron may be brought to
firing level (Hern *et al.,* 1962). It has not been determined whether, in this
circumstance, only the monosynaptic corticospinal connections are responsible;

interneurons, driven by corticospinal and other routes, may also be involved. Further, it is not known whether these other routes involve pyramidal tract activation of rubrospinal and reticulospinal pathways, though the most plausible interpretation of the work of Felix and Wiesendanger (1971) on cerebrally evoked muscle contractions in chronically pyramidotomized monkeys involves such activation.

All of the corticomotoneuronal EPSPs thus far studied have had latencies so short that only the largest fibers of the pyramidal system can be held responsible (Clough *et al.,* 1968; Landgren *et al.,* 1962a; Phillips and Porter, 1964). It is doubtful that the baboon possesses 2500 such fibers, which may explain why corticospinal convergence onto motoneurons is so restricted and the cortico-motoneuronal EPSP is so small (Phillips and Porter, 1964). This small collection of large fibers does not restrict its attention to motoneurons supplying muscles of the hand; many neurons of the dorsal column nuclei are driven by these large fibers (Harris *et al.,* 1965). In this case, the excitatory action provoked by a weak shock to the cerebral cortex is so powerful that the neuron promptly discharges. Unlike the corticomotoneuronal "potentiation" effect during iterative stimulation, the corticocuneate effect often shows evidence of transmitter depletion (Harris *et al.,* 1965). Thus, although the pyramidal system can influence alpha motoneurons quickly, it can do so only weakly; a high frequency barrage is required to adequately depolarize a motoneuron. How the system behaves in the intact, awake baboon is another story. The large pyramidal tract fibers are probably supplied by large cell bodies in the cerebral cortex, which are easily excited electrically but which require an intense synaptic bombardment. The smaller cell bodies, more readily driven to firing level by synaptic action, have slowly conducting axons and do not seem to be involved directly with the motoneurons supplying muscles of the baboon's hand. Thus, if a "hot line" exists to alpha motoneurons, it involves a negligible fraction of the massive, diffusely terminating pyramidal system—a fraction that is zero or close to that in a majority of mammals and that may be exactly zero in birds.

C. Chronic Unit Recording

The past decade has seen a surge of interest in the study of neuronal activity in waking and behaving animals. The studies to date have been primarily correlational with the relationships between unit activity and movement being surmised by visual inspection. The data that have been obtained through this experimental approach, when taken together with the intracellular findings concerning corticomotoneuronal EPSPs, demolishes the "hot line" notion and calls for a broader view of the mechanism of production of both learned and "voluntary" movements.

Neurons on either side of the central sulcus of the macaque monkey vary their discharge in relation to movement (Evarts, 1964, 1965, 1968, 1969; Fetz, 1969; Fetz and Finocchio, 1971; Hardin, 1965; Luschei, Johnson, and Glickstein, 1968). Some increase and others decrease their tonic discharge rate, the change bearing a fairly fixed relationship to the movement. In particular, most precentral neurons respond before and during the movement, whereas most postcentral neurons respond during and after the movement, thus eliminating most of the latter from direct involvement in production of the precentral neuron activity. Some are pyramidal tract neurons, and others are not. Among the pyramidal tract neurons, a few may have direct synaptic connections with the alpha motoneurons that are essential to the movement. The neurons that increase their discharge rates prior to and during the movement or sustained contraction reach average rates of 15-35/sec, with few exceeding 50/sec (Evarts, 1964, 1965, 1968, 1969; Fetz, 1969; Fetz and Finocchio, 1971). This condition led Evarts (1964) to postulate a frequency-limiting mechanism to prevent high-frequency discharge during the waking state. This same condition implies that "potentiation" of corticomotoneuronal synapses does not occur, for the firing rates are too low. Such values do not tell the whole story, however, for these same neurons may occasionally attain rates of 100/sec or more for brief periods, making a minor amount of "potentiation" possible (Porter, 1970). These higher rates occur near the time of maximal force output by the muscle (Evarts, 1968) and during the peak of a reinforced burst in an operant situation (Fetz, 1969). Inspection of the periods of higher firing rates in published records (Evarts, 1968, 1969) reveals a more complex situation, but shows clearly that during sustained contractions against a load, the unit firing frequency is much too low to produce any "potentiation." To obtain significant depolarization via this mechanism in the acute preparation, evoking D waves but not I waves, direct cortical stimulation at 500-700/sec must be used (Landgren et al., 1962a; Phillips and Porter, 1964; Porter, 1970). Even at the 660/sec rate associated with the I waves, the "potentiation" appears to plateau (Landgren et al., 1962a) as suggested in Fig. 8. This does not rest well with the "hot line" notion. The direct corticomotoneuronal route requires the cooperation of some additional set of fibers acting fairly powerfully on the motoneurons.

Another significant observation derives from chronic unit studies: the activity of any precentral neuron may be readily uncoupled from the muscle response through differential reinforcement in a free operant situation (Fetz and Finocchio, 1971). It takes fewer than 50 trials to get the animal to produce a burst of unit activity like that previously associated with movement, or with reciprocal isometric contraction, in the complete absence of an electromyographic response. The reverse procedure—that of producing the muscle contraction in the absence of cerebral unit firing—has not been sufficiently examined, though the suggestion is that such an uncoupling might also work (Fetz, personal communication). In these experiments, some units have attained firing rates above 100/sec near the peak of muscle contraction, again just beginning to encroach on rates where some minimal "potentiation" of corticomotoneuronal synapses is possible. That the proper neurons have not been sampled is a possibility; a rare neuron attains firing rates of 500-600/sec in association with a movement, only to transform into an "injury discharge" and die (Fetz, personal communication). Putting the known physiological data together, and then assuming the "hot line" notion to be true, the effects of any "injury discharge" should yield an easily observable muscle contraction involving more than a single motor unit.

Recording the activity of single pyramidal tract fibers in the bulb, Hardin (1965) observed low rates of discharge in quiet, awake animals and mild increases during movement as others have found (Evarts, 1965, 1968, 1969; Fetz, 1969; Luschei *et al.,* 1968). However, he also observed short bursts of activity attaining rates from 100 to 400 per second, the latter being well into the range where "potentiation" of corticomotoneuronal synapses occurs. This bursting occurs not only in the monkey but also in the cat, an animal which does not specialize in direct corticomotoneuronal connections. It also occurs in sleeping animals. It is often associated with phasic movements in the waking animal, but neither rhythmic bursts nor rhythmic variations in tonic activity occur during rhythmic movements such as walking—just a gentle rise in tonic firing rate as occurs during postural adjustments. One gets the impression from Hardin's paper of a less rigid coupling between pyramidal tract fiber activity and movement than appears in later work, which restricts the output of the animal to a few, discrete movements or sustained contractions. The system behaves as though it provides a slow and almost steady excitation onto motoneurons, the "final touch" being provided through some other route. Certainly, the data available on the issue suggest that the "potentiation" is considerably less when the motoneuron membrane voltage is low than when it is higher (Landgren *et al.,* 1962a).

D. The Idea of Motor Cortex

The expression "motor cortex" evokes nebulous images of "executive action," of autonomy, of initiation and direction of activity. Perhaps because of this, the knowledge that many corticospinal fibers originate in such tissue and that some terminate directly onto motoneurons seems to carry with it the "hot line" notion—the notion of an "upper motoneuron" that dutifully carries all commands from headquarters to the front lines. Yet, this notion finds no comfort or consolation in the wealth of data now available; these data must be pushed to the utmost in order to make the "hot line" notion barely tenable. No one would seriously contend that the pyramidal system has nothing to do with movement, but that it is the sole or principal actor is unlikely. It is perhaps the most diffuse and diverse system in the brain, yet it eschews any neurons having to do with the special senses and the vestibular system. In many mammals, it extends its influence right to the terminal junctions of primary afferent fibers and to the dendrites of primary efferent neurons. What selective pressures have molded this system in the arboreal primates may have more to do with readiness to act, as reflected in the disjunctive reaction time paradigm, than with the details of the act itself.

The existence of electrically excitable motor cortex leads inevitably to a focus on isolated movements or muscle contractions rather than on behavior, for fully integrated motor acts are not a conspicuous consequence of stimulation at a single site on the cerebrum. The degree of isolation of movements or muscle contractions, however, is widely variable both within and among species (Bates, 1960). Simpson and King (1911) found isolated movements of either forelimb or hindlimb following cerebral stimulation in the sheep, and could distinguish areas yielding flexion from those yielding extension, whereas Bagley (1922) often obtained combined movements such as contralateral hindlimb and ipsilateral forelimb.[21] On the other hand, Ruch, Chang, and Ward (1946) could map out cerebral points for activating individual muscles in the macaque monkey. Simpson and King (1911) state, with respect to the sheep, that "practically no motor disturbance follows the complete removal of the so-called motor area on one side. After losing the whole of the superior frontal convolution and frequently the greater part of the middle frontal convolution as well, the animal when lifted down from the table[22] would walk to its food-box without any trace of lameness and at once begin to eat." Bagley (1922) concurred in this observation and conclusion. If the sheep is said to possess "motor cortex," then what is the meaning of the term motor? How can images of "executive action" be associated with this tissue in the sheep? The situation is not so difficult with the primates, for unmistakable motor disturbance follows removal of the electrically excitable motor cortex. Yet, even the primates retain a large bag of tricks after such ablations, and may come out with much less motor disturbance if certain precautions are taken (Travis and Woolsey, 1956).

The idea of motor cortex derives neither form nor substance from the available experimental observations. Electrically excitable cortex is present in birds (Kalischer, 1905) and reptiles (Bagley and Richter, 1924; Dart, 1934; Johnston, 1916), as well as mammals, and its extent varies according to the criteria that are set. The lowest thresholds for evoking muscle contractions are usually in

---

[21] Bagley wisely avoided using the term coordination with respect to these combined movements.

[22] The authors apparently refer to the operating table, the animal having just aroused from the anesthetic condition!

the agranular tissue of the frontal lobes, but not always (Bautista and Matzke, 1965; Biedenbach and Towe, 1970; Gray, 1924; Martin and Fisher, 1968; Towe and Biedenbach, 1969). Whether this low threshold has any physiological significance is uncertain; it may be a consequence more of the structure of the tissue than of the magnitude of its influence on motor output. Strong stimulation of the postcentral gyrus of the monkey yields only I waves in the medullary pyramid, whereas stimulation deep in the tissue yields both D and I waves (Towe and Kennedy, unpublished observations). By raising the threshold criterion for electrically excitable motor cortex, the postcentral gyrus can readily be included (Foerster, 1936; Kennard and McCulloch, 1943; Welker, Benjamin, Miles, and Woolsey, 1957; Woolsey, 1958; Woolsey et al., 1953). Ablation studies yield equivocal results. Consider the recent work of Semmes, Mishkin, and Cole (1968), in which prefrontal, temporal, and occipital lobes of the macaque monkey were unilaterally ablated—leaving all of the "motor cortex" and essentially all of the pyramidal system intact. They describe the resultant contralateral abnormalities as "slight weakness, slight to moderate loss of speed and dexterity of movement and relative disuse of the upper limb especially for reaching and manipulation." Later, they elaborate on the abnormalities of the contralateral hand thusly: "inaccuracy of reaching (which improved gradually, at least in the particular situation), loss of delicacy and precision of grasp, impaired maintenance of grip." Who would have guessed that the "motor cortex" and the pyramidal tract were intact bilaterally in these animals?

We have yet to attain a clear idea of the role that neopallium plays in relation to muscle contraction, movement, behavior, and to life style. The lone overnight flight of a migratory hummingbird across the Caribbean Sea may be regarded as a single, prolonged motor act, its simple, repetitive nature demanding little of the nervous system. Yet, that flight is not only sustained but is also directed and accurate in orientation. We know nothing of the role that the telencephalon plays in perpetrating this feat. Cetaceans travel widely and fairly precisely around the oceans of the world, and pinnipeds move long distances with great accuracy. We know nothing of the role that "motor cortex" plays in these spectacular performances. Seals are famous for their aquatic and terrestrial balancing feats, behaviors which must be under fairly direct vestibular control. Yet the vestibular system affects the cerebral cortex only indirectly, and the pyramidal system ignores much of the vestibular system altogether. The globular summer nest of the harvest mouse, the mound house and dam of the beaver, the simple den of the rabbit, the labyrinthine burrows of prairie dogs—these, and a host of similar accomplishments, all require something of the nervous system. Our current concept of "motor cortex" is of no aid in understanding such behaviors—nor, for that matter, is our nebulous concept of a "motor system." Our strong Aristotelian view of the organism as a blank tablet upon which the experiences of life may be written precludes any further broadening or sharpening of our idea of "motor cortex" and any integration of "motor cortex" functions with brainstem mechanisms. With regard to the cerebral cortex, we seem destined to think exclusively in terms of the "initiation and control" of movement.

The pyramidal system, as the most conspicuous of corticofugal systems, is simply not understood. It has connections throughout the brainstem and spinal cord, and influences cells of both motor and sensory affinities. It is intimately involved in the somatic life of the animal and may have visceral interests as well. Its extreme anatomical variability both within and between species speaks for its lack of prime selective importance. It seems to have originated some 300 million years ago and yet has only recently discovered that motoneurons exist as potential direct targets for its influence. From the data now available, it is obvious that any mammal, man included (Bucy *et al.,* 1966; Maspes and Pagni, 1964; Nehlil, 1964), could survive as an individual without the pyramidal system, and many mammals could even get along without an electrically excitable motor cortex. However, whether any collection of mammals could survive as a species under such circumstances may be quite another matter; it probably could not. The pyramidal system probably adds the necessary "readiness to act" that makes all the difference in the selective process where speed and appropriateness of action are so important.

Chapter 4

Subcortical Mechanisms of Behavioral Plasticity

JENNIFER S. BUCHWALD AND KENNETH A. BROWN

DEPARTMENTS OF PHYSIOLOGY AND PSYCHIATRY, MENTAL RETARDATION
CENTER and BRAIN RESEARCH INSTITUTE, UCLA MEDICAL CENTER

I. Introduction

If complex forms of overt behavior, such as voluntary motor activity, are to be analyzed and understood, a clear distinction between integration and acquisition of behavior is desirable. Although, in practice, response integration and motor learning are profoundly intertwined, in principle the mechanisms underlying either function may be considered independently. For example, a conditioned leg flexion induced by a particular conditioning stimulus may involve only the simplest kind of motor activity. In contrast, a highly integrated form of somatic and visceral motor activity, sham rage, can be produced by electrical stimulation of the caudal hypothalamus. This response is not acquired and is triggered as a complex behavior pattern simply by virtue of the inherent neuroanatomical connections of the hypothalamus (Bard, 1928). Thus, in analyzing mechanisms of motor control, it may be advantageous to approach response *acquisition* separately from response *integration* and to abandon the notion that complexity of movement is a necessary concomitant of a learned response.

In considering the bases of acquired motor responses, the concepts of Hughlings Jackson (1898) related to the evolution of integrative motor activity are a helpful starting point. In this view, integration of local reflexes is accomplished at the spinal level by the relatively simple, automatic system of reciprocal and crossed inhibitory reactions seen in the spinal animal. The addition of the brainstem, cerebellum, and diencephalon allows more general motor patterns to emerge, including postural and locomotor reactions which require simultaneous integration of entire groups of spinal reflexes. Thus, a higher level of motor control is superimposed on the lower mechanisms which are used together in groups while still maintaining the selective, sequential inhibition and facilitation of the more primitive response mechanisms. Cortical influences constitute a still more general governing mechanism of motor function, and distance receptors as well as somatic exteroceptors and intero-ceptors furnish very broad stimulus patterns. The motor reactions mediated by the forebrain may involve orientation and movement of the entire organism, with muscular coordination characteristic of the intact, adult animal.

In parallel with the Jacksonian schema of response integration, Piaget (1952) has suggested a similar hierarchy for motor learning in which local, autonomous responses are the first to be acquired, e.g., the conditioned sucking response which is initially evoked by many sorts of tactile stimuli but is eventually triggered only by the nipple tegmentum. As higher brain levels become functional, these local responses become generalized and are incorporated into other more diffuse and complex acquired responses when these are added to the behavioral repertoire. It does not necessarily follow, however, that as this progressive accumulation of increasingly complex, learned responses evolves, the underlying mechanisms of motor learning concurrently become more complex.

The learning process, per se, which mediates a conditioned sucking reflex may be very similar to that which underlies more sophisticated forms of acquired behavior in the adult organism.

For a number of years our laboratory has been interested in general problems of motor learning, as distinct from motor integration, so it is to this aspect of overt behavior, i.e., motor response acquisition, that the present paper is addressed. Habituation of behavioral responses, which may be considered as representing the simplest form of motor learning (Thorpe, 1963), as well as behavioral conditioning will be utilized in this discussion as models of behavioral plasticity.

One approach to an understanding of motor learning is to determine whether a simple motor response can still be "learned," i.e., conditioned or habituated, after the cortex and successively lower levels of the neuraxis are deleted. Here it is important to recall that all neural levels become increasingly interdependent in the course of phylogeny and ontogeny, and deficits arising from damage to the central nervous system (CNS) are therefore dual in nature (Jackson, 1898). Removal of a part of the brain not only involves loss of the integrative functions performed by the deleted tissue but may also result in an imbalance of excitatory or inhibitory influences in the remaining parts of the brain. Clearly then, caution must be used when observing the effects of lesions or neuraxial transections of the CNS. Motor learning deficits in particular must be viewed with reservation in such situations, since excitatory or inhibitory imbalances and loss of integrative control mechanisms may completely obscure the fact that motor learning capacity is left intact.

Another approach to the problem of motor learning is the analysis of electrophysiological responses recorded from various brain sites during conditioned acquisition or habituation of a motor response. Plasticity of behavioral responses is ultimately a function of the motoneurons mediating the overt activity. However, between motoneuronal output, which signals such alterations in behavior, and the sensory stimulus that triggers the response, where is response plasticity initiated? This question is of fundamental importance to an understanding of causal processes in learning phenomena. Recordings from brain sites which indicate changes in neural activity prior to the appearance of a conditioned response can suggest loci of earliest conditioned associations which, subsequently, assist in the development of conditioned responses in other brain areas and, ultimately, in the conditioned discharge of appropriate motoneurons and muscles. During the simpler procedure of habituation, the most peripheral, or primary, locus of response plasticity can be determined by recordings throughout the pathway of the habituating stimulus. Although habituation occurs even in the spinal preparation, any contribution of the forebrain to this learning process can be suggested by comparing recordings in intact and decerebrate preparations.

In the following discussion we shall review data derived from these various kinds of experiments as they relate to mechanisms of motor learning. We shall attempt to determine what capacities for conditioning and habituation persist as higher levels of the neuraxis are progressively deleted by reviewing data from behavioral studies of decorticate, decerebrate, and spinal preparations. We shall then suggest systems which underlie the development of the overt conditioned response by indicating where early conditioned changes of neural activity develop prior to the appearance of the behavioral response, as indicated by electrophysiological recordings. Similarly, we shall suggest mechanisms basic to response habituation by indicating the primary neural level at which modulations occur and the extent to which these modulations differ in the intact *versus* decerebrate preparation. Finally, the implications of these data for motor response acquisition will be considered and possible substrates for the maintenance of motor learning will be suggested.

II. Behavioral Plasticity in Decorticate Preparations

The general behavior of chronically prepared "decorticate" cats (Bard and Rioch, 1937; Dusser de Barenne, 1920; ten Cate, 1934), dogs (Lebedinskaia and Rosenthal, 1935; Rothmann, 1923), and monkeys (Karplus and Kreidl, 1914) was observed in several laboratories early in this century. In some cases, conditioned responses were reported to develop in these preparations, but careful histological descriptions of remaining tissue rarely accompanied such observations. The interest of most investigators was directed primarily toward verifying neocortical removal, without much concern about the extent of additional subcortical damage. Thus, a difficulty often encountered with reports of conditioning or its absence in "decorticate" subjects, even in later studies, concerns the varying amount of subcortical damage which inevitably occurs with neocortical removal. In chronic "decorticate" preparations, there is also considerable, and usually unspecified, structural loss due to degeneration, e.g., in the corticofugal motor pathways and in the thalamic relay nuclei. Neither surgical nor degenerative damage is commonly described in adequate detail when the histology of a "decorticate" preparation is reported. The term decorticate, then, does not specifically denote removal of only neocortex, and the term has been applied generally to preparations with extirpation of all or most neocortex together with varying amounts of paleocortex and associated limbic lobe structures, portions of the striatum, and occasionally some thalamic tissue. It follows that functional deficits in such animals cannot be directly attributed to neocortical removal alone. A decorticate preparation is therefore interesting primarily with regard to behavioral capacities which are retained in spite of structural loss. Functional deficits are more difficult to interpret.

Behavioral plasticity was not in itself a major interest of most of the early investigators of these preparations. Instead, the postural, locomotor, and broad reactive tendencies of the decorticate animal were studied rather thoroughly while motor learning capacities were observed only casually if at all. In fact, the occurrence of conditioned responses was occasionally interpreted as a sign of incomplete neocortical ablation since, for much of this century, the cortex was assumed to be indispensable to conditioning (Lebedinskaia and Rosenthal, 1935; Zeliony, 1929). Thus, notions about the necessity of cortical participation in response lability and specificity existed for many years and became generally acknowledged without experimental support and in spite of data to the contrary.

A. CONDITIONING IN THE DECORTICATE PREPARATION

Cortical mediation of motor learning, or acquired behavior, has traditionally been identified with the "pyramidal system." Pyramidal section does not, in fact, abolish the execution of learned movements or voluntary behavior in chronic preparations (Bucy et al., 1966; Laursen and Wiesendanger, 1967; Lawrence and Kuypers, 1968; Denny-Brown, 1966; Mettler, 1948). Removal of the classical motor cortex in primates also does not eliminate initiation of learned responses in chronic preparations (Foerster, 1936; Lashley, 1924). Thus, identification of the "pyramidal system" or the motor cortex with motor learning phenomena may be misleading.

An artificial distinction between pyramidal and extrapyramidal mediation of acquired behavior and confusion about the functions of motor cortex in voluntary response control have perhaps tended to obscure the larger question of the role of the cortex as a whole in motor learning. A controversy about the particular cortical loci from which learned responses originate begs the question of whether such responses require cortical control at all. It has been shown repeatedly that discrete ablation of the primary cortical projection area of a conditioned or discriminative stimulus does not abolish the acquisition and maintenance of a conditioned reaction (Diamond and Neff, 1957; Diamond et al., 1962; Pennington, 1937; Lashley, 1929; Tunturi, 1955). Furthermore, evidence against a direct intracortical substrate for conditioning has been provided by experiments which demonstrate a persistence of conditioned reactions in the absence of transcortical connections. When the cortical primary projection area of a conditioned stimulus is isolated from adjacent cortex by a circular incision or by implanted barriers, elicitation of the conditioned response is essentially unaffected (Doty, 1961; Doty, Rutledge, and Larsen, 1956; Loucks, 1961; Sperry and Miner, 1955). Undercutting the tissue may eliminate the conditioned response, but relearning occurs, although it may take longer or require a higher stimulus intensity than before the undercutting operation (Loucks, 1961). Such evidence, based on limited cortical extirpation, seriously questions the notion of exclusive cortical mediation of learned behavior.

The classic study of behavioral capacities in the completely decorticate animal was carried out by Goltz (1892), with histology reported by Holmes (1901–1902). Goltz observed the chronically "decorticate" dog for several weeks and noted that reactions to auditory stimuli were present in this preparation; sounding a loud horn near the sleeping subject's head would awaken it, and sounds generated near the awake animal would evoke ear movements. Several years later, Zeliony (1911, 1913) attempted to establish a conditioned response in a chronic decorticate dog but was at first unsuccessful. Pavlov (1927) therefore suggested tentatively that some portion of the neocortex was essential to the formation of a true conditioned reflex. Subsequently, however, this doctrine was experimentally reexamined by Poltyrev and Zeliony (1929, 1930), who reported the establishment of differentially conditioned responses to auditory stimuli in decorticate dogs. Two subjects were successfully trained, about as rapidly as normals, to lift one forepaw to a whistle, the other forepaw to a sharp percussive sound, and to make no response to a tone. No histological verification of cortical removal was included in these reports. Shortly thereafter, Culler and Mettler (1934; Mettler, Mettler, and Culler, 1935; Girden, Mettler, Finch, and Culler, 1936) also obtained clear, though diffuse, conditioned leg flexions and reversible stimulus discrimination between a bell and a 1000-Hz tone in decorticate dogs, with careful histological verification of cortical removal. Although responses developed at approximately normal rates, the responses themselves were not localized to the shocked leg. The shock was delivered to only one hind paw, but the subject would lift both legs upon presentation of the conditioned stimulus. Consequently, the cortex was viewed by these investigators as requisite for development of an efficient, *localized* response, though not for conditioning of a diffuse response. The preparations all sustained some degree of striatal, thalamic, and rhinencephalic damage, but very detailed descriptions of remaining tissue and postoperative degeneration were not given.

By the late 1930's, it was thus clear that a form of conditioning could occur in the absence of neocortex. The classical experiments of Lashley (1929) with rats also helped to combat the concept of an exclusive cortical "switchboard" mechanism of response modification, although a satisfying alternative to cortical mediation of behavioral lability was not advanced. However, perhaps largely because of Pavlov's unwitting influence and the burgeoning popularity of behaviorism, which drew heavily on Pavlovian concepts, the cortex was still generally considered essential for localized behavioral response plasticity in higher mammals. Another possible reason for the enduring belief that cortical participation was required for the development of specific conditioned reactions may have been the hyperactive and sham rage tendencies of the decorticate preparations (Cannon and Britton, 1927; Bazett and Penfield, 1922; Bard and Mountcastle, 1948). Delivery of an unconditioned stimulus such as shock often causes prolonged struggling in the conditioning apparatus, disrupting performance on subsequent trials, thus making an adaptive acquired response improbable. Similar disruptive behavior also occurs spontaneously or in response to neutral stimuli or restraint (Bromiley, 1948; Cannon and Britton, 1927). The early successful attempts to condition decorticate preparations were thus confined to gross, diffuse responses which could be brought to criterion levels more easily than localized responses. Subcortical damage was also more extensive in the earlier decorticate preparations and may have limited the motor capacities of these subjects to gross movements.

Bromiley (1948), however, was able to obtain a discrete flexion of one foreleg to tone in a decorticate dog, with foot shock as the UCS, by limiting the number of trials to 15–25 per day and by terminating a series of trials when the preparation became too agitated to respond adaptively. In this case, in addition to complete neocortical removal, some bilateral damage was done to the striatum, particularly the putamen, but the amygdala and septal structures were intact, and hippocampal tissue was damaged only in caudal portions beneath the corpus callosum. Although there was no operative damage to the thalamus, subsequent degeneration of the dorsal thalamic nuclei was almost complete.

Bromiley's results illustrate the point that misconceptions of cortical function may arise from misinterpretation of functional deficits caused by partial destruction of the CNS. In earlier studies, the release of reactive tendencies incompatible with the development of a specific conditioned response might have masked the motor learning capacities of decorticate preparations, leading to the erroneous conclusion that the cortex was indispensable for such specific motor learning.

B. Conditioning in "Striatal" and "Thalamic" Preparations

Several investigators have attempted to compare the behavioral capacities of cats after decortication which spares the striatum, i.e., the caudate nucleus, putamen, and globus pallidus ("striatal" preparation) and after decortication and further removal of the striatum, sparing the thalamus ("thalamic" preparation). A primary object of such comparisons is to evaluate the contributions of the striatum to behavioral integration.

Chronic "striatal" cats are reported to feed spontaneously, to localize low-intensity auditory stimuli, to associate sounds or positions of a feeding dish with food, to clean and groom themselves, and to exhibit estrous, rage, and fear responses when stimulated appropriately (Bard and Rioch, 1937; Rioch and Brenner, 1938; Schaltenbrand and Cobb, 1931; Wang and Akert, 1962).

"Thalamic" animals, on the other hand, show few if any of these reactions. They are hyperactive, and their grooming, sham rage, and scratch reflex reactions are undirected. Complex behavior sequences appear to be disintegrated into individual response components (Bard and Rioch, 1937, Emmers, Chun, and Wang, 1965; Schaltenbrand and Cobb, 1930; Wang and Akert, 1962). Thus, Wang and Akert (1962) concluded that striatal influences are responsible for the integration of basic response sequences into the more adaptive and coordinated repertoire of the "striatal" animal. A problem with this interpretation, however, is the question of limbic lobe participation in the functions of "striatal" preparations. Since damage to the rhinencephalon is typically more severe in "thalamic" than in "striatal" subjects, differences in the behavioral capacities of the two groups may reflect differences in the integrity of limbic rather than striatal structures. Indeed, the degree of functional impairment within Wang and Akert's "striatal" group seems to correlate about as well with amount of limbic lobe destruction as with differences in striatal damage, in spite of extensive, though incomplete, limbic lobe "deafferentation" and "de-efferentation." For example, the "striatal" subject which showed the least behavioral impairment also sustained the least damage to the hippocampus and amygdala; both structures remained nearly intact and connected to the thalamus and to remaining frontal and basal temporal cortical fragments. The same question of striatal *versus* limbic lobe mediation of function exists for other studies comparing "striatal" and "thalamic" preparations (Bard and Rioch, 1937; Schaltenbrand and Cobb, 1931).

Although the "striatal" preparations were not studied specifically for signs of conditionability, Schaltenbrand and Cobb (1931) noted that their subject appeared to orient its head and position itself near a food dish when hungry; similarly, the "striatal" animals of Wang and Akert (1962) seemed to associate the sound of a feeding dish placed on the floor with food. It is interesting to note that in the latter case, the animals would not immediately find the food *unless* the sound cues were presented concomitantly. Such observations of conditioning like phenomena should not be surprising since these preparations are roughly equivalent to the decorticate subjects which have been shown to develop conditioned reactions in more controlled studies.

C. Habituation in the Decorticate Preparation

There are no direct observations of habituation in adequately controlled situations in either decorticate or "striatal" preparations. Thresholds for acoustic stimuli may be raised slightly after decortication (Girden *et al.*, 1936; Mettler *et al.*, 1935), but several reports state that behavioral orientation to sounds is well preserved (Rioch, 1938; Bard and Rioch, 1937; Lebedinskaia and Rosenthal, 1935; Schaltenbrand and Cobb, 1931; Wang and Akert, 1962). Habituation of orientation to auditory stimuli was mentioned by Lebedinskaia and Rosenthal (1935), who noted normal habituation but did not report terminal histology, by Rioch (1938), and by Bard and Rioch (1937). In these reports, habituation of acoustic orienting responses is mentioned only as an incidental observation. Behaviorally, the establishment of a conditioned response would seem to involve habituation to neutral stimuli, and Bromiley (1948) reported that the noises made in operating the conditioning apparatus, with the conditioning stimulus generators disconnected, "failed to produce any observable response" in his decorticate dog. The hyperactivity seen in decorticate animals during early chronicity is transient and appears to be a motor release effect rather than a failure in habituation causing increased "exploratory" activity. Thus, there is no evidence that habituation processes are affected in any obvious way by decortication, except in cases of such prepotent reactions as sham rage. The "sham rage" response is certainly released by cortical removal and may be elicited by the same *sort* of stimulus repeatedly for many months (Bromiley, 1948); in this sense, the reaction does not habituate. The effective stimuli, however, are diffuse and typically presented to different areas of the body surface on successive occasions. Because no one has specifically studied habituation of sham rage under reasonably controlled conditions, it is possible that the reaction does habituate in common with other reflexive reactions. This must, however, remain an open question until the matter is investigated experimentally.

D. SUMMARY

The establishment of conditioned responses after virtually complete neo-decortication confirms the existence of a subcortical mechanism of conditioning. Unfortunately, this early research has not been systematically followed up. Instead, investigation of subcortical learning mechanisms appears to have become diffused in a variety of techniques, indirect data, and methodological differences. Clearly, however, the decorticate brain is capable of supporting a very extensive behavioral repertoire, which can be modified to a considerable degree. Although habituation has not been carefully examined, there is no report of diminished capacity for habituation in the decorticate animal. There has been one demonstration of a discrete, localized conditioned response in the literature on decorticates (Bromiley, 1948) and it may be significant that the subject sustained minimal subcortical damage. Neocortical removal was, in this case, virtually complete. The available evidence thus indicates that motor learning capacities of decorticate or "striatal" preparations are rather more quantitatively than qualitatively different from normals. It is unfortunate that a wider spectrum of learned behavior has not been systematically investigated in decorticate animals, but the existence of some degree of specific response plasticity and stimulus discrimination has been demonstrated. The participation of individual subcortical structures in these functions is difficult to specify, since relevant terminal histology has not always been well documented, but the available information suggests that the striatum and/or the rhinencephalon or some portion thereof plays an important part in the motor learning of the decorticate animal. Rather than a *sine qua non* of acquired behavior, the cortex would appear to be required largely for discrimination of complex, subtle stimulus properties and for the integration of the organism's behavior tendencies in general. This view of cortical function in response plasticity, as a broad organizer of sensorimotor commerce instead of an elaborate switchboard for highly particular acquired connections, corresponds closely with the Jacksonian schema and with the results of a great many experiments concerning the role of the cortex in sensorimotor integration.

III. Behavioral Plasticity in Decerebrate Preparations

The term decerebrate, like decorticate, carries a certain amount of ambiguity. The chronic "thalamic" preparation, for instance, with degeneration of thalamic structures, could be described as decerebrate. Commonly, the term decerebrate is applied to animals with neuraxes sectioned above, at, or below the level of the superior colliculus dorsally and the hypothalamus ventrally. In chronic decerebrate preparations, as in chronic decorticates, degenerative changes occur over time and vary with the level of transection. Thus it is necessary to consider each preparation individually and to rely on adequate terminal histology for determining structural correlates of retained function. Again, as in the earlier decorticate preparations, some of the behavioral capacities of the decerebrate cat or dog have been investigated, but interest in this preparation was primarily directed at the origins of postural rigidity and the organization of sham rage or pseud-affective responses, i.e., aggressive or defensive responses apparently without accompanying affect. Little attention has been paid specifically to the learning capacities of the "thalamic" or midbrain decerebrate animal.

A. Acoustic Reactions in the Decerebrate Preparation

Since the lower relay nuclei of the auditory pathway are preserved in the decerebrate preparation, we have focused on responses to acoustic stimuli which could be related to decorticate behavior and to our own electrophysiological data. Forbes and Sherrington (1914) studied the acoustic reflexes in the acute, intercollicularly decerebrated cat and observed isolated movements of the extremities in response to auditory stimuli, which were present even in the midbrain cat with transection caudal to the hypothalamus. More prolonged, coordinated movements of progression were induced by whistles and handclaps in kittens decerebrated at an intercollicular level when a few days or weeks of age (Weed, 1917). Bazette and Penfield (1922) reported that acoustic reflexes could be elicited in acute and chronic adult decerebrated cats as long as the inferior colliculus and part of the prepontine brainstem, including a portion of the red nucleus, remained intact. More recently, Bard and Macht (1958) reported that "a slight noise" elicited head movements and righting in chronic mesencephalic and pontine cats while loud noises induced pseud-affective responses or possible components of a startle reaction but no obvious orientation. Villablanca (1971), however, has noted startle and orienting reactions in many "thalamic" and decerebrate cats. In decerebrate rats, Woods (1964) found orientation to auditory stimuli well preserved. He speculates that more highly evolved mammals may require telencephalic structures for directed responses to auditory or visual stimuli.

While several studies have included casual observations of acoustic reactions in decorticate or decerebrate cats and dogs, anatomical descriptions of remaining portions of the brain are usually inadequate, and in most cases it is difficult or impossible to draw firm inferences about minimal brain tissue required for auditory orientation and directed response. Indeed, relevant experimental inquiry appears to have stopped with the demonstration of conditioning in the absence of neocortex. Even when histological descriptions of tissue removal are detailed, differences between acute and chronic preparations and in the amount of postoperative degeneration in chronics confuse the picture.

One of the few transection studies which directly shed some light on thalamic and rhinencephalic contributions to auditory reflex responses was done by Bard and Rioch (1937). Unfortunately, their observations of acoustic reactions in four cats deprived of varying amounts of forebrain were made only in passing. Three of their subjects oriented and showed directed approach responses to low-intensity auditory stimuli; these animals had bilaterally or unilaterally intact medial geniculate bodies, and intact portions of the hippocampus and amygdala, although the fornix and stria terminalis were cut. Strident, high-pitched sounds evoked a "fear" reaction, distinct from the sham rage responses elicited in these preparations by cutaneous stimulation. All three subjects exhibited habituation and spontaneous recovery of both orientation and fear reactions when acoustic stimuli were repeatedly presented. In contrast to these "striatal" preparations, a fourth, practically decerebrate subject, whose rhinencephalon and thalamic nuclei were removed, exhibited "no very specific auditory responses" and no orientation to low-intensity sounds.

These findings suggest that the integrity of the medial geniculate bodies, limbic lobe structures, or both is essential for directed, localized responses to acoustic stimuli in the cat. It is well to remember, however, that most histological descriptions of chronically decorticate brains, often in subjects reported to orient to acoustic stimuli, mention severe or complete degeneration of the thalamic relay nuclei, e.g. (Bromiley, 1948; Gastaut, 1958a,b; Girden *et al.,* 1936; Holmes, 1901–1902). In summary, with the exception of Villablanca's (1971) report, behavioral orienting reactions have not been clearly demonstrated in the decerebrate cat; the marginally positive findings of Forbes and Sherrington (1914) may have resulted from asymmetrical transection of the brainstem, biasing the innervation of the musculature to produce lateral movement of the head when a startle reaction raised the tonus of the preparation briefly.

B. CONDITIONING IN THE DECEREBRATE PREPARATION

The combined data from several experiments strongly suggests that decerebrate animals are capable of developing conditioned reactions. Perhaps the most unequivocal description of conditioning in a decerebrate carnivore is provided by Bard and Macht (1958). A 3-sec tone (CS) was paired with an air puff to the eye (US), which produced an unconditioned blink response; conditioning of this response to the tone occurred in 15–30 trials. This conditioned response was obtained in the cat decerebrated at the pontine level, just rostral to the fifth motor nucleus, as well as in the cat transected rostral to the red nucleus and superior colliculus. Bard and Macht did not, however, describe the conditioned response in detail, and sensitization effects, although seemingly unlikely, were not necessarily eliminated. Gastaut (1958a,b) described conditioning in the decerebrate dog of a diffuse "vegetative-affective" reaction, i.e., global agitation, piloerection, mydriasis, tachypnea, and vocalization, when an auditory stimulus was paired with shock. Differential conditioning was obtained with markedly different stimuli. Above the brainstem, this preparation possessed only piriform lobes, olfactory bulbs, intralaminar and midline thalamic nuclei, and hypothalamus; the geniculate bodies were completely degenerated. Unfortunately, Gastaut's discussions of these findings are relatively brief. Villablanca (1971) has observed a conditioned salivation reaction in response to handling prior to tube feeding in chronic cats decerebrated at the level of the third nerve as well as in "thalamic" cats. Finally, conditioned ocular responses were reported to develop in two chronic cats with isolated hypothalamic midbrain segments, containing only wedges of tissue from the optic chiasm to the inferior colliculi when a subthreshold midbrain reticular CS was paired with more intense reticular stimulation, sufficient to produce an unconditioned response (Zernicki, Doty, and Santibanez, 1970). While the responses could not be conditioned to light flashes and were "weak and unstable," they nonetheless were induced when the final stimulus in a session was withheld for 10 min instead of for the usual intertrial interval of 3 min. After several days, however, the conditioned responses disappeared without any visible change in the vitality of the preparations; attempts to condition other such preparations with a similar paradigm were unsuccessful.

C. Habituation in the Decerebrate Preparation

A number of investigators have noted decrements of reflex reactions in the precollicular decerebrate cat with repeated acoustic stimulation (Bard and Rioch, 1937; Bazett and Penfield, 1922; Forbes and Sherrington, 1914; Villablanca, 1971). Depending on the level of transection and the chronicity of the preparation, a variety of responses can be induced which subsequently habituate, e.g., widening of the palpebral spaces, retraction of the nictating membranes, ear flicks, claw extrusion, movements of the head and neck, tail movements, and other widely scattered contractions of skeletal muscles. Forbes and Sherrington (1914), the first to study such reactions in detail, found gradual response decrements and spontaneous recovery after repeated acoustic stimulation in acute decerebrate cats. Bazett and Penfield (1922), working with chronic as well as acute decerebrate cats, were able to elicit reactions to acoustic stimuli of very low intensity. Although habituation per se was not investigated, background noise from laboratory equipment was reported to evoke no reaction except when turned on after an interval of relative quiet. The comments of Bazett and Penfield strongly suggest that their preparations habituated to background acoustic stimuli and exhibited spontaneous recovery to these sounds during intervals of relative silence. Bard and Rioch (1937; Rioch, 1938) examined acoustic reactions in chronic "striatal" cats deprived of neocortex and varying amounts of forebrain and described habituation and spontaneous recovery of both orientation and "fear" reactions during repeated acoustic stimulation. These phenomena were seen in at least three preparations; a fourth subject, with sufficient subcortical injury to be classified as decerebrate, did not orient to low-intensity stimuli and showed signs of sham rage responses (e.g., piloerection on back and tail) rather than "fear" to loud, high-pitched sounds. Response decrements, however, were not mentioned in connection with this preparation.

Habituation of the reflex reactions to acoustic stimuli should be contrasted with the sham rage or pseud-affective responses to *somatic* stimuli, which may be elicited repeatedly in the chronic animal over many weeks or months with no sign of habituation (Bard and Rioch, 1937; Bromiley, 1948). Sudden loud acoustic stimuli may also elicit sham rage reactions, extreme agitation, or "fear," but these responses do seem to habituate with repeated stimulation (Bard and Macht, 1958; Bard and Rioch, 1937).

Response decrements seem to progress relatively rapidly in the decerebrate animal. Forbes and Sherrington (1914) reported one preparation which showed no pinna response after 7 sec of acoustic stimulation at intervals of "somewhat less than one second." A similar rapid habituation of acoustic reflexes has been seen by Villablanca (1971).

These observations, reported only casually and largely uncontrolled, certainly require elaboration. Nevertheless, they indicate that acoustic reflex habituation occurs in the absence of the forebrain and even in preparations lacking all central neural tissue above the inferior colliculi. These findings support the notion that a simple form of response plasticity can be mediated by relatively low levels of the neuraxis.

D. SUMMARY

It should be mentioned that some of the "decorticate" subjects of early studies (e.g., Culler and Mettler, 1934; Goltz, 1892; Holmes, 1901–1902) were, in fact, nearly decerebrate, and it is not always easy to distinguish the two sorts of preparation either anatomically or functionally. Perhaps the marked differences in behavioral repertoire of decerebrate, or of "thalamic," versus decorticate, or "striatal" animals, provide the best criteria for classifying preparations as "decorticate" or "decerebrate."

Evidence of response plasticity is more difficult to summon with regard to decerebrate preparations than is the case with decorticates. The loss of higher inhibitory influences severely disrupts the spontaneous behavior of the decerebrate animal; removal of the hypothalamus renders maintenance of the preparation particularly difficult and causes a marked reduction in the behavioral repertoire. Investigation of response plasticity under these circumstances has been understandably meager. Although the reports of conditioning in decerebrate preparations are relatively brief and incomplete, the available evidence indicates that classical conditioning can occur in decerebrate subjects, even those as highly evolved as the cat. Habituation to acoustic stimuli has been well demonstrated in several kinds of decerebrate preparations. Retention of conditioning or habituation, on the other hand, has neither been studied specifically nor casually attributed to the decerebrate preparation. Thus, decorticate and decerebrate preparations are similar in their ability to support a degree of response plasticity, but they also differ in several ways. Conditioning effects appear to extinguish more quickly in the decerebrate than in the decorticate preparation, and retention of either habituation or conditioning from day to day does not seem to occur in the decerebrate animal. Also, habituation seems to progress more rapidly in decerebrate subjects than in decorticates.

IV. Behavioral Plasticity in Spinal Preparations

A. CONDITIONING IN THE SPINAL PREPARATION

The capacity of the isolated mammalian spinal cord to "learn a conditional response" has remained a subject of controversy for more than three decades since the experiments of Shurrager and Culler (1938, 1940, 1941). These investigators reported that in acutely spinalized dogs a twitch of the exposed semitendinous hindleg muscle developed to electrical stimulation of the tail (the conditioning stimulus, CS) after the initially ineffective CS had been repeatedly paired with stronger electrical shock to the hindpaw (the unconditioned stimulus, US). In addition to the development of this "conditioned" response, Shurrager and Culler also indicated that extinction could be demonstrated.

In an attempt to extend these observations, Kellog and co-workers (Kellogg, Deese, Pronko, and Feinberg, 1947; Kellogg, Pronko, and Deese, 1946) subsequently carried out behavioral training procedures on chronically spinalized dogs in which a weak electrical stimulus to one hindpaw was utilized as the CS and a strong electrical stimulus to the opposite hindpaw was used as the US. Consistent responses to the CS, however, did not develop and the erratic movements that did appear were attributed to a sensitization induced by the repeated electric shocks. Thus, it was concluded that in these chronically spinalized animals true conditioned responses had not developed.

Pinto and Bromiley (1950) next attempted to reconfirm the original findings of Shurrager and Culler by duplicating their acute training procedures. From among the 27 acutely spinalized dogs that were utilized, 10 failed to develop any response to the CS. The other dogs showed such varied and inconsistent muscle twitches during CS presentations that these responses were interpreted as either coincidental or a result of increased muscle excitability following surgical exposure or of sensitization following the repeated electrical stimulations. Thus, it was again concluded that true conditioning had not occurred in the isolated spinal cord.

Since both the electrical stimulation used as CS and the surgical exposure of the muscle to be "conditioned" had been suggested as undesirable sources of hyperexcitability, a final attempt was made by Dykman and Shurrager (1956) to circumvent all objections. In these experiments a behavioral training procedure was carried out on chronically spinalized animals with a brush stroke utilized as the CS. As Kellogg had previously been unsuccessful in training chronic adult spinal animals, Dykman and Shurrager used only *kittens* and the CS brush stroke along one hindleg was paired with shock to the ipsilateral paw as US. Out of 15 kittens spinalized and behaviorally trained in this regimen, 12 were reported to develop consistent hindleg responses to the CS which could be extinguished by withholding US reinforcement and subsequently reestablished by replacement of the US. Thus, Dykman and Shurrager concluded that conditioned responses could be established in the isolated spinal cord of the kitten.

Subsequent studies utilizing other paradigms have resulted in conflicting conclusions concerning the conditionability of the isolated spinal cord. In the adult spinal dog, the development of a "conditioned" leg flexion response to stimulation of the tail was reported to develop but only when sensitization of the flexor motoneurons, produced by the US hindlimb stimulation, was still present (Koyasu, 1957). This study concluded that the spinal neurons have a

sensitizing capacity whereby reflexes more complicated than those inherent to the cord can be induced but that "conditioned connections" which are easily established in higher centers are essentially absent. In a somewhat similar conditioning study on the adult spinal dog, completely negative results were reported (Lloyd, Wikler, and Whitehouse, 1969) and similarly negative results were reported after attempts were made to condition the adult spinal cat (Forbes and Mahan, 1963). In spinalized adult rats, a conditioning experiment was carried out (Buerger and Fennessy, 1970) in which the experimental animal was shocked each time his foot, with electrode attached, extended into an electrolyte solution; the yoked control was shocked each time the experimental animal was shocked regardless of leg position. After a 10 to 30-min training period, the animals were tested individually, i.e., each animal received a shock whenever his foot extended into the solution. The experimental animals were reported to develop and maintain a flexed leg position, i.e., with the foot above the solution, sooner and for a longer period of time than did the controls. Similar results were obtained when, 2 days after the initial observation, two experimental animals were used as controls, while their original yoked controls became the experimental subjects. In a study utilizing spinalized kittens, semitendinosus muscle contractions induced by tail pinches were compared when the tail pinch was paired with a toe pinch ("conditioning routine") and when 10 sec intervened between the two stimuli ("pseudo-conditioning routine") (Buerger and Dawson, 1968). Although habituation of the flexion response induced by the tail pinch continued to occur in both training regimes, the tail pinch response significantly increased over a 5-day period in the conditioned animals but not in the pseudoconditioned animals.
animals utilized, two were subjected to both the "conditioning" and "pseudoconditioning" routine with results similar to those noted above.

Since the positive data of Dykman and Shurrager, which indicated the clear development of a specific conditioned flexion response in spinalized kittens, had neither been confirmed nor invalidated by any of the above studies, a replication of this study was initiated in our laboratory with the same conditioning paradigm, experimental preparation, and postoperative ages at training (Buchwald and Schramm, 1965). Twenty-four kittens ranging in age from 1 day to 3 weeks were utilized; littermates were divided into spinalized and intact groups. Since Dykman and Shurrager studied only spinalized kittens subjected to the conditioning routine without additional control groups, the kittens utilized in our study were divided into four groups, i.e., intact control, intact experimental, spinalized control, and spinalized experimental. The experimental, or conditioning, paradigm consisted of presentations of a brush stroke across the skin of the hamstring muscles, which produced no initial response, paired with shock to the hindpaw, which produced a hindleg flexion; the control paradigm simply consisted of presentations of the hamstring brush strokes. Two training sessions of 35 trials each were carried out daily on each kitten.

Among the nonspinalized, intact kittens, responses did not develop to the brush stroke regardless of whether or not it was reinforced by shock. In contrast, flexion responses to the brush stroke developed among all 13 spinalized kittens trained to brush stroke reinforced with shock (Fig. 1). Thus, replication of the spinal conditioning procedures of Dykman and Shurrager produced results similar to those obtained by the earlier workers. However, similar flexion responses developed within a 3-day period in the eight spinalized kittens presented with *brush stroke alone.* The appearance of these responses to the nonreinforced paradigm indicated the development of a postoperative supersensitivity (Stavraky, 1961). Under conditions of such supersensitivity, or lowered excitability threshold, response patterns developed in the spinalized kittens which never appeared in their littermates with nonlesioned spinal cords. A unique feature of the reinforced trials, however, was the disappearance of the brush stroke response when the reinforcing shock was withheld (Fig. 1); when the hindpaw shock was subsequently paired again with the brush stroke, the brush stroke response returned. Thus, presentations of the combined CS-US induced a different response than the CS alone.

These results indicate that in the chronically spinalized kitten, supersensitivity gradually develops, so that 2 or 3 days after spinal transection an initially neutral stimulus, i.e., a brush stroke, may begin to elicit a hindleg flexion response. Against such a background of supersensitivity, other acquired response patterns can be demonstrated. Thus, the brush stroke response that developed coincident with presentations of the paired CS-US was extinguished when the reinforcing US was withheld. When the CS was once again paired with the US, the brush stroke response returned. Although we would hesitate to identify these responses as examples of classical conditioning, the present data indicate that *under conditions of supersensitivity* behavioral response patterns may be modified by conditioning procedures in the isolated spinal cord.

B. HABITUATION IN THE SPINAL PREPARATION

Habituation, spontaneous recovery, and dishabituation have been clearly and indisputably shown both in the behavior of chronic spinal animals, e.g., the flexion reflex habituation resulting from repeated cutaneous stimulation, and in the central reflex pathway of acutely spinalized preparations. These data have been recently reviewed (Kandel and Spencer, 1968; Groves and Thompson, 1970) and thus will not be treated further herein. The relative ease with which this form of response plasticity can be induced in the isolated spinal cord is indeed in contrast with the conflicting mixture of experimental data concerning spinal conditioning.

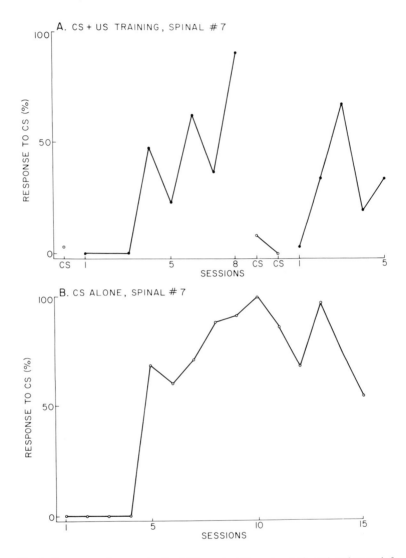

Fig. 1. Responses of two spinalized littermate kittens to reinforced and nonreinforced CS presentations. Open dots indicate training sessions in which only the CS, a light brush stroke across the hamstring muscles, was presented; solid dots indicate sessions in which the CS was paired with the US, a brief shock train delivered to the hindpaw of the same leg. Each session represents 35 trials; two training sessions were carried out daily. In A, after eight reinforced training sessions, two "extinction" sessions of CS alone are carried out and are subsequently followed by five retraining sessions. In B, the brush stroke is presented without shock reinforcement.

C. SUMMARY

The capacity of the isolated spinal cord to develop conditioned responses has been a subject of considerable experimental scrutiny, more intense than that directed to learning capacities of the decerebrate animal although somewhat surpassed by the investigations of decorticate learning. Interestingly, the positive report of specific conditioning in the completely decorticated animal by Bromiley (1948) was followed, 2 years later, by his study of spinal conditioning with negative results (Pinto and Bromiley, 1950). Inability to condition the isolated spinal cord has likewise been reported in numerous other studies. Although several studies have reported the development of responses in spinal preparation during conditioning procedures, the most suggestive of these data have been obtained from kittens and rats. Minimal encephalization and background supersensitivity may be important factors promoting the positive data in these experimental preparations.

Although an unequivocal demonstration of classical conditioning has not yet been shown for the spinal mammalian preparation, marked reflex habituation has repeatedly been found to develop rapidly, to show spontaneous recovery, and under certain circumstances to display dishabituation.

V. Electrophysiological Studies of Response Plasticity

The preceding data have indicated that even in the most simplified mammalian nervous system, i.e., the spinal preparation, some capacity for learning is still present. This can be most clearly demonstrated for the habituation of motor responses mediated by the isolated spinal cord. More complex forms of learning, i.e., conditioned motor responses, have also been demonstrated in the truncated nervous system; acquisition of a classical conditioned response has clearly been demonstrated in the decorticate prepara-tion, as well as in the decerebrate animal; the case for conditioning in the isolated spinal cord remains equivocal. The significance of these studies, taken together, is that considerable capacity for behavioral plasticity remains intact after deletion of much of the machinery of the central nervous system.

In an attempt to determine where and how the capacity for response plasticity originates, electrophysiological recordings have been carried out in our laboratory during behavioral conditioning and habituation procedures. Common to these studies has been a search for neural loci of primary changes in response to the training paradigm. The conditioning studies have focused on defining systems in which earliest response modulations develop during training, far in advance of the conditioned motor response. The habituation studies have carried a slightly different emphasis; an attempt has been made to define the neuronal locus closest to the stimulus input at which response plasticity occurs. At such sites, primary mechanisms might be expected. While neither of these studies has focused on the motor aspect of the learning process, per se, they have been directed toward questions which are fundamental to an understanding of motor learning.

A. TECHNIQUES OF UNIT RECORDING AND ANALYSIS

In our recordings of neuronal unit activity, both single and multiple unit techniques have been utilized. The advantages of the multiple unit technique, particularly at the descriptive level, as well as some of the disadvantages of this technique, have been discussed in detail elsewhere (Buchwald, Weber, Holstein, and Schwafel, 1969; Buchwald and Grover, 1970). While multiple unit activity cannot be equated with the precise behavior of a single discharging neuron, it is believed to represent primarily the action potential discharge of cells and fiber elements around the recording electrode and, where comparable studies have been carried out, close correspondences between multiple unit and single unit data have been reported. Thus, multiple unit recordings provide a summary of activation at the recording site based primarily upon net change in discharge frequency of local action potentials.

In our experiments, multiple unit data were analyzed by first integrating the activity through an R-C or a frequency integration system (Weber and Buchwald, 1965; Buchwald *et al.,* 1969), and then measuring the area of each response. In many cases the integrated activity was computer-averaged over five-trial series before such areal measurements were made. These measurements were then used for regression and variance analyses to determine whether progressive response modulations were significant. Where single unit activity was recorded, similar statistical analyses were carried out, based on interspike intervals.

The data which are presented below have been drawn from a number of experimental series, aspects of which have been previously published (Buchwald and Eldred, 1961; Buchwald, Beatty, and Eldred, 1961; Buchwald, Standish, Eldred, and Halas, 1964; Buchwald, Halas, and Schramm, 1965; Holstein, Buchwald, and Schwafel, 1969; Kitzes and Buchwald, 1969; Buchwald and Humphrey, 1971; Humphrey, Kitzes, and Buchwald, 1970).

B. CONDITIONING STUDIES

In an attempt to determine within what systems changes in neural activity occurred prior to the appearance of the conditioned motor response, a series of electrophysiological recordings were carried out on cats during behavioral conditioning procedures. The location of such early changes in neural response would suggest loci of primary conditioning mechanisms which might then be subjected to more analytical scrutiny. Of particular interest to us were the auditory system (the central pathway of the conditioning stimulus), the somatosensory system (the central pathway of the unconditioned stimulus), and the midbrain reticular formation.

In the conditioning experiments, a 1.5-sec tone was used throughout as the conditioning stimulus (CS) and a 0.5-sec shock train to the hindpaw was used as the unconditioned stimulus (US). Prior to conditioning, the CS alone was presented over several sessions as an habituating stimulus. Thus, at the onset of conditioning the CS induced an habituated response. Conditioned leg flexion responses generally appeared by 150 conditioning trials and reached an 80% level of performance by approximately 400 trials.

After the cats had reached and maintained a performance level of approximately 80% for 3 consecutive days, they were trained under complete Flaxedil paralysis for two sessions which were alternated with normal training sessions. In this way, unit responses to the CS which were independent of sensory feedback effects from the conditioned movements could be determined as well as unit responses which were completely dependent on feedback from the motor response. Moreover, in the normal training sessions interposed between paralytic sessions, the animals continued to respond at an 80% performance level, indicating that no severe impairment of function had been incurred during the paralytic sessions.

1. Somatosensory Pathway (US)

In the somatosensory relays of the US, no conditioned responses to the tone stimulus developed prior to the actual performance of the conditioned leg flexion (Fig. 2). Recordings from the medial lemniscus, ventrobasal thalamus, or somatosensory cortex indicated that only when the CS began to induce conditioned flexion responses did responses occur at these sites. During subsequent paralytic training these responses disappeared, which indicated that they were simply a reflection of sensory feedback from the conditioned limb movement rather than the representation of a primary conditioning process within the somatosensory pathway.

2. Auditory Pathway (CS)

Conditioned discharge patterns did develop very early in conditioning, however, in the CS relay nuclei, i.e., in the auditory pathway. Prior to the reinforced training trials, at the end of habituation, responses to bilateral tones recorded from the inferior colliculus, medial geniculate body and posterior ectosylvian cortex presented the appearance of an inhibition of unit discharge

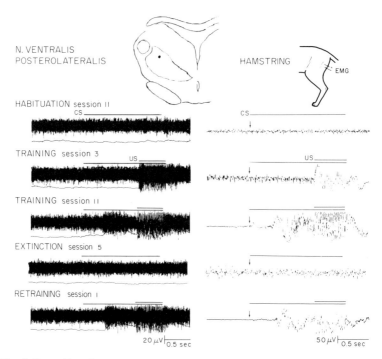

Fig. 2. Recordings from the nucleus ventralis posterolateralis of a normal waking cat. Paired traces to the left indicate the multiple-unit activity (above) and its integration (below) for the training sequence and sessions indicated. Traces to the right indicate EMG activity during corresponding trials recorded from the hamstring muscles of the reinforced leg. Bars and arrows above the traces indicate onset and duration of CS and US. Electrode placement for unit recordings is illustrated by the diagrammatical insert. (From Buchwald, Halas, and Schramm, 1966.) Reprinted by permission of Pergamon Press, Elmsford, New York.

(Fig. 3, first trace). Following the first pairings of tone with shock, "dishabituation" occurred which abolished the precedent inhibition (Fig. 3, second trace); further pairings of tone and shock resulted in the gradual development of an accelerated unit discharge to the tone. This response was never induced by the tone alone and during subsequent extinction the accelerated discharge rapidly disappeared (Fig. 3, third trace). This sequence of response alterations, i.e., the inhibition characteristic of the habituated responses, the loss of inhibition during "dishabituation," and the accelerated discharge induced by conditioning, developed at all levels of the auditory pathway studied in these experiments; the sequence developed well in advance of the conditioned motor response, but the conditioned acceleration continued to occur as the behavioral response became established. Moreover, during paralytic training the conditioned

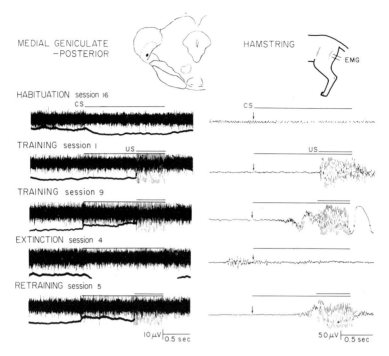

Fig. 3. Recordings from the medial geniculate body of a normal waking cat. The traces and markers for this figure are as previously described for Fig. 2. Electrode placement is indicated on insert. (From Buchwald *et al.,* 1966.) Reprinted by permission of Pergamon Press, Elmsford, New York.

acceleration remained intact and was essentially the same response as that which occurred in the nonparalyzed animal.

3. Midbrain Reticular Formation

In the midbrain reticular formation, similarly early responses were recorded which were short latency bursts of discharge (Fig. 4, second trace); with additional conditioning, the onset bursts became progressively longer in duration, paralleling the increasingly prominent sustained acceleration in the auditory pathway (Fig. 4, third trace). In the reticular formation, after the overt conditioned response developed, an increased unit discharge occurred which corresponded in time to the EMG of the conditioned flexion response (Fig. 4, third trace). During paralytic training, the conditioned onset burst and sustained acceleration remained intact while the late phasic response correlated with leg movement no longer occurred; thus, this component simply reflected sensory discharge produced by the motor response.

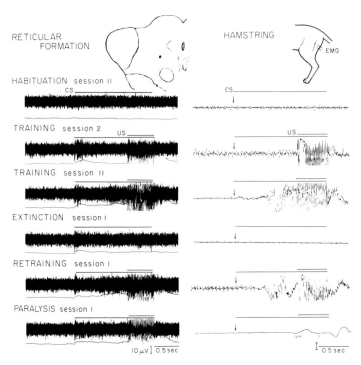

Fig. 4. Recordings from the mesencephalic reticular formation of a normal waking cat. The traces and markers for this figure are as previously described for Fig. 2. Electrode placement is indicated on insert. (From Buchwald *et al.*, 1966.) Reprinted by permission of Pergamon Press, Elmsford, New York.

4. Spinal Motor Neurons

Conditioned responses of spinal cord gamma motoneurons also appeared early in conditioning, many trials before the development of the conditioned flexion response mediated by the alpha motoneurons. Gamma motoneuron discharge was initially habituated to the tone CS or the tone intensity was adjusted so as to induce no initial response [Fig. 5(A)]; the hindpaw shock US either accelerated or inhibited the gamma discharge depending upon whether it was a flexor or extensor motoneuron. After several conditioning trials of tone paired with shock, the tone began to induce a unit discharge which generally replicated the response induced by the shock [Fig. 5(B,C,D)]. These conditioned responses showed all the characteristics of "true" conditioning in that they could be extinguished and reconditioned; they developed only when the CS and US were paired, i.e., they did not develop when the CS and US were alternated; they showed specificity to the conditioning tone frequency and were not induced by other, "neutral" acoustic stimuli.

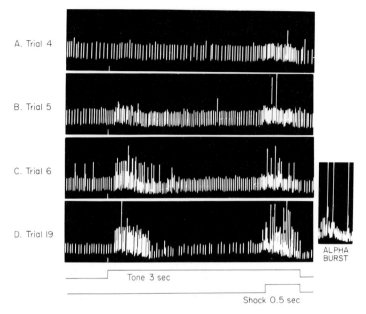

A. Trial 4

B. Trial 5

C. Trial 6

D. Trial 19

ALPHA
BURST

Tone 3 sec

Shock 0.5 sec

Fig. 5. Conditioning a response in a tonically discharging gamma efferent fiber recorded from a lumbar ventral root filament. A 1000-Hz tone of 3 sec duration (CS) was paired with 0.5 sec shock train to the ipsilateral hind paw (US). Bars at bottom indicate stimulus durations. Intertrial interval was 3 min. Conditioning was not apparent on the first to fourth trials (A), but conditioned acceleration was seen in the fifth trial (B) and became marked on the sixth (C). Additional spike of moderate height giving conditioned response in tracings C and D may also be that of a gamma fiber. By comparison, potential amplitudes of alpha fibers elicited by pinching the toe extended off the oscilloscope face (insert to right). (From Buchwald and Eldred, 1961.) Reprinted by permission of The Williams and Wilkins Company, Baltimore, Maryland.

After the conditioned flexion response was established, conditioned gamma discharge continued to occur and to commence at a much shorter latency, i.e., 20 to 25 msec, during each trial than the conditioned alpha discharge with a latency of 80–100 msec, as illustrated in Fig. 6. If nonreinforced presentations of the CS were repeatedly made, the alpha response rapidly extinguished, whereas the more resistant, lower threshold gamma response persisted for an additional 100 to 200 trials.

5. Summary

The early development of the conditioned gamma response indicated that a process sufficiently precise to produce the characteristics of true conditioning had developed very quickly in the training procedure, far in advance of the total excitation necessary to induce the overt conditioned response.

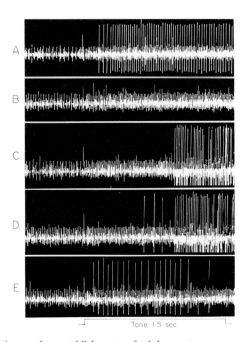

Fig. 6. Extinction and reestablishment of alpha motoneuron conditioned response recorded from a lumbar ventral root filament. At the beginning of the extinction trials (A), the tone CS elicited acceleration of the tonically discharging low amplitude gamma unit and initiated discharge of the high amplitude alpha unit. Onset of CS is indicated by artifact on the trace and duration of CS by bar at bottom of figure. After repeated unreinforced presentations of the CS, alpha discharge was abolished, leaving only the gamma-fiber acceleration (B). When the first US reinforcement was given (C), alpha potentials appeared during the 0.5-sec shock period at the right end of the trace, but not during the CS period preceding the shock. On the next trial, a feeble alpha-fiber discharge occurred during the CS period preceding the second shock reinforcement (D). After five reinforcements the alpha-fiber response to the CS alone (E) had been reestablished. (From Buchwald *et al.,* 1961.) Reprinted by permission of The Williams and Wilkins Company, Baltimore, Maryland.

Responses in the auditory pathway and those which developed at approximately the same time in the reticular formation may have been mutually reinforcing through collaterals from brainstem to auditory nuclei and from auditory nuclei to brainstem. In either case, early conditioned discharge of the reticular formation could, in turn, trigger the gamma motoneurons, known to be highly sensitive to reticular activation. During additional conditioning, discharge of the conditioned gamma response through the muscle spindle circuits with feedback into the central nervous system, as well as the continued reinforcement of brainstem processes, would facilitate the development of conditioned excitation sufficient to discharge the higher threshold alpha motoneurons and to induce an overt conditioned response.

C. Habituation Studies

Because of the relative simplicity of the habituation paradigm, as compared with that of conditioning, loci of primary mechanisms could be sought simply by determining the level at which neural responses began to show alterations during repetitions of the habituating stimulus. Habituation sessions consisted of 200 stimulus presentations repeated at 5-sec intervals; 1.5-sec duration tone or white noise was used throughout as the habituating stimulus and 0.5-sec shock train to the paw was used as the dishabituating stimulus. Two types of experimental subjects were studied, the paralyzed decerebrate cat and the intact cat, examined both during normal wakefulness and during Flaxedil paralysis. Any differences in the responses of these preparations at loci of primary change would suggest the extent to which basic habituation processes are similar in the complex and simplified system.

1. Auditory Pathway, Decerebrate Preparation

In a series of paralyzed decerebrate cats, recordings were made peripherally from the round window, as well as centrally from the acoustic relay nuclei, in order to determine at which level neural response decrements developed as a function of tone repetitions. From the round window, recordings were made of the cochlear microphonic potential, which is a reflection of hair cell receptor discharge in the cochlea. During acoustic habituation, the cochlear microphonic potential did not develop decrements as a function of acoustic stimulation. However, responses simultaneously recorded from the cochlear nucleus showed marked reductions during the habituation procedure (Fig. 7, series I); the cochlear nucleus response decrements were reversible and spontaneous recovery to the initial response level was usually complete after a 10-min rest period (Fig. 7, series II). Thus, changes in cochlear receptor activity did not occur during acoustic habituation but at the level of the primary central relay, i.e., the cochlear nucleus, marked response decrements did develop in the decerebrate animal.

2. Auditory Pathway, Intact Preparation

In general, response decrements which developed during repeated tone presentations in the intact cat were less marked, less rapid, and more irregular in progression than those of the decerebrate cat. At the level of the cochlear nucleus, a progressive enhancement of unit activity often occurred in the nonparalyzed cat due to the gradual relaxation of the middle ear muscles, as decrements to the repeated tone developed in the motoneuron-acoustic reflex responses. When the same cats were subjected to acoustic habituation during neuromuscular paralysis, i.e., with ear muscle effects deleted, decrements in the

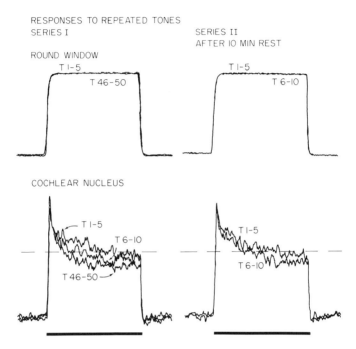

RESPONSES TO REPEATED TONES
SERIES I

SERIES II
AFTER IO MIN REST

ROUND WINDOW

COCHLEAR NUCLEUS

Fig. 7. Integrated round window microphonic (top) and cochlear nucleus multiple unit activity (bottom) during presentations of a 1250 Hz, 70 db tone to a paralyzed, decerebrate cat. Tones were repeated at 5-sec intervals; a 10-min rest period separated series I from series II. During both series the microphonic response remained constant while the neural activity progressively diminished (*P* < 0.05). Bars below traces represent duration of the 1.5-sec tone; RC integration was utilized. (From Buchwald and Humphrey, 1972.)

cochlear nucleus tone responses were generally clearer although distinctly less marked than in the decerebrate cat.

These differences between intact and decerebrate preparation reflect, we believe, the competing, dishabituating effects of arousal mechanisms. In intact, paralyzed cats specifically examined for dishabituation characteristics, shock to the hindpaw was found to produce an immediate, marked dishabituation of the habituated acoustic responses in the cochlear nucleus, inferior colliculus, and medial geniculate body. In the nonparalyzed, intact cats, such stimulation was accompanied by behavioral arousal. In contrast, the same shock stimulus in paralyzed decerebrate cats induced little or no dishabituation of the habituated cochlear nucleus response.

In spite of the somewhat erratic development of response decrements in the intact experimental animals, the development and retention of such acquired nonresponsiveness is a characteristic of successful behavioral adaptation. An electrophysiological reflection of retained habituation effects is suggested by recordings from the inferior colliculus and medial geniculate body made over consecutive days of habituation to a particular tone frequency. As indicated in Fig. 8, some carryover of response habituation appears to occur from one day to the next. Each trace represents a frequency integration of unit activity averaged for five trials. Although the ongoing activity levels remain approximately the same, some savings or retention can be observed in the initial and final tone responses as the habituation is repeated over 6 days.

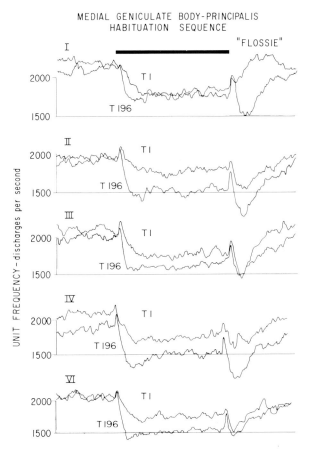

Fig. 8. Multiple unit responses of the medial geniculate body in a normal waking cat during acoustic habituation over 6 consecutive days. Sessions are indicated by I–VI; frequency integration of five trial blocks has been averaged and trials 1–5 are indicated by T1, trials 196–200 by T196. Note that the background activity changes very little over the 6-day period while both the initial and final five trial blocks show progressive alterations.

D. SUMMARY

The appearance of response decrements in the cochlear nucleus but not in the cochlear microphonic potential indicates that a capacity for response plasticity exists at the level of the first sensory relay nucleus but not in the peripheral receptor mechanism. In the decerebrate animal the cochlear nucleus response decrements showed the same temporal characteristics as those of motoneuron habituation and, thus, of an overt motor response. A comparison of these data with those obtained from the intact cat indicates that while response decrements develop rapidly in the cochlear nucleus of the decerebrate cat, these decrements occur much more erratically in the intact cat. Similarly, shock to the paw induces little or no dishabituation of cochlear nucleus response decrements in the decerebrate cat but marked dishabituation, accompanied by behavioral arousal, in the intact animal. On the basis of these results, we have suggested that arousal, or dishabituatory influences, mediated primarily by the reticular formation, are to some extent reflected within the specific auditory pathway. Thus, in the intact cat the erratic response decrements would correlate with constantly fluctuating arousal levels whereas, in the decerebrate cat with arousal mechanisms truncated, this influence is largely deleted. In the intact subject, as generalized arousal to the novel stimulus, e.g., a tone, diminishes, the sensory nuclei receive less dishabituating excitation so that subsequent to habituation of the arousal response, response decrements develop by virtue of local mechanisms similar to those of the decerebrate preparation. An additional difference between responses of the decerebrate and intact preparations to habituation procedures was that essentially no retention could be demonstrated in the decerebrate, so that responses not only decremented rapidly but also recovered rapidly and completely. In contrast, the intact cat showed some day-to-day savings of habituation effects. This difference, we feel, may largely be attributed to the presence or absence of the limbic lobe, and in particular to the hippocampus. Support for this notion will be presented in the next section.

VI. Retention

The development of motor learning has been discussed in the preceding sections both from the point of view of electrophysiological origins of neural response modulation and by an analysis of behavioral learning capacity in the progressively truncated neuraxis. Development of response plasticity, i.e., the acquisition of a conditioned response or the appearance of response habituation, is, however, only one aspect of motor learning. In order for the acquired response to be usable and incorporated into other response patterns, there must be retention of the specific information generated by specific learning processes.

A mechanism underlying retention and consolidation of habituation or conditioning effects may be considered separately from the nature and locus of information storage itself. A large body of evidence indicates that long-term memory is not confined to a single brain structure or group of structures (Lashley, 1929, 1950) but rather seems to be widely distributed throughout the brain (Gaito, 1966). Once stored, information is relatively impervious to disruption short of lethal insult to the brain and it may remain at least potentially accessible to recall processes for very long periods of time. Immediate memory, on the other hand, can be abolished by several sorts of interventions (Glickman, 1961; Grossman, 1967; Deutsch, 1962). Although the literature is somewhat incomplete and contradictory, it is fairly clear that until consolidation occurs, information is vulnerable to disruption or decay but subsequently it is relatively stable. Thus, "memory" appears to involve several processes, including short-term retention, consolidation, long-term storage, and recall, each of which may be mediated separately. A general discussion of this topic is well beyond the scope of this paper but the evidence concerning possible neural substrates of short-term retention and consolidation, as related to motor learning is of interest. Based on the behavioral and electrophysiological data provided by studies of learning in the truncated preparation, and other pertinent investigations, the following discussion will suggest a possible substrate for retention of information resulting from habituation and conditioning procedures.

The demonstration of retention over several days in the conditioned responses of decorticate dogs clearly points to a subcortical mechanism of consolidation. Establishment of stable conditioned responses, i.e., leg flexions to a tonal CS, in these preparations required training in short blocks of trials spread over several days because the subjects' behavior was so susceptible to disruption by diffuse sham rage responses. Examination of the percentages of correct responses obtained during trials on successive days reveals a gradual improvement in performance until complete savings are seen from day to day (Bromiley, 1948; Girden *et al.*, 1936). Moreover, after a 43-day interval without trials, Bromiley's preparation relearned a discrete leg flexion conditioned response within 75 to 100 trials, whereas the response had originally developed over approximately 500 trials. These findings indicate that the effects of conditioning can be held for long periods of time in a highly developed, adult nervous system lacking neocortex.

On the other hand, although habituation and conditioning have been reported in the decerebrate preparation, maintenance of such learning over hours or days does not seem to occur. Bard and Macht (1958) were able to develop conditioned eye blink responses to a tonal CS in their chronic decerebrate cats, but there was no evidence that conditioning endured from one day to the next. Furthermore, extinction of the response occurred almost immediately, within one or two trials. Gastaut (1958b) has described a similarly abrupt extinction after conditioning of a diffuse "vegetative-affective" response to tone in the decerebrate dog. In agreement with this behavioral literature, differences in the retention capacity of the decerebrate animal, as compared with the intact, are suggested by our own electrophysiological habituation data. In the intact animal, increasingly rapid response decrements appeared in the inferior colliculus and medial geniculate body over repeated days of acoustic habituation trials. After similar acoustic habituation procedures in the decerebrate preparation, which lacks the inferior colliculus and medial geniculate body, the cochlear nucleus response decrements showed rapid and complete recovery within 10 min with no indication of savings.

Since maintenance of learning is apparently lost or severely attenuated by decerebration yet endures after decortication, it seems likely that consolidation is mediated by some subcortical forebrain mechanism. The major structural losses of the decerebrate preparation, as compared with the decorticate, are the striatum, the thalamus, and the limbic lobe. Although maintenance of acquired responses has not been studied specifically in preparations lacking various combinations of neocortex and subcortical structures, some inferences may be made from experiments involving discrete lesions in these areas. Such studies are abundant in the literature, and we can only mention some of the data that seem to be particularly significant, referring the interested reader to a more thorough review elsewhere (Grossman, 1967). It is worth reemphasizing, at this point, that apparent deficits in both acquisition and retention after subcortical lesions may arise secondarily from other effects, such as sensory or perceptual impairment, motivational or emotional changes, or damage to motor integrative systems.

A. THE STRIATUM

Although there are a few examples of conditioned response disruption following lesions in the striatum, this literature is still relatively small and undeveloped. Some studies have demonstrated that caudate lesions adversely affect delayed response performance and response alternation tasks (Battig, Rosvold, and Mishkin, 1960, 1962; Rosvold and Delgado, 1956), which might be interpreted as a deficit in short-term retention. On the other hand, these effects resemble the results of prefrontal cortical lesions, which have been related to response perseveration rather than failure of retention (Mishkin, 1964). The caudate nucleus and frontal cortex have, in fact, been implicated as parts of a single system mediating response inhibition in general (Battig *et al.*, 1960, 1962; Nauta, 1964). Supporting evidence for this view is provided by experiments involving stimulation of the caudate nucleus during ongoing behavior, which causes an abrupt cessation of responding that persists for the duration of stimulation (Buchwald, Weyers, Lauprecht, and Heuser, 1961; Rosvold and Delgado, 1956). Since Bromiley's decorticate dog suffered bilateral removal of the putamen but showed a retention of conditioning, a significant memory function for the putamen seems unlikely. Damage to the globus pallidus has been reported to affect acquisition and retention of conditioned learning (Gambarian, Garibian, Sarkisian, and Garibian, 1971; Laursen, 1962), but a primary result of pallidal lesions is hypokinesia (Carey, 1957) which may underlie most or all of these deficits. Taken together, these results seem to implicate the striatum primarily in motor control rather than in information storage.

B. THE THALAMUS

A role for the thalamus in learning was suggested by Brown and Ghiselli (1938), who found that complex operant response acquisition was impaired by large thalamic lesions. These effects, however, may simply have been due to interruption of primary sensory pathways. Smaller lesions in the dorsomedial thalamus have been shown to disrupt performance of preoperatively acquired discriminative responses (Knott, Ingram, and Correll, 1960; Schreiner, Rioch, Pechtel, and Masserman, 1953; Thompson and Massopust, 1960; Warren and Akert, 1960), but they also produce marked changes in affect. Other investigators have found little or no impairment of learned response performance after lesions of the pulvinar or of the anterior, medial, or dorsomedial thalamic nuclei (Chow, 1954; Brown and Ghiselli, 1938; Dahl, Ingram, and Knott, 1962; Peters, Rosvold, and Mirsky, 1956). In general, the literature concerning thalamic mediation of information storage is inconclusive and, as Grossman (1967) has pointed out, some or all of the deficits derived from thalamic damage may be primarily related to affective changes.

C. THE LIMBIC LOBE

In the decorticate preparations previously described which exhibited day-to-day retention of conditioning, the limbic lobe was largely intact. In view of their very close functional, anatomical, and phylogenetic relations, it is perhaps somewhat artificial to consider the limbic lobe structures as separate entities. Nevertheless, lesions, stimulation, and recordings in these areas show different effects and indicate different degrees of involvement in memory functions.

Septal lesions selectively disrupt performance of preoperatively acquired passive avoidance (McCleary, 1961, 1966), and, as in the caudate, stimulation of the septum inhibits performance of ongoing operant responses (Ingram, 1958; Knott et al., 1960). Affective changes, however, are a confounding variable in most septal lesion studies (McCleary, 1961), as are deficits in motor performance (Butters and Rosvold, 1968; Kleiner, Meyer, and Meyer, 1967), either of which might well account for apparent deficits in retention.

Amygdaloid lesions impair acquisition of a variety of tasks but do not prevent the recovery of preoperative learning (Brady, Schreiner, Geller, and Kling, 1954; Weiskrantz, 1956). Motivational and emotional changes also occur with amygdaloid lesions, so that it is difficult to evaluate performance deficits. Furthermore, the position of the amygdala in the brain is such that access to it for lesioning or stimulation usually involves damage to adjacent structures which may be more directly involved in retention. Some amygdaloid units have been found to respond optimally to complex, motivationally significant stimuli, such as "meows" or the sight of a rat (O'Keefe and Bouma, 1969; Sawa and Delgado, 1963), suggesting that the amygdala performs higher-order sensory integration and/or evaluation. A memory function of the amygdala, however, has not been strongly proposed.

The hippocampus, on the other hand, appears to be a very likely substrate for storage of learned information. A number of studies involving lesions of the hippocampus in animals indicate that this structure is necessary for maintenance of habituation, data which have recently been summarized in two lengthy reviews (Douglas, 1967; Kimble, 1968). In humans, hippocampal lesions or disruptive stimulation are known to abolish memory consolidation (Milner, 1958; Milner and Teuber, 1968; Penfield and Milner, 1958; Scoville and Milner, 1947).

The capacity of the hippocampus to hold sensory input for long periods of time might support a mechanism for storage of the significance of stimuli during conditioning and habituation. Responses of hippocampal cells to sensory stimuli exhibit uniquely extended durations (e.g., Green and Machne, 1955; Vinogradova, 1966), and the network of closed loops within the hippocampus (McLardy, 1959, 1963; Turner, 1969), or between the hippocampus and other brain areas (e.g., Green, 1960; Nauta, 1958), could well support short-term retention of afferent impulses prior to consolidation. Olds and his associates (Hirano, Best, and Olds, 1970; Olds and Hirano, 1969) have found that, during conditioning, hippocampal units in the rat exhibit larger relative changes in firing rates and more marked discrimination between neutral and reinforced stimuli than do units sampled in the hypothalamus and midbrain. They regard their data as evidence for hippocampal participation in storage of conditioning effects.

Thus, several lines of evidence favor the view that hippocampal influences are of primary importance to the retention or storage of habituation and conditioning effects.

In the case of habituation, the initial arousal responses induced by the first presentations of the habituating stimulus would gradually tend to disappear due, at least in part, to hippocampal blockade of reticular formation activation (Grastyan, Lissak, Madarasz, and Donhoffer, 1959). It is perhaps significant that electrical stimulation of the hippocampus has been shown to inhibit conduction through the polysynaptic relays of the reticular formation (Adey, Segundo, and

Livingston, 1957). Eventually, the habituating stimulus would become efficiently "recognized" by the hippocampus, i.e., associated with stored effects of previous stimulus presentations, and its arousal effects would be quickly damped. In this view, the hippocampus is offered as an alternative substrate for Sokolov's (1963) stimulus "model" formed in the cortex during habituation. Incoming stimuli would be compared with stored hippocampal models containing stimulus-response information. When stimulus and model of stimulus-habituation coincided, the arousal response mediated by the reticular formation would be blocked. Novel stimuli, which would have no stimulus-response model, would not be "recognized," and therefore would induce a more prolonged arousal.

Habituated stimuli might subsequently become blocked within the sensory pathways themselves, once the stimuli were identified as nonsignificant and no longer induced arousal. Without the dishabituating excitation of arousal influences, responses in the sensory relay nuclei would decrement rapidly, as seen in the later stages of habituation in sensory nuclei in intact cats and in the cochlear nucleus of the decerebrate cat. Additional data in support of this concept have been reviewed elsewhere (Buchwald and Humphrey, 1971). The sensory pathway would thus provide the specificity of input needed for the formation of a selective hippocampal model for each habituated, or nonsignificant, stimulus; such a stimulus recognition function seems unlikely to be supported by the nonspecific arousal responses mediated by the reticular formation. In addition to this indirect effect on sensory transmission, resulting from blockade of arousal influences, a more direct action on the sensory pathways might occur through projections from the hippocampus to the sensory relay nuclei (Cazard and Buser, 1963; Douglas, 1967; Fox, Liebeskind, O'Brien, and Dingle, 1967; Parmeggiani and Rapisarda, 1969; Pribram, 1967; Redding, 1967), once the stimulus recognition model became well established.

Such mechanisms for blockade of incoming sensory information could serve to reduce the "noise" of nonsignificant sensory stimuli and to facilitate transmission of significant input. A change in the significance of a previously habituated stimulus by a dishabituating stimulus would reverse the habituation process and arousal would reappear. Pairing a dishabituating, or unconditioned stimulus, with an habituated, or conditioning stimulus, would evoke an appropriate response more and more efficiently, as the hippocampal holding mechanism blocked nonsignificant stimulus-response sequences and established a new stimulus-recognition model for the significant stimulus-response sequence. This process, as in habituation, could include selective changes in the facility of transmission in sensory pathways, so that information would ultimately be conveyed more efficiently to efferent systems mediating the specific learned response.

VII. Summary

Overt behavior may be thought of as the net product of two interacting systems, one of which serves to promote motor integration, e.g., postural stabilization and complex movements, the other of which underlies motor learning, e.g., acquired responses and volitional actions. In analyzing mechanisms of motor control, it may thus be advantageous to study response acquisition separately from response integration. Just as integrated motor activity is believed to develop as a hierarchy of increasingly complex motor patterns, beginning with localized spinal reflexes and developing into diffuse, complex patterns of activity, learned behavior may similarly evolve from local conditioned responses, such as conditioned sucking, to the increasingly generalized and interrelated acquired responses characteristic of the adult organism. In an attempt to analyze the basic units of the learning hierarchy, motor learning data derived from animals with chronic deletions of higher neuraxial levels has been reviewed; additionally, in an attempt to suggest neural loci of primary change during the development of specific types of motor learning, such as conditioning or habituation, electrophysiological data derived from experiments carried out in our own laboratory have been reviewed.

It seems clear that the simplest form of motor learning, i.e., motor response habituation, is present in decorticate, decerebrate, and spinal preparations; in fact, with progressive deletion of the higher levels, habituation seems to become increasingly easy to observe. Thus, in the decerebrate preparation, motor responses induced by acoustic stimuli habituate almost immediately, as do somatic reflex responses in the spinal preparation. Similarly, electrophysiological responses recorded from the cochlear nucleus of the decerebrate animal show more rapid and consistent response decrements to repeated acoustic stimulation and less dishabituation than do similar responses in the intact animal. Thus, the ease with which response decrements develop seems to be directly related to deletion or depression of higher influences. Electrophysiological studies of acoustic habituation have further indicated that response modulations which eventually appear as an habituated motor response may begin very close to the level of stimulus input; thus, although response alterations do not develop at the cochlear receptor level, i.e., the hair cell, marked decrements can be recorded at the level of the first central relay, i.e., the cochlear nucleus, during repeated stimulation procedures.

With respect to more complex learning, the behavioral literature provides convincing evidence that rather specific conditioned responses, i.e., a conditioned leg flexion to tonal CS, can be established in the decorticate preparation. In the decerebrate animal, fewer observations have been made but the data are nonetheless indicative that specific conditioned responses can be developed. In the spinal animal, the evidence relating to conditioning remains equivocal. In many of these studies, negative results have been reported, while in other studies various forms of response alteration have been reported during conditioning, particularly when "lower" mammals or immature subjects are utilized. Thus, the capacity for acquiring a simple conditioned response, although possible in the absence of forebrain structures, seems to diminish as the neuraxis is progressively truncated, in contrast to the increasing ease with which habituation develops as higher levels are progressively deleted.

Prior to the appearance of the overt conditioned response, early electrophysiological alterations of unit activity were found to develop in the subcortical pathway of the conditioning stimulus as well as in the midbrain reticular formation; at approximately the same time in the conditioning procedures, conditioned responses of the gamma motoneurons were recorded at spinal cord levels. The enhanced activity of the CS pathway, reticular formation, and gamma motoneurons continued to be induced by the CS after the behavioral conditioned response appeared. These subcortical systems are thus suggested as early, possibly primary, mediators of conditioned associations which facilitate the subsequent conditioning of other brain areas and the ultimate appearance of the overt motor conditioned response.

The changes observed in the primary afferent pathways during both habituation and conditioning imply that the significant events of the S-R sequence may take place very close to the stimulus receptor. A capacity for response plasticity at such "peripheral" loci could explain the survival of habituation and conditioning after drastic neuraxial transection and encourages the view that plasticity in the CNS can be studied in a relatively well-defined, restricted, accessible part of the brain. Once identified, such a site of primary change in the CNS could be further scrutinized with a variety of techniques, such as intracellular recording, chemical analysis, and electron microscopy, to determine cellular and subceullular mechanisms of plasticity.

Although the nature of habituation and conditioning seems essentially similar in the intact and truncated preparation, certain differences are of interest. The differences in plasticity which appear as higher neural levels are progressively deleted, largely reflect an increasing bias toward response decrement in the case of habituation and an increasing bias against convergence and response increment in the case of conditioning. Of particular significance in this regard would seem to be the progressive deletions of the ascending activating system of the reticular formation. The studies which have been reviewed here suggest that deletion or depression of reticular activity promotes the development of response habituation. On the other hand, alterations in reticular activity which develop early in conditioning trials suggest that facilitatory reticular influences play a role in conditioning. While much of the evidence for participation of the reticular formation in learning phenomena is controversial, we would suggest that the reticular formation is a preeminent mediator of altered capacities for habituation and conditioning as the neuraxis is progressively truncated. We suggest that arousal influences initially tend to oppose habituation and to facilitate conditioning.

Although retention of habituation in the intact animal is a commonplace behavioral observation and was noted electrophysiologically as an increased rate of unit response habituation in the medial geniculate and inferior colliculus during acoustic habituation on successive days, there is presently no evidence, either behaviorally or neurophysiologically, that habituation effects are stored in the decerebrate preparation. Several lines of evidence from the literature suggest that the limbic lobe, particularly the hippocampus, provides a mechanism for retention and consolidation of both habituation and conditioning effects, so that stimuli are more efficiently "recognized," assigned significance, and channelled appropriately to efferent systems as a result of repeated training trials.

We feel that an approach which combines the advantages of simplified behavioral paradigms, electrophysiological analysis, and simplified nervous systems is most promising. By examining the same sorts of response plasticity in both intact and truncated preparations and by recording concurrent neurophysiological changes occurring in both sorts of system, a clearer understanding of basic mechanisms of learning may be obtained without sacrificing relevance to the normal, adult animal.

Acknowledgement

This work has been supported by USPHS Grants NB 05437 and GM 0048. Bibliographic assistance was obtained from UCLA Brain Information Service Supported by NIH Grant 70-2063. Computing assistance was obtained from the Health Sciences Computing Facility, UCLA, sponsored by NIH Special Research Resources Grant RR-3.

The authors would like to thank Mrs. Glow Holland for her assistance in the preparation of this manuscript.

Chapter 5

Comparisons of the Efferent Projections of the Globus Pallidus and Substantia Nigra in the Monkey

MALCOLM B. CARPENTER

COLLEGE OF PHYSICIANS AND SURGEONS
COLUMBIA UNIVERSITY

I. Introduction

Considerable evidence from a variety of disciplines suggests that the globus pallidus and substantia nigra each play an important role in neural mechanisms responsible for human dyskinesias. The precise role played by these nuclei remains to be defined. The substantia nigra is implicated primarily in the metabolic disturbances which underlie Parkinsonism and appears to be the principal source of striatal dopamine (Dahlström and Fuxe, 1964; Andén, Carlsson, Dahlström, Fuxe, Hillarp, and Larsson, 1964; Poirier and Sourkes, 1965; Hornykiewicz, 1966). Although direct evidence that the globus pallidus may be involved in Parkinsonism is less clear, this structure may be involved in some way in all forms of basal ganglia dyskinesia for two reasons: (1) it is the source of the principal output of the basal ganglia, and (2) it is the only part of the basal ganglia that projects to the thalamic nuclei that in turn project to the motor cortex. While the precise functions of each of these nuclear masses are unknown, it seems certain that accurate data concerning their efferent connections would contribute to the unraveling of a puzzle which has long constituted one of the great enigmas of neurology.

This comparative study of the efferent projections of the globus pallidus and substantia nigra in the monkey was the outgrowth of attempts to determine the connections of the subthalamic nucleus (Carpenter and Strominger, 1967). In the course of this study it became evident that no valid conclusions could be reached without precise data concerning the projections of the globus pallidus and substantia nigra. Because of the great significance of the globus pallidus and substantia nigra in concepts of neural mechanisms underlying the most prevalent of all human dyskinesias, namely Parkinsonism, remarks will be confined to these nuclear masses.

II. Material and Methods

This study was based upon the analysis of anatomical data taken from 42 monkeys in which discrete lesions were produced in the globus pallidus and substantia nigra. Lesions in the globus pallidus were produced by electrodes introduced into the lateral surface of the brain at various angles. These electrodes traversed the insular cortex and the putamen. Lesions in the substantia nigra were produced by three different stereotaxic approaches. Electrodes used to produce lesions in the substantia nigra were introduced: (1) through the frontal cortex into the rostrocaudal axis of the nigra, (2) laterally at an angle conforming to the lateromedial axis of the nucleus, and (3) posteriorly through the cerebellum in the caudorostral axis of the nigra.

Degeneration resulting from lesions in the globus pallidus was studied in transverse, sagittal, and horizontal sections stained by the Nauta-Gygax (1954) technique. Sections through the lesions in all animals were evaluated in Nissl and Weil stained sections. Degeneration resulting from nigral lesions also was studied by the Nauta-Gygax technique except in one recent series in which sections were stained by the Wiitanen (1969) technique. The thalamic terminology and cytological delineations of Olszewski (1952) were used throughout these studies.

A. GLOBUS PALLIDUS

Although certain studies (Kleist, 1934; Alexander, 1942; Hassler, 1961) suggest a definite somatotopic representation within the basal ganglia, anatomical and physiological support for this concept is meager. There is evidence which indicates that striatal afferent and efferent fiber systems are topographically organized. The neostriatum receives fibers from broad areas of the cerebral cortex and from the intralaminar thalamic nuclei, both of which are topographically organized (Powell and Cowan, 1956; Webster, 1961; Carman, Cowan, and Powell, 1963; Kemp and Powell, 1970). Although biochemical data indicate that nigrostriatal fibers exist (Fuxe and Andén, 1966), anatomical information based on fiber degeneration has been meager. Striatal efferent fibers projecting to both the globus pallidus and the substantia nigra are topographically organized (Voneida, 1960; Szabo, 1962, 1967, 1970; Cowan and Powell, 1966). Striopallidal fibers are organized in both dorsoventral and rostrocaudal sequences and radiate like spokes of a wheel into both segments of the pallidum.

The globus pallidus gives rise to the ansa lenticularis, the lenticular fasciculus, and the pallidosubthalamic projection. These three distinct bundles are arranged in a rostrocaudal sequence, but fibers of the ansa lenticularis and the lenticular fasciculus merge in Forel's field H. The extent to which pallidal efferent fibers may be topographically organized is unknown and relatively unexplored. However, it would be surprising if the high degree of topographical organization seen in the neostriatum were not continued in some way in the pallidofugal fiber system. There is some evidence that the pallidosubthalamic projection may be systematically organized (Papez, Bennett, and Cash, 1942; Nauta and Mehler, 1966).

Data concerning pallidofugal fiber systems were based upon 22 discrete pallidal lesions in 20 monkeys (Carpenter, Fraser, and Shriver, 1968). These lesions involved the lateral pallidal segment, the medial pallidal segment, and both medial and lateral pallidal segments. None of these lesions involved the internal capsule.

To facilitate descriptions, the lateral pallidal segment was divided into three parts by two hypothetical planes perpendicular to a midsagittal plane that passed through the most rostral and caudal borders of the medial medullary lamina of the pallidum (Fig. 1). These hypothetical planes divided the lateral pallidal segment into three unequal parts which could be defined accurately in transverse, horizontal, and sagittal sections. Portions of the lateral pallidal segment in front of the most rostral hypothetical plane were designated as the *rostral part*. Portions of the lateral pallidal segment between the two hypothetical planes, and lateral to the medial pallidal segment, were designated as the *central part*. The portion of the lateral pallidal segment caudal to the second hypothetical plane was referred to as the *caudal part*.

1. Lateral Pallidal Segment

Twelve lesions in 10 animals destroyed localized portions of the lateral pallidal segment. These lesions were unilateral in eight animals and bilateral in two. Degeneration from these lesions was entirely ipsilateral and projected only to the subthalamic nucleus.

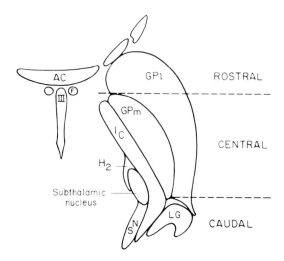

Fig. 1. Schematic diagram of a horizontal section through the globus pallidus and subthalamic region illustrating the division of the lateral pallidal segment into three parts, designated as rostral, central, and caudal. Abbreviations used here and in subsequent figures follow: AC, anterior commissure; AV, anterior ventral nucleus; CG, central gray, CI, inferior colliculus; CL, subthalamic nucleus; CM, centromedian nucleus; CS, superior colliculus; DM, dorsomedial nucleus; Fx, fornix; GPl, globus pallidus, lateral segment; GPm, globus pallidus, medial segment; H, Forel's field H; H_2, lenticular fasciculus; Hb, habenular nuclei; IC, internal capsule; LD, lateral dorsal nucleus; LG, lateral geniculate body; LL, lateral lemniscus; ML, medial lemniscus; MM, mammillary body; MTT, mammillothalamic tract, OT, optic tract; Pf, parafascicular nucleus; PPN, pedunculopontine nucleus; Pul, pulvinar, Py, pyramid; RN, red nucleus; SCP, superior cerebellar peduncle, SI, substantia innominata; SN, substantia nigra; STN, subthalamic nucleus; VA, ventral anterior nucleus, principal part; VAmc, ventral anterior nucleus, magnocellular part; VLc, ventral lateral nucleus, caudal part; VLm, ventral lateral nucleus, medial part; VLo, ventral lateral nucleus, oral part, VPM, ventral posterior medial nucleus; ZI, zona incerta. III, third ventricle; III N, oculomotor nerve; IV N, trochlear nerve; VI, abducens nucleus. Reprinted by permission of Elsevier Publishing Company, Amsterdam, Holland.

a. Rostral Part. Lesions in three animals destroyed dorsal, ventral, and intermediate portions of the rostral part of the lateral pallidal segment near levels where the anterior commissure passes through the pallidum. Degeneration from these lesions projected exclusively to the subthalamic nucleus (Figs. 2 and 3) except for that resulting from striatal injury due to electrode passage. Fibers from the lesion projected medially and caudally within the medial pallidal segment, traversed central parts of the peduncular part of the internal capsule, and entered the subthalamic nucleus. Comparisons of the pallidosubthalamic projection in these three animals revealed common features and some differences. In none of the animals was degeneration unusually profuse in rostral

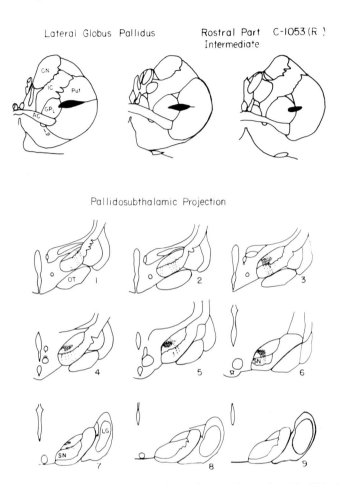

Fig. 2. Rhesus C-1053. Diagrams illustrating an intermediate lesion (black) in the rostral part of the lateral pallidal segment at three levels. Pallidosubthalamic degeneration resulting from this pallidal lesion is shown below in nine successive levels through the subthalamic nucleus. These levels represent the rostral (1–3), middle (4–6), and caudal (7–9) thirds of the subthalamic nucleus. Degeneration is indicated by dashes (fibers of passage) and stipples (terminal). Reprinted by permission of Elsevier Publishing Company, Amsterdam, Holland.

parts of the subthalamic nucleus. The most significant common feature was the predominant, selective termination of fibers in the medial half of the subthalamic nucleus. The more ventral the lesion in the rostral part of the lateral pallidal segment, the more medial was the degeneration in the subthalamic nucleus. Thus pallidosubthalamic fibers from the rostral part of the lateral pallidal segment were found to terminate in the medial half of the rostral two-thirds of the subthalamic nucleus, and in no other locations.

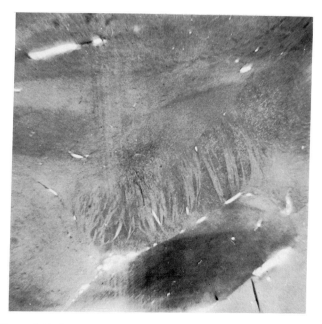

Fig. 3. Rhesus C-1053. Photomicrograph of terminal degeneration in the medial half of the right subthalamic nucleus. Nauta-Gygax, ×11. Reprinted by permission of Elsevier Publishing Company, Amsterdam, Holland.

b. Central Part. Eight lesions in six monkeys destroyed localized regions in central parts of the lateral pallidal segment. These lesions, involving predominantly rostral portions of this subdivision, were classified as dorsal, ventral, and intermediate. Dorsal lesions in two animals produced degeneration that projected medially and caudally into the medial pallidal segment where it occupied only dorsal regions (Figs. 4 and 5). At levels of the subthalamic nucleus degenerated fibers crossed through lateral regions of the peduncular part of the internal capsule at a steep angle. The bulk of these fibers terminated in the dorsolateral part of the subthalamic nucleus where they filled a triangular-shaped area in the rostral third of the nucleus. In the middle third of the nucleus degeneration shifted medially, but remained dorsal in location; the entire ventral border of the nucleus was free of degeneration. Degeneration in the above position diminished in the caudal third of the nucleus but remained in its lateral half. No degeneration was seen in either the ansa lenticularis or the lenticular fasciculus.

Five lesions in three monkeys selectively destroyed ventral portions of the lateral pallidal segment in its central part (Fig. 6). Degeneration from these lesions projected medially and caudally into the medial pallidal segment and was concentrated in a ventral location. Fibers traversed the peduncular part of the

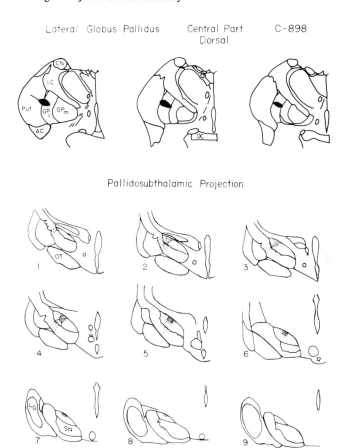

Fig. 4. Rhesus C-898. Diagrams illustrating a dorsal lesion (black) in the central part of the lateral pallidal segment at three levels. Pallidosubthalamic degeneration resulting from this lesion is plotted below. Degeneration was localized primarily to dorsal regions of the lateral half of the rostral two-thirds of the nucleus. Reprinted by permission of Elsevier Publishing Company, Amsterdam, Holland.

internal capsule and entered the ventral part of the rostral two-thirds of the subthalamic nucleus. These fibers terminated predominantly in the lateral half of the nucleus. Lesions involving ventral portions of the central part of the lateral pallidal segment at more rostral levels projected to more medial regions of the subthalamic nucleus than similar lesions in more caudal regions.

c. Caudal Part. One lesion studied in horizontal sections destroyed part of the lateral pallidal segment caudal to the medial pallidal segment. This extreme caudal part of the lateral pallidum lies rostral to the lateral geniculate body. Degeneration from this lesion traversed the peduncular part of the internal capsule caudal to the medial pallidal segment and entered the junctional zone

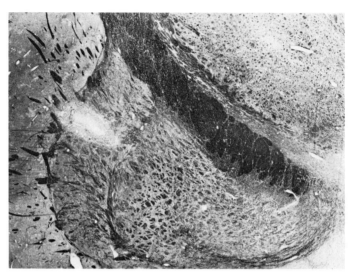

Fig. 5. Rhesus C-894. Photomicrograph of a dorsal lesion in the central part of the left lateral pallidal segment. Weil, ×8.

between the subthalamic nucleus and the substantia nigra. Fibers passing into the substantia nigra were considered to be strionigral fibers degenerated as a consequence of passage of the electrode through the striatum. Pallidosubthalamic fibers projected to a small caudal portion of the nucleus located dorsally. These observations were interpreted to mean that the extreme caudal part of the lateral pallidum projects to the dorsolateral and caudal pole of the subthalamic nucleus, a region to which no other portion of the lateral pallidal segment was found to project.

Data concerning the projections of the lateral pallidal segment support the concept that pallidosubthalamic fibers have a specific topographic organization. Observations suggest that the most medial and lateral regions of the lateral pallidal segment project fibers respectively to the medial and lateral parts of the subthalamic nucleus. This generalization takes into account the fact that the subdivision designated as the rostral part of the lateral pallidal segment is also the most medial, and the subdivision designated as the caudal part is also the most lateral part. Pallidosubthalamic fibers arising in the lateral pallidal segment are organized so that: (1) rostral and central portions of the lateral pallidal segment project fibers to the rostral two-thirds of the subthalamic nucleus, and (2) the rostral part projects fibers to the medial half of the nucleus and the central part to the lateral half of the nucleus. Caudal parts of the lateral pallidal segment project fibers to dorsolateral and caudal regions of the subthalamic nucleus. These fibers also are arranged in a dorsoventral sequence so that: (1) fibers from dorsal regions of the rostral part terminate in more lateral parts of

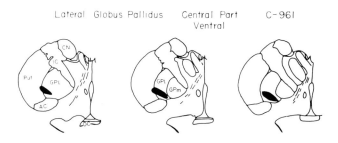

Lateral Globus Pallidus   Central Part   C-961
Ventral

Pallidosubthalamic Projection

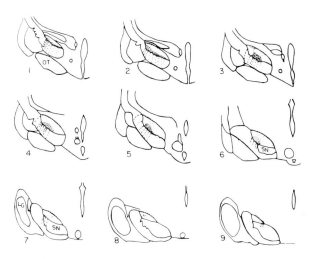

Fig. 6. Rhesus C-961. Diagrams illustrating a ventral lesion (black) in the central part of the lateral pallidal segment at three levels. Pallidosubthalamic degeneration plotted below was localized mainly to ventral and lateral parts of the rostral two-thirds of the nucleus. Reprinted by permission of Elsevier Publishing Company, Amsterdam, Holland.

the medial half of the nucleus than fibers originating from more ventral regions of this part, and (2) fibers from dorsal and ventral regions in the central part of the lateral pallidum project to corresponding dorsal and ventral regions of the lateral half of the subthalamic nucleus.

It is notable that none of the lesions in the lateral pallidal segment produced degeneration in the ventromedial and caudal parts of the subthalamic nucleus. This same observation was made by Nauta and Mehler (1966) who suggested that this region of the subthalamic nucleus received fibers from the substantia innominata.

2. Medial Pallidal Segment

Lesions in six animals were confined to the medial pallidal segment. In three
of these animals lesions localized to dorsal or ventral regions produced
degeneration in (1) the pallidosubthalamic projection and (2) either the ansa
lenticularis or the lenticular fasciculus. Three other lesions, confined to
intermediate regions of the medial pallidal segment, produced degeneration in all
pallidofugal fiber systems.

One lesion in the dorsal part of the medial pallidal segment produced (1)

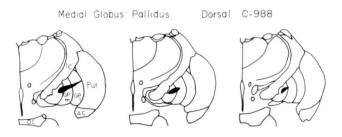

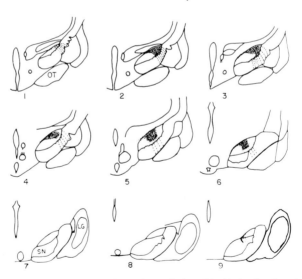

Fig. 7. Rhesus C-988. Diagrams illustrating a lesion (black) in the dorsal part of the
medial pallidal segment. Degeneration resulting from this lesion was present in the lenticular
fasciculus and the pallidosubthalamic projection. Pallidosubthalamic fibers terminated
primarily in dorsal and lateral parts of the rostral two-thirds of the subthalamic nucleus. In
the caudal part of the middle third of the nucleus (5 and 6) terminal degeneration occupied
a dorsal and central region. Terminal degeneration also was seen in the caudomedial part of
the subthalamic nucleus (9), but sections at levels 7 and 8 were not available for study.

profuse degeneration in the lenticular fasciculus, and (2) degeneration in the pallidosubthalamic projection. Degeneration within the subthalamic nucleus was essentially the same as that associated with dorsal lesions in the central part of the lateral pallidal segment, except for the addition of a small number of fibers projecting to the ventromedial and caudal pole of the nucleus (Fig. 7).

In two animals lesions destroyed ventral portions of the medial pallidal segment at levels near the optic chiasm (Fig. 8). In these animals degeneration emanating from the globus pallidus was seen only in the ansa lenticularis and the pallidosubthalamic projection. Fibers projecting to the subthalamic nucleus were most concentrated in ventral regions of the nucleus, close to the internal capsule and were greatest in the rostral two-thirds of the nucleus. In these animals degeneration extended further medially in the subthalamic nucleus than with lesions confined to the lateral pallidal segment.

Lesions in three animals confined to intermediate regions of the medial pallidal segment produced degeneration in all pallidofugal fiber systems. Degeneration in the subthalamic nucleus was more profuse than that associated with any other pallidal lesions, and while greatest in the lateral half of the rostral two-thirds of the nucleus, it extended into the medial half of the caudal third of the nucleus.

Lesions involving portions of both the medial and lateral pallidal segments confirmed the above observation with respect to the pallidosubthalamic projection and provided certain data concerning pallidal efferent fibers originating from the medial pallidal segment.

As might be expected, lesions involving the medial pallidal segment produced quantitatively more degeneration in the subthalamic nucleus than lesions

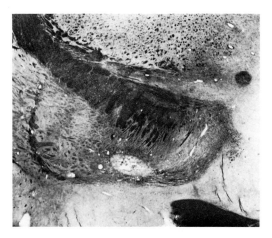

Fig. 8. Rhesus C-983. Photomicrograph of lesion in the ventral part of the medial pallidal segment. This lesion was medial to the accessory medullary lamina of the pallidum and directly destroyed part of the ansa lenticularis. Nauta-Gygax, x7.

confined to the lateral pallidal segment. Quantitative differences appeared due to interruption of larger numbers of efferent fibers from the lateral segment converging and traversing the medial pallidal segment. The outstanding qualitative difference was that lesions involving the medial pallidal segment were associated with greater terminal degeneration in the medial half of the caudal two-thirds of the subthalamic nucleus. These data have been interpreted to mean that pallidosubthalamic fibers from the medial pallidal segment project to a small ventromedial and caudal part of the subthalamic nucleus (Fig. 9).

Pallidosubthalamic projections

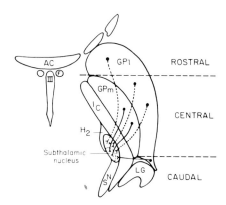

Fig. 9. Composite diagram illustrating the topographical organization of pallido-subthalamic fibers in a schematic drawing of a horizontal section. Pallidosubthalamic fibers arising from the lateral pallidal segment are indicated by dotted lines while those from the medial pallidal segment are indicated by solid lines. Rostral and central parts of the lateral pallidal segment project fibers to the rostral two-thirds of the subthalamic nucleus; rostral parts of this segment project fibers to the medial half of the nucleus, while central parts of this segment project fibers to the lateral half of the nucleus. The caudal part of the lateral pallidal segment projects fibers to the caudal and lateral parts of the subthalamic nucleus. Portions of the medial pallidal segment project a modest number of fibers to medial and caudal parts of the subthalamic nucleus. Pallidosubthalamic fibers also are organized in a dorsoventral sequence not shown in this figure. Reprinted by permission of Elsevier Publishing Company, Amsterdam, Holland.

Ansa Lenticularis and the Lenticular Fasciculus. The most widely distributed pallidofugal fibers arise exclusively from the medial pallidal segment. Data based on isolated lesions of the medial pallidal segment and lesions involving both pallidal segments suggest that fibers of the lenticular fasciculus arise mainly from dorsal portions of the medial pallidal segment. In five animals, lesions involving ventral portions of the medial pallidal segment produced degeneration in the ansa lenticularis but not in the lenticular fasciculus. These data suggested that fibers of the ansa lenticularis arise from ventral portions of the medial pallidal segment and that a significant part of these fibers originated from neurons lateral to the accessory medullary lamina of the medial pallidal segment (Fig. 10). Thus pallidal efferent fibers arising from the medial pallidal segment displayed a dorsoventral organization with respect to origin. This topographic organization could be followed only as far as Forel's field H where fibers of the ansa lenticularis and lenticular fasciculus merged and could no longer be identified as separate bundles. The bulk of these pallidofugal fibers curved laterally dorsal to the zona incerta and entered the thalamic fasciculus

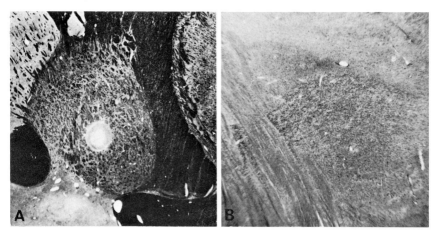

Fig. 10. A. Rhesus C-960. Photomicrograph of a combined lesion involving portions of the left medial pallidal segment situated lateral to the accessory medullary lamina of the pallidum. Sagittal section. Weil, ×6. B. Photomicrograph of pallidal degeneration traversing the internal capsule in its projection to the subthalamic nucleus. No degeneration was present in the lenticular fasciculus (LF), but degeneration was seen in the ansa lenticularis. Nauta-Gygax, ×65.

(Nauta and Mehler, 1966; Carpenter and Strominger, 1967). Pallidofugal fibers in the thalamic fasciculus coursed dorsolaterally and rostrally to enter the ventral tier thalamic nuclei (Fig. 11). Profuse terminations were seen in the ventral lateral nucleus in the pars oralis [VLO; Fig. 12(A, B, and C)] and the lateral part of the pars medialis (VLm). At more rostral levels, fibers of this system projected to the principal part of the ventral anterior nucleus (VApc; Fig. 13). No pallidofugal fibers appeared to project to the magnocellular part of the ventral anterior nucleus (VAmc) or to Olszewski's (1952) cell group X. Some pallidofugal fibers separated from the thalamic fasciculus fairly far caudally, curved medially and dorsally from the principal bundle, traversed the ventral posterior medial nucleus (VPM) of the thalamus and terminated in the centromedian nucleus [CM; Figs. 11 and 12(D)]. Fibers entering the centromedian nucleus appeared most concentrated ventrally and rostrally and were less numerous than those projecting to the rostral ventral tier thalamic nuclei.

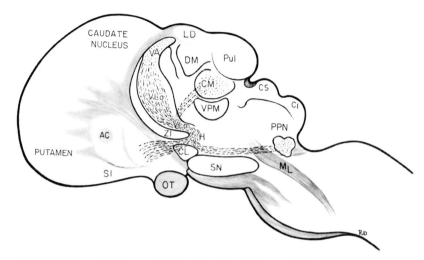

Fig. 11. Schematic diagram of the efferent projections of the medial pallidal segment. Fibers of the ansa lenticularis and lenticular fasciculus merge in Forel's field H. Most of these fibers pass in the thalamic fasciculus to the ventral lateral (VLo and VLm) and ventral anterior (VA) thalamic nuclei. Some fibers separate from this bundle and project to the centromedian (CM) nucleus. Pallidotegmental fibers descend to cells of the pedunculopontine (PPN) nucleus. See page 140 for list of abbreviations used. Reprinted by permission of Elsevier Publishing Company, Amsterdam, Holland.

A small bundle of pallidofugal fibers separated from Forel's field H, medial to the subthalamic nucleus and descended as a distinct *pallidotegmental bundle* (Fig. 11). In their course these fibers descended along the ventrolateral border of the red nucleus and moved laterally and dorsally at more caudal levels. As these fibers shifted dorsally and laterally in the caudal midbrain tegmentum, they became partially intermingled with fibers of the medial lemniscus. At levels of the inferior colliculus the fibers swept dorsally to arborize about the large cells of the pedunculopontine nucleus, a cell group traversed by fibers of the superior cerebellar peduncle (Olszewski and Baxter, 1954). No pallidofugal fibers were found to descend in the brainstem caudal to isthmus levels.

There are a number of other small pallidofugal projections described in the literature (see Nauta and Mehler, 1966), one of which is a projection to the hypothalamus. Fibers regarded as pallidohypothalamic project medially from Forel's field H, loop over the fibers of the fornix and course ventromedially toward the hypothalamus. According to Nauta and Mehler (1966) and our own findings (Carpenter and Strominger, 1967), no distinct terminations were seen in the ventromedial nucleus or elsewhere in the hypothalamus. Nauta and Mehler described fibers, which appeared directed toward the hypothalamus, that looped back to join the main bundle of pallidofugal fibers. These fibers looping ventral toward the hypothalamus were considered to be composed of aberrant fibers of

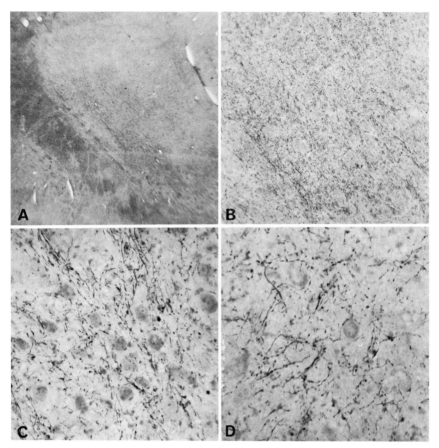

Fig. 12. Rhesus C-980. A, B, and C. Photomicrographs of degeneration projecting from the medial pallidal segment to the ventral lateral (VLo) thalamic nucleus. Nauta-Gygax, x8, x52, x133. D. Photomicrograph of terminal degeneration in the centromedian (CM) nucleus. Nauta-Gygax, x325. Reprinted by permission of Elsevier Publishing Company, Amsterdam, Holland.

the ansa lenticularis. They were not observed in our material. Since all areas of the globus pallidus have not been explored, it cannot be stated flatly that no pallidal fibers project to the hypothalamus, but it seems likely that if they exist, they are not numerous.

In all animals with lesions in the medial pallidal segment and in some with lesions in the lateral segment, some degenerated fibers were found in the lateral part of the stria medullaris which terminated in the lateral habenular nucleus. The significance of this projection is unknown.

The most prominent negative findings were absence of pallidofugal fibers in the zona incerta, the red nucleus, and the inferior olivary complex.

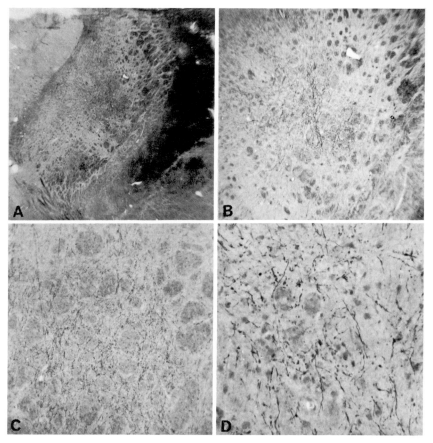

Fig. 13. A, B, and C, Rhesus C-988. Photomicrographs of degeneration from the medial pallidal segment projecting to the principal part of the ventral anterior (VApc) thalamic nucleus. Nauta-Gygax, ×8, ×22, ×52. D, Rhesus C-983. Degeneration resulting from lesion in Fig. 8, terminating in VApc. Nauta-Gygax, ×325. Reprinted by permission of Elsevier Publishing Company, Amsterdam, Holland.

B. Substantia Nigra

Two previous attempts were made to determine the efferent projections of the substantia nigra in the monkey using the Nauta and Gygax (1954) technique (Carpenter and McMasters, 1964; Carpenter and Strominger, 1967). In the first of these attempts electrodes were introduced into the nigra by a frontal approach which damaged thalamic nuclei, the internal capsule, and sometimes interrupted pallidofugal fibers. In spite of these compromising circumstances, well-localized lesions in the substantia nigra in nine monkeys indicated that ascending fibers from the nigra entered Forel's field H and projected laterally along the dorsal border of the subthalamic nucleus, traversed the internal capsule at a steep angle, and entered the medial segment of the globus pallidus. These nigral efferent fibers seemed to be intermingled with fibers of the lenticular fasciculus but coursed in the opposite direction. In the globus pallidus most fibers were distributed within the medial pallidal segment, but a considerable number of degenerated fibers were concentrated near the medial and lateral medullary laminae. These presumed nigropallidal fibers were scattered in the neuropil and did not seem to end directly upon pallidal neurons. A few degenerated fibers seen in the lateral medullary lamina of the pallidum entered the most medial part of the putamen, but none extended for any distance.

A more complete and valid analysis of nigral efferent fibers, based on the Nauta technique, was obtained from animals in which lesions were produced via electrodes introduced: (1) in a coronal plane (lateromedial axis of the nigra) or (2) via a posterior infratentorial approach (caudorostral axis of the nigra). Neither of these stereotaxic approaches was perfect. Electrodes inserted at an angle in a coronal plane traversed retrolenticular parts of the internal capsule, the brachium of the superior colliculus, and parts of the medial geniculate body. With the posterior infratentorial approach the electrode interrupted fibers of the superior cerebellar peduncle, but because all fibers in this bundle decussate, they did not present a problem at diencephalic levels. With both of these approaches some fibers of the medial lemniscus and spinothalamic tract were invariably interrupted.

Lesions in six animals were produced by these stereotaxic approaches. Three lesions were produced by electrodes introduced in a coronal plane. In two animals the lesions destroyed large parts of the pars compacta and pars reticularis in the medial part of the nigra. The other lesion destroyed the lateral part of the substantia nigra (mainly pars compacta). Lesions produced by the posterior infratentorial approach involved both pars compacta and pars reticularis in central parts of the nigra.

Degeneration resulting from these lesions was remarkably similar and can be described synthetically. Ascending degeneration passed lateral to the red nucleus and entered the prerubral area (Forel's field H). From this location fibers projected dorsally and rostrally into the medial part of the ventral lateral nucleus (VLm) of the thalamus where fibers closely surrounded individual cells in a manner characteristic of fiber terminations. Part of these fibers projected rostrally and dorsally into the magnocellular part of the ventral anterior nucleus (VAmc). Terminal degeneration in VAmc was not as profuse as in VLm but was substantial. None of the degenerated fibers were distributed to the principal part of the ventral anterior nucleus (VApc) or to oral parts of the ventral lateral nucleus (VLo). In all these animals a relatively smaller number of nigral efferent fibers passed laterally from Forel's field H along the dorsal and rostral borders of the subthalamic nucleus. These fibers penetrated the internal capsule lateral to the subthalamic nucleus and entered the globus pallidus. Most of these degenerated fibers did not pass beyond the medial pallidal segment, but degeneration in some animals was seen in the medial and lateral medullary laminae of the pallidum. None of these nigral efferent fibers could be followed into the putamen or caudate nucleus.

In only one of these animals were degenerated fibers seen in the subthalamic nucleus, and these were sparse. Considerable degeneration was seen in the red nucleus and in the prerubral area. Degenerated fibers from the lesion area projected dorsally through lateral parts of the tegmentum into the superior colliculus. Fibers projecting to deep layers of the superior colliculus appeared to be corticotectal fibers from the crus cerebri interrupted in their dorsal projection by the nigral lesions. Degeneration in superficial layers of the superior colliculus appeared related to interruption of fibers of the brachium of the superior colliculus. In some animals a few degenerated fibers, descending ventrolateral to the red nucleus, could be followed into the pedunculopontine nucleus. The precise origin of these fibers remains in doubt, but it is possible that they might be either pallidotegmental or corticotegmental fibers (Cole, Nauta, and Mehler, 1964; Knook, 1965; Kuypers and Lawrence, 1967).

The above observations are basically the same as reported by other investigators who have used the Nauta technique in studies on the cat and rat (Cole, Nauta, and Mehler, 1964; Afifi and Kaelber, 1965; Faull and Carman, 1968). All of these investigations, including our own, indicated that the principal projections of the substantia nigra were to the thalamus and that these fibers terminated in a selective manner about cells of VLm and VAmc. Cole, Nauta, and Mehler (1964) and Afifi and Kaelber (1965) reported that in the cat degenerated fibers could be followed into the entopeduncular nucleus and the globus pallidus, but such fibers were extremely sparse and did not appear terminal. A few fibers were seen in the putamen (Cole, Nauta, and Mehler, 1964), but these were not impressive. Faull and Carman (1968) made a careful study of nigral efferent fibers in the rat employing multiple controls in the form of lesions which destroyed adjacent structures. In some animals nigral lesions were predominantly in either the pars reticularis or the pars compacta. The major projection from both parts of the nigra was described as a nigrothalamic system passing into the ventrolateral border of the ventral medial (VM) nucleus, a subdivision of the thalamus considered the homolog of the ventral lateral and ventral anterior thalamic nuclei in the primate. No evidence was found of a nigrostriatal or nigropallidal pathway.

There are other kinds of evidence, anatomical and biochemical, which suggest that data concerning nigral efferent fibers, obtained by the Nauta technique, may be incomplete. In the older literature there are many reports (von Monakow, 1895; Holmes, 1901; Dresel and Rothman, 1925; Ferraro, 1925;

Morrison, 1929; Mettler, 1943) which indicate that lesions destroying portions of the striatum produce retrograde cell changes and cell loss in the substantia nigra. These anatomical studies support the existence of a nigrostriatal pathway. Mettler (1970) recently confirmed the above observation, and presented new data suggesting that an even larger number of primary efferent fibers project to the globus pallidus. This conclusion was reached by comparing the cell loss in the nigra following striatal and pallidal lesions. Biochemical evidence suggests that nigrostriatal fibers are profuse and through their terminals transmit and maintain normal concentrations of catecholamines (Dahlström and Fuxe, 1964; Andén, Dahlström, Fuxe, and Larsson, 1964; Poirier and Sourkes, 1965; Hornykiewicz, 1966). In view of the obvious discrepancies presented by these data when compared with those obtained by the study of anterograde degeneration with the Nauta technique, it has been suggested that nigrostriatal fibers may be refractory to the Nauta method (Faull and Carman, 1968), or that the terminals may be too fine to be resolved by the light microscope. Electron microscopic observations (Fuxe, Hökfelt, and Nilsson, 1964; Mori, 1966) indicate that axon terminals in the striatum are exceedingly fine (i.e., 0.1 to 0.4 μ). In spite of this possibility, it seemed worthwhile to attempt a study of nigral efferent fibers based upon one of the recently developed silver impregnation methods. The method most suitable for the monkey in our experience is the Wiitanen (1969) technique. This method stains fine fibers and terminals and has been most successful following relatively short survival periods (i.e., 4-6 days). It is our impression that most of these fine fibers and terminals disappear and are no longer stainable after survival periods of 14 days.

1. Unilateral Nigral Lesions

Lesions well localized to the substantia nigra were produced in monkeys by electrodes inserted at an angle of 44° from the horizontal in a coronal plane [Fig. 14(A, B, and C)]. In our stereotaxic instrument, electrodes were introduced into the brain 11 mm anterior to the interaural line and traversed the retrolenticular part of the internal capsule, portions of the lateral and medial geniculate bodies, and the brachium of the superior colliculus. The electrode entered the lateral part of the substantia nigra and passed ventromedially in nearly the axis of the nucleus. This approach made it possible to produce lesions in the lateral, middle, and medial thirds of the substantia nigra, but with medial lesions an electrode track was present in lateral portions of the nucleus. Most of the lesions involved portions of both the pars compacta and pars reticularis. In those instances when the animal's head was unknowingly shifted toward the side on which the electrode would be inserted, lesions were dorsal to the substantia nigra; if the animal's head was shifted in the opposite direction, lesions were produced in the crus cerebri [Fig. 14(D)]. Lesions mainly in the medial

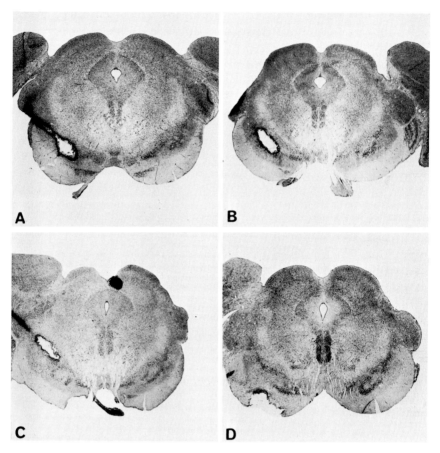

Fig. 14. Photomicrographs of lesions in the substantia nigra. A. Rhesus C-1152. B. Rhesus C-1173. C. Rhesus C-1146. D. Rhesus C-1180. The lesion in rhesus C-1180 mainly involved portions of the crus cerebri, but selectively destroyed a small part of the pars reticularis of the nigra which produced degeneration of nigrothalamic fibers. No degeneration projected to the striatum. Nissl, x3.4.

lemniscus dorsal to the substantia nigra selectively involved small parts of the pars compacta, and lesions mainly in the crus cerebri frequently involved portions of the pars reticularis. All lesions produced in the substantia nigra by this stereotaxic approach produced degeneration in the lateral and medial geniculate bodies, the brachium of the superior colliculus, the superior and inferior colliculi and in various parts of the medial lemniscus. It seems likely that these lesions also involved some spinothalamic and spinotectal fibers. In spite of this unavoidable parasurgical trauma, this stereotaxic approach resulted in cleaner, more specific lesions than any method we have used.

Observations were made in five animals with discrete lesions in the substantia nigra. Part of the pattern of nigral efferent projections was constant in all animals and will be presented synthetically. Degeneration which varied in location and appeared dependent upon the position of the lesion within the substantia nigra will be considered separately.

At the level of the lesion, degeneration was profuse in all parts of the substantia nigra surrounding and lateral to the lesion. Portions of the nigra medial to the lesion were free of degeneration, although degenerated fibers were seen along the superior surface of the uninvolved part.

2. Midbrain

At midbrain levels a large number of fibers projected dorsally from the lesion into the lateral tegmentum. These fibers, traversing the medial lemniscus and parts of the red nucleus, projected profusely to lower layers of the superior colliculus where many fibers appeared to terminate. A modest number of these fibers crossed in the commissure of the superior colliculus to enter deeper layers of the opposite superior colliculus. Transtegmental projections to the superior colliculus were joined by degenerated fibers of the brachium of the superior colliculus which were entirely ipsilateral and terminated mainly in the stratum opticum and stratum cinereum.

3. Basal Ganglia

Degeneration considered to arise from cells of the substantia nigra projected rostrally and dorsally into Forel's field H. Caudally it formed an impressive collection of fibers dorsal to the oral pole of the nigra and medial to the subthalamic nucleus. Where the subthalamic nucleus was fully developed, the principal concentration of fibers was seen dorsal to the medial part of this nucleus, but less dense degeneration extended medially toward the mammillo-thalamic tract. A large part of these fibers projected laterally along the superior and rostral borders of the subthalamic nucleus [Fig. 15(A)]. These fibers followed a course somewhat similar to that of the lenticular fasciculus, but in an opposite direction. Some of the fibers coursed through the dorsolateral parts of the subthalamic nucleus. When these laterally projecting fibers reached the internal capsule, they appeared to divide into two main bundles: Fibers of the more dorsal bundle entered the reticular nucleus of the thalamus and passed dorsally and rostrally [Fig. 15(B)]; the other bundle divided into a spray of fibers that crossed through the internal capsule over a fairly broad region [Fig. 15(C)]. These fibers entered the medial segment of the globus pallidus. In the medial pallidal segment the most profuse degeneration was seen at levels rostral to the subthalamic nucleus; here the fibers coursed laterally and

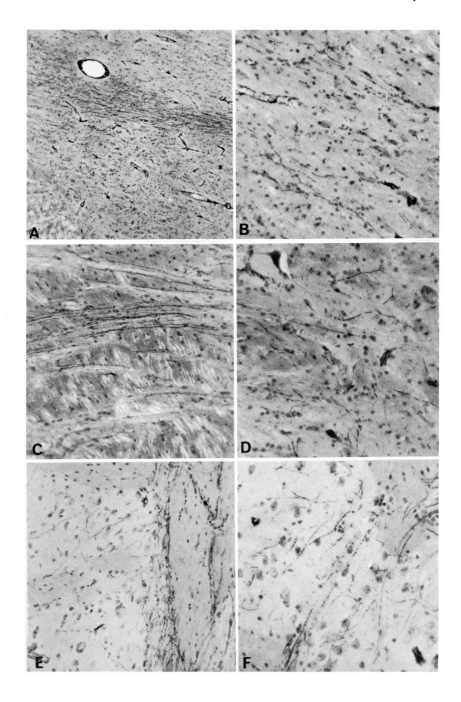

ventrolaterally within this segment. Most of these degenerated fibers passed into the medial medullary lamina and into the lateral pallidal segment. The lateral pallidal segment contained degenerated fibers part of which came from the medial pallidal segment and part of which crossed through more lateral and rostral parts of the internal capsule from the reticular nucleus of the thalamus. Nigral efferent fibers entered the globus pallidus by traversing the internal capsule over an extensive distance. Throughout all thalamic levels rostral to the lenticular fasciculus small bundles of fibers, contained within the reticular nucleus of the thalamus, crossed through the posterior limb of the internal capsule and entered the globus pallidus. These fibers seemed to become concentrated about the medial and lateral medullary laminae of the pallidum. In sections throughout the globus pallidus degenerated fibers appeared to be in passage [Fig. 15(D)]. Many of these fibers could be followed for some distance within the pallidum, but none were seen to establish close relationships to pallidal neurons or their processes.

Degenerated fibers, concentrated in great profusion on both sides of the lateral medullary lamina of the pallidum, projected into the putamen [Fig. 15(E and F)]. Degenerated fibers in the putamen were fine disintegrated axons that radiated laterally, dorsally, and ventrally [Fig. 16(A and B)]. These degenerated fibers were independent of the adventitial perivascular elements and did not bear any relationship to the bundles of myelinated striatal fibers that course ventromedially toward the pallidum, commonly referred to as Wilson's pencils (Nauta and Mehler, 1966). Degeneration in these myelinated fiber bundles was seen only in small localized regions of the putamen traumatized by the electrode. This degeneration represented putaminofugal fibers. A number of degenerated corticostriate fibers (Carman, Cowan, and Powell, 1963; Carman, Cowan, Powell, and Webster, 1965; Kemp and Powell, 1970) entered the lateral margin of the putamen from the external capsule. Some of these fibers were interrupted by passage of the electrode through cortex and white matter. There is evidence that corticostriate fibers in the cat terminate upon dendritic processes and cell somata (Kemp, 1968).

Nigrostriatal fibers project to both the putamen and the caudate nucleus in profusion, and the location of the degeneration within these structures seemed related to the part of the substantia nigra destroyed. Degeneration projecting to the caudate nucleus appeared to reach this structure via the bridges of striatal

Fig. 15. Rhesus C-1146, photomicrographs. A. Degenerated fibers projecting laterally from Forel's field H in the dorsal capsule of the subthalamic nucleus. Wiitanen, x52. B. Nigral efferent fibers in the thalamic reticular nucleus. Wiitanen, x133. C. Nigral efferent fibers traversing the internal capsule toward the globus pallidus. Wiitanen, x133. D. Nigral fibers in passage within the globus pallidus. Wiitanen, x210. E and F. Degenerated fibers concentrated along the lateral medullary lamina of the globus pallidus and projecting into the putamen. Wiitanen, x133, x210.

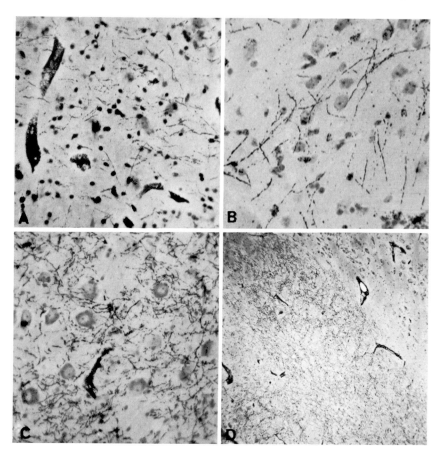

Fig. 16. A. Rhesus C-1187. Photomicrograph of degenerated fibers in the medial segment of the globus pallidus. Wiitanen, x325. B, C, and D. Rhesus C-1146. Photomicrographs. B. Degenerated fibers in the putamen. C. Terminal degeneration in the medial part of the ventral lateral nucleus (VLm) of the thalamus. D. Nigrothalamic degeneration in the magnocellular part of the ventral anterior nucleus (VAmc). Wiitanen, x325, x325, x52.

tissue that cross the anterior limb of the internal capsule and similar bridges that interconnect dorsal parts of the putamen with the body of the caudate nucleus. Our data further suggest that some nigral efferent fibers may reach both the body of the caudate nucleus and dorsal parts of the putamen via rostral projections that pass in the reticular nucleus of the thalamus. On the basis of the data available it seems that lateral parts of the nigra project predominantly to dorsal parts of the putamen and that central regions project to middle regions of the putamen. Medial portions of the nigra appeared related to ventral portions of the putamen. A lesion in the lateral third of the central part of the substantia nigra did not produce any degeneration in the rostral part of the head of the caudate nucleus, but at the fornix level degeneration in the head of the caudate nucleus was seen laterally close to the anterior limb of the internal capsule. In the body of the caudate nucleus, degeneration remained ventrolateral in location but virtually disappeared at levels where the dorsomedial nucleus of the thalamus appeared. The tail of the caudate nucleus was free of degeneration. Lesions involving predominantly the middle third or the lateral two-thirds of the substantia nigra produced some degeneration in the caudate nucleus, but not in parts rostral to the putamen. At levels where fibers of the anterior limb of the internal capsule separated the putamen from the head of the caudate nucleus, degeneration in the caudate nucleus occupied regions close to the internal capsule. Degeneration diminished greatly in the body of the caudate nucleus, where it was localized mainly to a small lateral zone. No degeneration was seen in the tail of the caudate nucleus.

4. Subthalamic Region

As mentioned above, a number of degenerated fibers projecting laterally from Forel's field H traversed rostral portions of the subthalamic nucleus before crossing the internal capsule and entering the globus pallidus. These fibers, probably *en passage*, formed radiating fascicles unrelated to cells of the nucleus. In caudal parts of the subthalamic nucleus a smaller number of degenerated fibers were seen in the nucleus; these fibers did not appear to terminate in the subthalamic nucleus, but they could not be followed in continuity through the internal capsule. The fact that degenerated fibers were seen emerging from the peduncular part of the internal capsule lateral to the subthalamic nucleus suggested that these fibers also were in passage. It was our impression that few, if any, nigral efferent fibers terminated in the subthalamic nucleus, but these results were not as definite as those obtained with the Nauta-Gygax method (Carpenter and McMasters, 1964; Carpenter and Strominger, 1967). No degeneration was seen in the zona incerta.

5. Thalamus

A considerable number of ascending nigral efferent fibers from Forel's field H projected to the thalamus (Fig. 17). These fibers projected dorsally and rostrally lateral to the mammillothalamic tract. In their trajectory these fibers followed a medial course into the medial part of the ventral lateral nucleus (VLm) where terminal arborizations intimately surrounded cells of this thalamic subdivision [Fig. 16(C)]. Fibers of this same bundle extended rostrally into the magnocellular part of the ventral anterior nucleus (VAmc) of the thalamus where terminations were seen [Fig. 16(D)]. No degeneration was seen in the principal

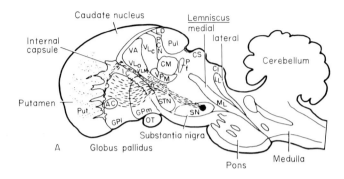

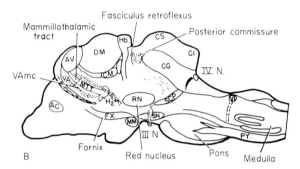

Fig. 17. Schematic drawings of the efferent projections of the substantia nigra in sagittal section. A. Drawing through basal ganglia, thalamus, and lower brainstem lateral to that shown in B. Fibers arising from the substantia nigra project rostrally and dorsally into Forel's field H. In A fibers of the principal lateral projection traverse the subthalamic nucleus, the thalamic reticular nucleus, and the internal capsule to enter the globus pallidus. These fibers project through the pallidum to enter parts of the putamen. Part of the medial nigral projection to the thalamus is shown in A; these fibers terminate in medial parts of VLm. In B, nigrothalamic fibers are shown projecting to the magnocellular part of the ventral anterior nucleus (VAmc). Some degenerated fibers in passage are shown in the thalamic reticular nucleus. (See list of abbreviations.)

part of the ventral anterior nucleus (VApc) or in either the oral or caudal parts of the ventral lateral nucleus (VLo or VLc).

Considerable additional thalamic degeneration was seen in sections stained by the Wiitanen technique. This degeneration was seen in parts of the paracentral nucleus (PCN), the dorsomedial nucleus (DM), and in the centromedian nucleus (CM). A number of fibers from the region of the VLm entered the internal medullary lamina of the thalamus and passed dorsolaterally and caudally. Although most of these fibers projected beyond the paracentral nucleus into lateral parts of the dorsomedial nucleus, several islands of degeneration closely surrounded cells in this nucleus, suggesting regional terminations. Fibers passing caudally in the internal medullary lamina projected into the paralaminar region of the dorsomedial nucleus throughout its extent with variations in intensity. Most of this ipsilateral degeneration was seen in the pars multiformis and densocellularis (Olszewski, 1952), but it was not confined to these cytological subdivisions. Fibers entered lateral and ventral parts of DM from ventromedial regions of the internal medullary lamina. A small number of fibers in both the paracentral and dorsomedial nuclei were seen to cross the midline near the rostral part of the centromedian nucleus. These fibers entered corresponding portions of PCN and DM on the opposite side.

Part of the profuse degeneration seen in the region of VLm projected dorsally and caudally in the internal medullary lamina to enter ventromedial parts of the centromedian nucleus. These fibers appeared to course caudally and laterally in the ventral lamella of the internal medullary lamina and at various levels projected into ventral parts of CM. Additional fibers coursing dorsomedially from Forel's field H traversed medial and caudal parts of the ventral posterior medial nucleus (VPM) and entered the centromedian–parafascicular (CM-PF) complex. Degeneration within the ipsilateral CM-PF complex was impressive, especially in ventral and caudal regions and extended the rostrocaudal extent of the complex. Although many fibers appeared in passage near the ventral lamella of the internal medullary lamina, a number of convincing terminal arborizations were seen in all parts of CM and in parts of PF lateral to the fasciculus retroflexus. Some degenerated fibers projected from lateral parts of CM into ventral portions of the central lateral nucleus (CL). At levels of the thalamic adhesion a few fibers crossed the midline and entered ventral parts of the opposite centromedian nucleus.

Additional thalamic degeneration was seen in the ventral posterior lateral nucleus (VPL) and was quantitatively related to encroachment of the lesion upon portions of the medial lemniscus. In some instances fibers of the spinothalamic tract also may have been involved. Degeneration in VPM appeared to be mainly fibers of passage, although some terminal degeneration may have been present in the lateral portions of the nucleus. Direct electrode trauma was responsible for degeneration in the medial and lateral geniculate bodies.

6. Control Lesions

Observations in two other animals with lesions considered at first inappropriate for study yielded important data. The lesion in one animal was situated in the medial lemniscus along the dorsal border of the substantia nigra. This lesion selectively involved a small part of the pars compacta of the nigra. Degeneration resulting from the lesion was profuse in VPL, moderate in the CM-PF complex and in VLm and VAmc. Moderately profuse degeneration was seen in the putamen, especially in the middle and dorsal thirds.

In another animal, the lesion involved the crus cerebri and a small adjacent part of the pars reticularis of the nigra [Fig. 14(D)]. Thalamic degeneration resulting from this lesion was less profuse in VLm and VAmc than in animals with more extensive nigral lesions, but degeneration in DM and the CM-PF complex was similar. The most important finding was the absence of degeneration in the caudate nucleus and putamen.

III. Discussion

The efferent projections of the globus pallidus and the substantia nigra are distinctive even though fibers from these nuclei are intermingled at some sites.

A. GLOBUS PALLIDUS

The efferent projections of the globus pallidus, representing the principal output of the basal ganglia, are profuse, widespread, entirely ipsilateral, and consist of both ascending and descending components. The projections of the medial and lateral segments of the globus pallidus are so different that it seems unlikely that these segments can be concerned with the same functions. The lateral pallidal segment projects exclusively and topographically upon the subthalamic nucleus. The medial pallidal segment projects a small number of fibers to the ventromedial and caudal pole of the subthalamic nucleus; these fibers are distributed to a region that seems unrelated to the lateral pallidal segment. These data suggest that the subthalamic nucleus resembles a miniature globus pallidus in which there is a correspondence between: (1) the lateral pallidal segment and the rostrolateral part of the subthalamic nucleus, and (2) the medial pallidal segment and the caudomedial part of the subthalamic nucleus (Fig. 9).

The interrelationships between the subthalamic nucleus and the globus pallidus appear highly significant. While the principal input to the subthalamic nucleus is derived from the lateral pallidal segment, the output of the subthalamic nucleus is fed back primarily to the medial pallidal segment. Previous studies have shown that lesions destroying significant parts of the medial pallidal segment can abolish, or greatly reduce, subthalamic dyskinesia in the monkey resulting from localized lesions of the subthalamic nucleus (Carpenter, Whittier, and Mettler, 1950). Lesions involving the lateral pallidal segment do not ameliorate this form of dyskinesia. Current interpretation of evidence suggests that subthalamic dyskinesia due to lesions in the subthalamic nucleus is a consequence of removal of inhibitory influences which normally act upon the medial pallidal segment. It seems likely that impulses arising from the "released" medial pallidal segment are relayed to the motor cortex via thalamic relays in the ventral lateral nucleus (VLo). This thesis is supported by data indicating that lesions in the medial pallidal segment or in VLo can ameliorate this form of dyskinesia without producing paresis (Carpenter, Whittier, and Mettler, 1950; Talairach, Paillas, and David, 1950; Roeder and Orthner, 1956; Cooper, 1957; Martin and McCaul, 1959; Andy and Brown, 1960).

There is some evidence that certain lesions causing severe degeneration of neurons in the lateral pallidal segment may produce a choreoid dyskinesia virtually identical with that resulting from discrete lesions in the subthalamic nucleus (Carpenter and Strominger, 1967). These findings have been interpreted to mean that extensive interruption of subcortical afferent systems to the subthalamic nucleus can produce the same disturbances as localized lesions in the subthalamic nucleus. The hypothesis that severe choreoid dyskinesia may occur from disruption of either afferent or efferent subthalamic fibers is not new (Moersch and Kernohan, 1939; Papez et al., 1942; Whittier and Mettler, 1949), but the functional integrity of the medial pallidal segment and its efferent systems must be preserved. Anatomical, physiological, and clinical data concerning the subthalamic nucleus and its connections represent one of those rare occasions where there seems to be mutual concurrence of fact and theory.

The principal outflow of the globus pallidus arises from the medial pallidal segment, emerging via the ansa lenticularis and the lenticular fasciculus. There is a suggestion that these efferent bundles have a topographic origin within the medial pallidal segment, but so far it has not been possible to determine if these separate efferent fiber bundles have distinctive terminations in cytological subdivisions of the thalamus. It might be possible to obtain these data by careful systematic studies, provided enough material of an appropriate nature could be produced. At this juncture it can only be said that the medial pallidal segment projects profusely upon the lateral part of VLm, large regions of VLo, large parts of VApc, and that a recurrent division of pallidofugal fibers separates from the thalamic fasciculus and projects to the centromedian nucleus (CM).

Pallidofugal fibers ending in VLo appear to be overlapped by cerebellar projections largely from the dentate nucleus (Clark, 1936; Walker, 1938; Olszewski, 1952; Jansen and Brodal, 1954, 1958; Carpenter, 1967). The nature of the presumed interaction of pallidofugal and cerebellofugal fibers upon cells of VLo is unknown, but its importance is obvious. In the monkey VLo projects in a topical fashion to area 4 (Walker, 1938, 1949); area 6 is said to receive a relatively small number of fibers from VL (Mettler, 1947; Walker, 1949). Since thalamocortical fibers from VL constitute a major projection system that influences pyramidal tract neurons, it might be expected that alterations in activity of VL neurons would be reflected in marked changes in discharges in the pyramidal tract (Purpura, Frigyesi, McMurtry, and Scarff, 1966). Thus pallidofugal fibers projecting to VLo convey impulses which are one of the major subcortical determinants that underlie motor activity.

The nature of the impulses which pallidofugal fibers convey to VApc is conjectural. Physiological data link VA to systems that produce synchronous cortical activity (see review in Carmel, 1970). The elicitation of recruiting responses from VA tends to activate the nonspecific thalamic nuclei and to exert effects upon widespread regions of the frontal cortex.

Pallidofugal fiber systems projecting to the centromedian nucleus (CM) appear to constitute part of a feedback system by which some of the output from the medial pallidal segment can be returned to the putamen (Mettler, 1947; Nauta and Whitlock, 1954; Powell and Cowan, 1956; Powell, 1958). It would appear that this feedback circuitry might influence the levels of activity in both the striatum and the pallidum and in some manner control pallidal impulses that impinge upon thalamic relay nuclei.

Pallidotegmental fibers were first demonstrated experimentally by Nauta and Mehler (1966), although their careful search of the literature identified this bundle in earlier studies where it was designated as the "subthalamicotegmental" tract (Papez, 1942). In normal monkey brains Woodburne, Crosby, and McCotter (1946) traced fibers, considered to be a component of the ansa lenticularis, caudally to the nucleus mesencephalicus profundus. In spite of many reports of descending pallidal fibers in the brainstem, the only projection which can be substantiated is that passing to the pedunculopontine nucleus, a cell group which is partially embedded in the superior cerebellar peduncle at levels of the inferior colliculus. The efferent connections and function of this nucleus are not known and appear difficult to resolve because cells of the nucleus bear intimate relationships to numerous fiber systems that traverse this tegmental area. From the work of Kuypers and Lawrence (1967) it is known that fibers from the precentral gyrus also project to the pedunculopontine nucleus.

B. Substantia Nigra

Observations of nigral efferent projections obtained with the Wiitanen technique have confirmed findings established with the Nauta method, provided new data relative to nigrostriatal fibers, and raised certain questions with respect to the centromedian-parafascicular (CM-PF) complex and the subthalamic nucleus.

It is doubtful if very many of the degenerated fibers reaching the superior colliculus arise from the substantia nigra. Those that reach the superior colliculus via a transtegmental approach are probably corticotectal fibers given off from the crus cerebri and interrupted as they traverse the nigra (Kuypers and Lawrence, 1967). Fibers reaching the superior colliculus via its brachium are known to arise from the optic tract, the striate cortex, and the lateral geniculate body (Altman, 1962; Garey, Jones, and Powell, 1968).

The extent to which nigral efferents project to the midbrain tegmentum could not be determined in the presence of extensive degeneration of corticotectal and corticotegmental fibers. Although degeneration was seen in the red nucleus, especially in rostral parts, it was impossible to determine if these fibers originated from the substantia nigra. It seems likely that most of the degeneration seen in the red nucleus represented corticorubral fibers from the precentral gyrus which descend in the crus cerebri and traverse portions of the nigra *en route* to the red nucleus (Kuypers and Lawrence, 1967).

The most interesting new observation concerns the demonstration of a profuse nigrostriatal projection that appears to be topographically organized. Part of the pathway by which these fibers project to the putamen has been previously described, but data were inconsistent and not convincing (Carpenter and McMasters, 1964; Cole, Nauta, and Mehler, 1964; Afifi and Kaelber, 1965; Carpenter and Strominger, 1967; Faull and Carman, 1968). Current findings indicate that nigrostriatal fibers from Forel's field H cross through the internal capsule in large numbers lateral and rostral to the subthalamic nucleus and follow a course similar to that of the lenticular fasciculus, but in a reverse direction. A large number of fibers from Forel's field H pass dorsally and rostrally in the thalamic reticular nucleus and traverse more rostral regions of the posterior limb of the internal capsule. Fibers that cross the internal capsule rostral and lateral to the subthalamic nucleus enter the medial pallidal segment, except for its most medial part. Fibers that course in the thalamic reticular nucleus mainly enter more rostral parts of the lateral pallidal segment and the medullary laminae of the pallidum. While our data indicate that virtually all of these fibers are in passage within the globus pallidus and the medullary laminae of the pallidum, this observation must be regarded as an interpretation until confirmed by valid electron microscopic techniques. In the light microscope degenerated fibers in the pallidum appeared relatively coarse and did not arborize about pallidal neurons or their processes. The lateral medullary lamina of the pallidum appears to serve as a channel for the distribution of fibers to various parts of the putamen. In this lamina fibers passed dorsally, ventrally, rostrally, and caudally.

Degeneration seen in the putamen contrasts sharply with that seen in the pallidum. These degenerated fibers are very fine, long, and radiate in many directions from the medial margin of the putamen. These fibers, distributed fairly evenly over large areas, rarely formed discrete islands of degeneration. None of these degenerated fibers could be detected at low magnifications. It was not possible to determine the manner in which these fibers terminated in relation to cells; these data must await electron microscopic determinations.

The location of our lesions in central and caudal parts of the substantia nigra appears to account for the predominant degeneration in the putamen. Available data suggest that lateral parts of the nigra at these levels project primarily to dorsal parts of the putamen. The middle third of the nigra appears related to the middle regions of the putamen and there is a suggested correspondence between the medial part of the nigra and ventral parts of the putamen. All animals with lesions in the nigra had some degeneration in the head and body of the caudate nucleus, but it tended to occupy lateral and ventrolateral regions close to the internal capsule. None of these lesions produced degeneration in the most rostral part of the head of the caudate nucleus or in the tail of this nucleus. These findings suggest that nigrostriatal fibers probably are topographically organized in a fashion reciprocal to that of putamino-nigral fibers (Szabo, 1967). The fact that none of these lesions destroyed rostromedial parts of the substantia nigra (Voneida, 1960; Szabo, 1962) probably accounts for the absence of nigrostriatal degeneration in the most rostral part of the head of the caudate nucleus.

Data from control animals indicate that large cells of the pars compacta are the principal, if not the exclusive, source of nigrostriatal fibers. This observation is consistent with biochemical evidence (Dahlström and Fuxe, 1964; Poirier and Sourkes, 1965; Fuxe and Andén, 1966; Hornykiewicz, 1966; Andén, Dahlström, Fuxe, and Larsson, 1966). Physiological studies by Frigyesi and Purpura (1967) differ in that they conclude that the small caliber direct nigrocaudate fibers probably arise from the pars reticularis.

The question as to whether nigral efferent fibers project to the subthalamic nucleus or not is difficult to answer in studies based on the Wiitanen technique. Most of the earlier studies indicated that no nigral efferent fibers end in the subthalamic nucleus (Carpenter and McMasters, 1964; Cole, Nauta, and Mehler, 1964; Carpenter and Strominger, 1967), but Afifi and Kaelber (1965) reported that nigral fibers ended throughout the ipsilateral subthalamic nucleus. Faull and Carman (1968) merely mentioned that some nigral fibers traverse this nucleus in their passage to the thalamus. Current observations revealed large numbers of nigral efferent fibers that traversed dorsolateral parts of the rostral subthalamic nucleus and could be followed in continuity through the internal capsule to the medial pallidal segment. Middle and caudal regions of the subthalamic nucleus contained degenerated fibers mainly in the dorsal capsule of the nucleus, but occasional fibers were seen in those parts of the nucleus which could not be traced in continuity to the pallidum. These fibers did not appear terminal, but they raise a suspicion not previously entertained. The possibility that these fibers in the subthalamic nucleus might be of pallidal origin has been excluded.

The nigrothalamic projection to the medial part of the ventral lateral nucleus (VLm) and to the magnocellular part of the ventral anterior nucleus (VAmc) confirms observations in all previous studies based on anterograde degeneration using silver methods (see p. 154). Current data suggest that nigrothalamic fibers arise from the pars reticularis [Fig. 14(D)], since lesions in this part of the nigra do not give rise to fibers that cross through the internal capsule, traverse the globus pallidus, or end in the neostriatum. Nevertheless the possibility that some of these nigrothalamic fibers might arise from, or be collaterals of, large cells in the pars compacta cannot be excluded because fibers from the pars reticularis course through the pars compacta.

One of the most interesting observations in this study was the consistent presence of profuse terminal degeneration in the centromedian-parafascicular nuclear complex. The question is raised as to whether fibers projecting to this nuclear complex arise from the substantia nigra. Although there is a long-standing controversy concerning afferent projections to the CM-PF complex, a succinct and careful review of this subject has been made by Mehler (1966). According to Mehler (1966), the only significant terminal projections to CM arise from the motor cortex and the globus pallidus. As previously discussed, the medial pallidal segment projects fibers to CM (Nauta and Mehler, 1966; Carpenter and Strominger, 1967; Carpenter, Fraser, and Shriver, 1968). In animals with lesions in the substantia nigra no pallidofugal fibers were interrupted by either the lesion or the electrode track. Histological proof that pallidofugal fibers were not involved is provided by the absence of degeneration in the ansa lenticularis, the lenticular fasciculus, and the subthalamic projection, as well as by the absence of degeneration in VLo and VApc of the thalamus.

Projections from the motor cortex to CM have been reported by Auer (1956), Niimi, Katayama, Kanaseki, and Morimota (1960), and Petras (1964, 1966, 1969). According to Petras, area 4 projects terminal fibers which are distributed throughout CM (Petras, 1964), and area 6 projects fibers to PF (Petras, 1965). The possibility that corticofugal fibers from the motor cortex may have been concomitantly interrupted by either the electrode track or the lesion must be examined carefully. At first consideration this seemed unlikely since areas 4 and 6 project profusely to the ventral lateral nucleus of the thalamus, the thalamic reticular nucleus, and to parts of the caudate nucleus and putamen as well as to the CM-PF complex (Auer, 1956; Niimi, Katayama, Kanaseki, and Morimota, 1960; Petras, 1965). The critical consideration is how lesions in the substantia nigra could interrupt selectively only those fibers issuing from the motor cortex that project to CM-PF and leave other projections intact. The explanation appears to have been provided by a meticulous and brilliant analysis of corticothalamic projections in the cat done by Rinvik (1968). According to this author, corticothalamic fibers which arise in the pericruciate and coronal gyri follow different routes before terminating in the thalamus. The majority of corticofugal fibers to VL and the ventrobasal (VB) complex of the thalamus leave the posterior limb of the internal capsule, enter the reticular nucleus of the thalamus and its external medullary lamina, and course caudally and medially to be distributed to restricted areas of VL and the VB complex. These corticothalamic fibers were not interrupted by our lesions in the substantia nigra. The corticothalamic pathway described by Rinvik (1968) pertinent to the current study is circuitous and has been referred to as the "cerebral peduncle loop." Fibers following this pathway descend in the internal capsule and leave the "cerebral peduncle" at the mesencephalic-diencephalic junction and project rostrodorsally toward basal and inferior thalamic regions. Corticothalamic fibers projecting to the CM-PF complex, parts of PCN, and the paralaminar part of DM are described as following this route, along with fibers projecting to VPM, the small-celled part of VPM (VPMpc), and the ventral posterior inferior nucleus (VPI) of the thalamus. Kuypers and Lawrence (1967) have described similar fibers projecting to CM in the monkey.

In the light of these critical observations by Rinvik (1968), it is apparent that our lesions in the substantia nigra at levels of the superior colliculus have interrupted corticothalamic fibers, probably mainly from areas 4 and 6, that course in the so-called "cerebral peduncle loop." The presence of degeneration in the CM-PF complex, lateral to the fasciculus retroflexus, in parts of PCN and in the paralaminar part of DM leaves little doubt that fibers ending in these nuclei probably arise in the motor cortex. The fact that a lesion mainly in the crus cerebri [Fig. 14(D)] produced degeneration in CM-PF and in paralaminar parts of DM tends to support this thesis even though such degeneration was not as profuse as that associated with lesions confined to the substantia nigra. The only deviation of our data from that of Rinvik (1968) is that a small number of fibers in DM and CM-PF were observed to cross the midline and enter corresponding sites in these same nuclei on the opposite side. Rinvik observed contralateral degeneration only in PCN, as reported in this study.

The above discussion raises the question as to whether the degeneration in the medial part of VLm and in VAmc seen in the monkey after nigral lesions might also represent part of a corticothalamic projection. This seems unlikely since corticothalamic fibers to VLm (VM in the cat), and VA do not reach these nuclei via the so-called "cerebral peduncle loop" (Rinvik, 1968). Very few corticofugal fibers from the precruciate and rostral coronal gyri end in VA in the cat, and these fibers end in parts of VA near the reticular nucleus of the thalamus. However, coarse fibers do traverse VA *en route* to more caudal thalamic structures (Rinvik, 1968, 1968a). In the cat VM (the equivalent of VLm in the monkey) receives no fibers from the postcruciate gyrus, only a few from the precruciate gyrus, and some fibers from the gyrus proreus which reach the lateral part of VM by traversing VL. None of these cortical lesions produced terminal degeneration in the most medial parts of VA (i.e., VAmc) or in rostral or medial parts of VM (i.e., VLm in the monkey). These observations support the conclusion that nigral efferent fibers in substantial numbers terminate in VLm and VAmc.

Electrodes used to produce these nigral lesions entered caudal parts of the temporal lobe in the region of the superior temporal sulcus (von Bonin and Bailey, 1947). According to Whitlock and Nauta (1956) and DeVito (1969), no corticofugal fibers from these parts of the superior or middle temporal gyri project to the intralaminar thalamic nuclei. While it is conceivable that the electrode in the white matter could have interrupted fibers passing from the somatic sensory or auditory cortex, there is no evidence that these cortical areas distribute any fibers to the CM-PF complex in the thalamus (Kuypers and Lawrence, 1967; Jones and Powell, 1968; Diamond, Jones, and Powell, 1969).

Although some fibers of the medial lemniscus were involved in all of these nigral lesions, there is no experimental evidence that ascending fibers of this system project to the CM-PF complex (Clark, 1936; Walker, 1938; Rasmussen and Peyton, 1948; Matzke, 1951; Bowsher, 1958, 1961). The now classic study of Mehler, Feferman, and Nauta (1960) indicated that following anterolateral cordotomy in the monkey no terminal degeneration was distributed to the CM-PF complex, although degeneration was seen bilaterally in the central lateral (CL) nucleus and in paralaminar portions of the dorsomedial nucleus (DM).

One other ascending system which could have been interrupted and escaped recognition was the ventral trigeminothalamic tract, known to ascend in association with the medial lemniscus. Studies on the cat and monkey indicated that no ventral trigeminothalamic fibers projected to the CM-PF complex (Carpenter and Hanna, 1961; Mizuno, 1970). Stewart and King (1963) reported that some fibers from the pars caudalis of the spinal trigeminal nucleus passed *through* the CM-PF complex to terminate in more rostral intralaminar nuclei. Mehler (1966) reported similar observations.

There was no evidence in this study of nigral efferent fibers that the superior cerebellar peduncle was involved by our lesions or that cerebellofugal fibers were degenerated at any level. While some authors have suggested that cerebellofugal fibers may project to CM, critically evaluated evidence indicates that such fibers merely course *through* CM to be distributed to nuclei in, or adjacent to, the internal medullary lamina of the thalamus (Clark, 1936; Walker, 1938; Mehler, Vernier, and Nauta, 1958; Mehler, 1966).

The above discussion makes it seem unlikely that nigral efferent fibers project to the CM-PF complex. Current data support Mehler's (1966) thesis that the only significant afferent connections to CM originate from forebrain structures.

C. Comparisons of the Globus Pallidus and Substantia Nigra

There appear to be many similarities between the globus pallidus and the substantia nigra even though the pallidum is considered a forebrain derivative and the substantia nigra is said to arise from the midventral proliferation of the basal lamina of the midbrain (Cooper, 1946). It is first of interest that neither of these nuclei seems to receive an afferent input directly from the cerebral cortex. Although evidence indicating that the pallidum does not receive corticofugal fibers cannot be regarded as unquestioned, it is interesting that in the long series of papers establishing the topographical organization of corticostriate projections hardly any mention is made of corticopallidal fibers (Carman, Cowan, and Powell, 1963; Webster, 1965; Carman, Cowan, Powell, and Webster, 1965; Cowan and Powell, 1966; Kemp and Powell, 1970). Since the pallidum forms the medial border of the putamen for long distances, it seems unlikely that these investigators did not examine at least portions of the globus pallidus. Two authors (Webster, 1961; Petras, 1965, 1969) reported no evidence of a corticopallidal projection in studies of corticofugal fibers, but both admit that the problem requires further investigation.

For at least seven decades the cerebral cortex has been considered a major source of nigral afferent fibers, mainly on the basis of Marchi degeneration studies in man and animals (see reviews, Carpenter, 1961; Rinvik, 1966). A systematic investigation of corticonigral fibers in the cat based upon silver impregnation techniques indicated that only a few corticofugal fibers terminate in the substantia nigra (Rinvik, 1966). No corticonigral fibers were evident in silver-stained preparations in human cases with frontal lobotomy (Meyer, 1949; Smythies, Gibson, Purkis, and Lowes, 1957). Critical electron microscopic observations in the cat failed to disclose degenerated boutons in the substantia nigra following a variety of large cortical lesions (Rinvik and Walberg, 1969). The presence of enormous numbers of normal boutons in the nigra of these operated animals suggested that the cerebral cortex does not give rise to a functionally important nigral projection. These data seriously question the existence of corticonigral fibers in all mammals.

The second similarity between the globus pallidus and the substantia nigra is that both of these nuclear masses receive topographically organized projections from the neostriatum (Voneida, 1960; Nauta and Mehler, 1966; Cowan and Powell, 1966; Szabo, 1962, 1967, 1970). Striopallidal fibers project radially like the spokes of a wheel and terminate in both pallidal segments. Efferent projections from the head of the caudate nucleus (Szabo, 1962) are organized so that: (1) lateral parts project predominantly to the lateral pallidal segment, (2) middle parts send fibers to both pallidal segments equally, and (3) medial parts project mainly to the medial pallidal segment. Fibers from the head and body of the caudate nucleus terminate in the dorsomedial one-third of both pallidal segments, while fibers from the putamen end in remaining ventrolateral parts (Szabo, 1967, 1970). There are some regional differences in the putamen in that the precommissural putamen projects exclusively upon the globus pallidus, while other regions send fibers to both the pallidum and posterior parts of the substantia nigra. The mode of termination of striopallidal fibers appears to be predominantly axodendritic (Szabo, 1970). Thus, striopallidal fibers are topographically organized in both dorsoventral and anteroposterior sequences.

Strionigral fibers are topographically organized so that fibers from the head of the caudate nucleus project to the rostral part of the nigra and have a mediolateral correspondence with portions of the caudate nucleus (Szabo, 1962). The body of the caudate nucleus sends fibers to the most ventrolateral region of the nigra (Szabo, 1970). The putamen projects fibers to portions of the substantia nigra posterior to frontal levels through the oculomotor roots. Putaminonigral fibers are organized so that: (1) dorsal parts of the putamen project to dorsal and lateral parts of the nigra, (2) ventral parts of the putamen project to ventral and medial nigral areas, and (3) central, or intermediate, portions of the putamen send fibers to central portions of the substantia nigra (Szabo, 1967). Most of the strionigral fibers end in the pars reticularis, but some are seen in the pars compacta. No definitive statement can be made concerning the mode of termination of strionigral fibers. The majority of fibers seem to end in the neuropil, but axodendritic terminations are suggested (Szabo, 1970). Thus, strionigral fibers have a topographic organization comparable to that of striopallidal fibers.

The globus pallidus receives afferent fibers from the subthalamic nucleus which project mainly to the medial segment (Carpenter and Strominger, 1967). There is no reliable information concerning projections from the subthalamic nucleus to the substantia nigra.

Although the efferent fibers of the globus pallidus and substantia nigra are intermingled in Forel's field H, the projections of these nuclear masses are distinctive. The projections from the globus pallidus are more widespread, entirely ipsilateral, and consist of a major ascending component and a minor descending component. The lateral pallidal segment projects exclusively to the subthalamic nucleus. The medial pallidal segment projects predominantly to ipsilateral thalamic nuclei [i.e., the lateral part of the pars medialis of the ventral lateral nucleus (VLm), the oral part of the ventral lateral nucleus (VLo), the principal part of the ventral anterior nucleus (VApc), and the centromedian nucleus (CM)]. In addition, the medial pallidal segment gives rise to a relatively small pallidotegmental bundle which terminates in the pedunculopontine nucleus at caudal midbrain levels.

The substantia nigra, the largest single nuclear mass in the midbrain, gives rise to a profuse nigrostriatal projection which appears to be reciprocally related to the strionigral system. This system probably arises mainly from the pars compacta. The pars reticularis seems to give rise to nigrothalamic projections which end in the medial part of the pars medialis of the ventral lateral nucleus (VLm) and in the magnocellular part of the ventral anterior nucleus (VAmc). It seems likely that the reciprocal connections between the striatum and the substantia nigra must be concerned with mechanisms that control the transport of a primary catecholamine, dopamine. Strionigral fibers ending in the pars reticularis may constitute the afferent limb of this system (or feedback circuit), while nigrostriatal fibers arising from cells of the pars compacta actually convey dopamine to terminals in the striatum.

While direct nigrothalamic fibers may convey impulses involved in the subcortical integration of motor activity, it seems likely that the quantitatively larger nigrostriatal-dopamine system exerts much more potent effects upon motor function. The major outflow from the substantia nigra is to the striatum. The principal output of the striatum is conveyed to the globus pallidus. Pallidofugal fiber systems, especially those arising in the medial pallidal segment, appear to constitute the final link in the complex pathways by which impulses from the basal ganglia are delivered to thalamic relay nuclei that can modify the activity of cortical neurons concerned with motor function.

The hypothesis is presented that the major output of the substantia nigra is conveyed to the neostriatum. The major output of the basal ganglia is via pallidofugal fiber systems that convey impulses to thalamic relay nuclei which have access to cortical motor neurons.

LIST OF ABBREVIATIONS

AC	anterior commissure	Pul	pulvinar
AV	anterior ventral nucleus	Py	pyramid
CG	central gray	RN	red nucleus
CI	inferior colliculus	SCP	superior cerebellar peduncle
CL	subthalamic nucleus	SI	substantia innominata
CM	centromedian nucleus	SN	substantia nigra
CS	superior colliculus	STN	subthalamic nucleus
DM	dorsomedial nucleus	VA	ventral anterior nucleus,
Fx	fornix		principal part
GPl	globus pallidus, lateral segment	VAmc	ventral anterior nucleus,
GPm	globus pallidus, medial segment		magnocellular part
H	Forel's field H	VLc	ventral lateral nucleus, caudal
H_2	lenticular fasciculus		part
Hb	habenular nuclei	VLm	ventral lateral nucleus, medial
IC	internal capsule		part
LD	lateral dorsal nucleus	VLo	ventral lateral nucleus, oral
LG	lateral geniculate body		part
LL	lateral lemniscus	VPM	ventral posterior medial nucleus
ML	medial lemniscus	ZI	zona incerta
MM	mammillary body	III,	third ventricle
MTT	mammillothalamic tract	III N	oculomotor nerve
OT	optic tract	IV N	trochlear nerve
Pf	parafascicular nucleus	VI	abducens nucleus
PPN	pedunculopontine nucleus		

Acknowledgment

This work was supported by research grant NS-04082-08 from the National Institute of Neurological Diseases and Stroke of the National Institutes of Health.

Chapter 6

The Role of Prefrontal Control in the Programming of Motor Behavior

JERZY KONORSKI

DEPARTMENT OF NEUROPHYSIOLOGY
NENCKI INSTITUTE OF EXPERIMENTAL BIOLOGY, WARSAW, POLAND

I. General Considerations

Almost all studies on conditioning and learning begin with establishing the programs of training to which the animals are subjected. Thus, in classical conditioning we pair in various ways two variables, conditioned stimuli (CSs) and unconditioned stimuli (USs). According to the program of the experiment, we may establish various excitatory conditioned reflexes (CRs), or transform them into inhibitory CRs, or introduce differentiations, and so on. In instrumental conditioning the scope of possible programs is much larger, because here we deal with three variables, namely the CSs, the USs, and the instrumental responses. Whereas in humans such programs can be (at least in instrumental conditioning) carried over to the subject by oral instruction, in animals they must be trained by repeating the appropriate combinations of stimuli and provoking, by various techniques, the required instrumental responses. When a subject succeeds in mastering the task, this means that we have "inscribed" that program in his brain, so that he is able to accomplish it correctly. Of course we do not assume that the design of the program in our own brains and in those of the experimental animals is identical. It is certain, however, that the animal's program of fulfilling a given task corresponds to that which we have established for him, since the responses of the animal are predictable. It happens, however, that the subject may establish a quite different program from that which we tried to teach him; in that case the subject's responses will become unpredictable for us, until we find out the program which he has developed.

Studies concerned with the actual designs of programs inscribed in the animal's brain can be carried out in various ways. First, we can reach conclusions about these designs by varying the stimuli impinging upon the animal (and/or his internal environment) and observing changes which occur in his responses to these modified stimuli. Second, we can influence directly the animal's brain by ablation or stimulation techniques and observe the effects of these operations on the fulfillment of the program.

In this paper we shall narrow the scope of our discussion by dealing exclusively with instrumental conditioning based on alimentary (food) reinforcements. This means that we shall leave out classical conditioning, as well as conditioning based on noxious reinforcements.

We can roughly classify programs used in instrumental alimentary conditioning into the following groups:

1. The most elementary programming occurs when the animal is required to perform a given movement (R) to obtain continuous or intermittent reinforcement. No specific CSs are present.

2. A more complex program results when an instrumental response is linked to one or more controlling discriminative stimuli. The response is thereafter emitted only in the presence of these CSs.

3. R–no R Pavlovian differentiation: R–no R programming is defined by a situation in which the animal is differentially trained to perform an instrumental movement (R) to a CS_1, while in the presence of a CS_2 (a discriminative stimulus somewhat similar to CS_1) the instrumental act is not reinforced. This is analogous to an S^D–S^Δ situation. The stimulus controlling instrumental responding is called the positive CS (CS^+) and that presented without reinforcement is the negative CS (CS^-).

4. R–no R, both reinforced differentiation: In this program the CS_1 is followed by food if the animal does perform the movement R, whereas in the presence of a CS_2 (similar to CS_1) reinforcement occurs only if the animal does not perform this movement.

5. R_1–R_2 differentiation: In this program the animal is trained to perform movement R_1 in response to CS_1 and movement R_2 in response to CS_2.

6. R_1–R_2 delayed response program: This may be regarded as a variation of the R_1–R_2 program, in that the animal is allowed to react not to the actual CSs but to their traces.

It is easy to notice that programs 3 through 6 are parallel programs, since they are concerned with the formation of various responses to be performed to various stimuli, respectively. We have, however, left out sequential programs in which the subject is trained to perform a sequence of movements in a definite order. Since experiments on sequential programs have been not very numerous, they are not yet suitable to our analysis.

Many experimental studies (to be quoted further in the text) have shown that parallel programs are largely under the control of the prefrontal region of the cerebral cortex. Moreover, recent experiments (to be quoted below) have established that the prefrontal cortex is not functionally "equipotential," since particular parts of this region are related to particular programs. The aim of this article is to present experimental evidence demonstrating the functional heterogeneity of the prefrontal cortex and to draw conclusions about the functional organization of this region.

Generally, the behavioral experiments dealing with the above programs were systematically carried out on dogs and monkeys. Since only these materials are comparable, we shall limit our discussion mainly to these two species.

Since we shall base our discussion largely on the data obtained on dogs in our own laboratory, we present, for the reader's convenience, two experimental situations in which the corresponding experiments have been conducted. One situation is a Pavlovian soundproof chamber with the dog placed on a stand and the experimenter controlling the course of the experimental session from the prechamber (Fig. 1). The animal is usually trained to lift his left or right foreleg and place it on the feeder, or press a pedal situated nearby. The second situation is a compartment with three feeders and a starting platform situated in front of the experimenter's table (Fig. 2).

II. Simple S–R Conditioning

We cannot enter here into a full discussion of the central mechanism of instrumental conditioning either to the environment as a whole (Σ S), or to sporadic CSs. This problem was discussed in great detail in the author's recent book (Konorski, 1970, Chapters 8–10). Briefly, we have good reason to believe that the instrumental CR is based on two lines of connections (Fig. 3). One line goes "directly" from the central representation of the CS (further denoted as the "CS center") to the central representation of kinesthesis produced by instrumental movement (further denoted as the "movement center"). The other line goes from the CS center to the movement center through the central representation of drive—in our discussion, of hunger (further denoted as the

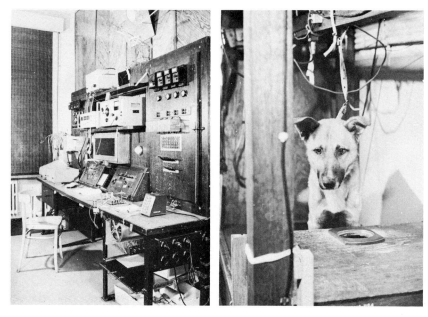

Fig. 1. The CR chamber. Left side: pre-chamber. Right side: the soundproof chamber with a dog on the stand.

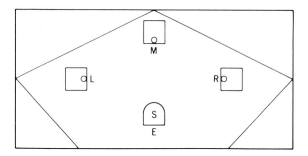

Fig. 2. Experimental room for locomotor CRs. S, starting platform; L, M, R, feeders; E, experimenter's seat. Reprinted by permission of McGraw-Hill, New York.

"hunger center"). Both of these lines must be jointly activated to produce the instrumental response. Thus, when the hunger center is inhibited by full satiation, or when in the presence of hunger the CS is not given, the instrumental response will not be produced. The indispensable condition for the formation and performance of an instrumental alimentary CR is that the motor response be reinforced by presentation of food, provoking the consummatory reaction and partially inhibiting the hunger drive.

It should be noted that in the first stage of CR training the animal performs the instrumental movement not only to the CS but also during the intertrial intervals. This means that the CR is first formed to the environmental compound stimulus (ΣS). Only in the next stage of training are the intertrial movements extinguished because of lack of reinforcement, while the CS acting within that environment instigates the instrumental response. In other words, the instrumental CR is established to ΣS + CS, while the CR to the ΣS operating alone is inhibited. The significance of this fact will be seen in the next section.

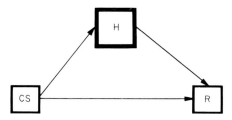

Fig. 3. Model of the instrumental CR. CS, R, and H denote the centers of CS, kinesthesis of instrumental response, and hunger drive, respectively. (Based on the model of W. Wyrwicka, *Acta Biol. Exp.,* 1952, **16,** 131-137.)

If our model of the instrumental CR represented in Fig. 3 is correct, then it must be predicted that by destroying particular parts of this model the CR should be impaired or abolished.

This in fact occurs. The destruction of the hunger system on both its levels (lateral hypothalamic lesion, Rozkowska and Fonberg, 1970, or medial amygdalar lesion, Fonberg, 1969) abolishes the instrumental CR for shorter or longer periods.

Similarly, lesions sustained in the motor, or rather kinesthetic, centers also affect the instrumental CRs to various degrees and in different ways (Konorski, 1970, Chapter 11). Without going deeper into this subject we should stress only that the "movement center" in our model represents that area of the brain in which the kinesthetic pattern of the trained movement is being formed. In fact, we have good evidence to show that lesions in the premotor area have detrimental effects on the performance of manipulatory instrumental movements (Stepien, Stepien, and Konorski, 1960, Stepien, Stepien, and Kreiner, 1963; Gerbner, and Pásster, 1965, and others).

To end this discussion on simple instrumental conditioning programming, Stepien and Stepien (1965) and Stepien, Stepien, and Sychowa (1966) have shown that after the removal of a small area in the posteromedial part of the precruciate area [Fig. 4, according to the myeloarchitectonic map of Kreiner (1966)], a curious symptom may be observed: in experiments with locomotor CRs in which the source of the CS is noncontiguous to the feeder, the lesioned

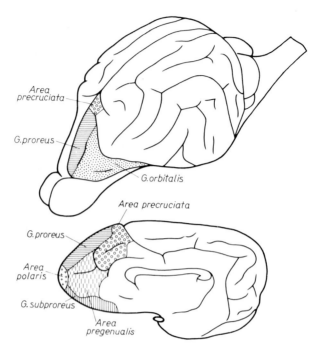

Fig. 4. The surface of the dorsolateral and medial aspects of the cerebral cortex of the dog, indicating those areas which are dealt with in this chapter.

dogs, in response to the CS, approach the source of the CS and not the feeder. The authors have called this symptom "magneto-reaction." It is interesting to note that this reaction is elicited only by positive alimentary CSs, but not by neutral stimuli, nor by the negative (nonreinforced) CSs.

The phenomenon of magneto-reaction may be understood if we realize that in natural life the signals of food (such as its sight, smell, or sounds produced by a prey) operate from the very place of food and only in our "artificial" experimental situations are they separated. Accordingly, in our CR training the animal must inhibit the normal tendency to approach the signal of food and learn to go straight to a feeder. Consequently, we are confronted here again with some inhibitory process which is included in the learned program and impaired after the appropriate cortical lesion. In other words, the magneto-reaction may be regarded as an early established natural CR, which may be suppressed by special training during the formation of an instrumental CR to noncontiguous CS.

To sum up, we may see that this "simple" program of instrumental conditioning to sporadic stimuli noncontiguous to the place of feeding is in the animal's brain more complex than in the experimenter's brain: quite unexpectedly for us it includes the act of suppressing a natural tendency to approach the source of the CS, as well as the tendency to perform the trained movement in response to the whole environment.

III. Pavlovian R−no R Differentiation

We began to study the effects of prefrontal lesions on Pavlovian differentiation in dogs in the early 1950's (Konorski, Stepien, Brutkowski, Lawicka, and Stepien, 1952; Brutkowski, Konorski, Lawicka, Stepien, and Stepien, 1956). We used as positive CSs auditory stimuli—metronomes, bells, tones, etc. As negative CSs, either stimuli similar to the positive CSs were presented, or an inhibitory compound composed of a stimulus quite different from the CS+ (the so-called conditioned inhibitor, CI) followed by the positive CS. The CI-CS+ interval was usually protracted to 5 sec or more. The instrumental response was lifting the right foreleg and placing it on a feeder situated in front of the animal. The food was presented by using remote control to move into position a bowl in the feeder. In some experiments vocal CRs were used, the dog being required to bark in response to the CS (Lawicka, 1957b).

When the training of both excitatory and inhibitory CRs was completed [as seen in Fig. 5(A)], the prefrontal regions of the cerebral cortex up to the presylvian sulcus were bilaterally removed. One week after surgery the experiments were resumed, and the following picture was observed. The positive CRs were completely preserved. As to the no−R responses to the CS−, they were strongly disinhibited. Moreover, the animals performed many instrumental movements in the intertrial intervals, thus manifesting that the instrumental CR established originally to the environment was also disinhibited (cf. Section II). The no−R response to the inhibitory CI−CS+ compound was also completely disinhibited, but the no-response to the conditioned inhibitor was unaffected. It should be recalled that CI, usually being quite distinct from the CS+, never evoked the instrumental response preoperatively. The dog's performance after prefrontal ablation is represented in Fig. 5(B).

When the animals were retrained, their instrumental responding gradually improved. At first the intertrial responses ceased to occur, then the dogs stopped responding to the (differentiated) CS−. Next the response to the CS+ immediately following the CI became inhibited, and only much later was the inhibitory response to the CI-CS compound with the 5-sec interval restored [Fig. 5(C)]. Usually the number of trials required for inhibitory responses to the (differentiated) CS− were equal to or less than that for original training, while the retraining of inhibition to the CS following CI by 5 sec was much more protracted.

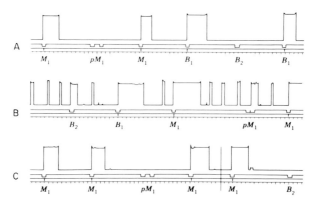

Fig. 5. Records of the experimental sessions with R—no R Pavlovian differentiations. Each record from top to bottom: lifting the foreleg and placing it on the feeder, CSs, presentation of food, time marker (in 5 secs). M_1, B_1, positive CSs; B_2, negative CS; pM_1, M_1 preceded by CI. (A) Correct responding. (B) Responding after prefrontal lobectomy. (C) Responding after recovery. Note that in (A) pM_1 with 5 sec CI-CS interval as well as B_2 elicits inhibitory response; in (B) many intertrial movements are seen; the responses to B_2 and M_1 preceded immediately by CI, but not CI itself, are disinhibited; (C) again completely normal responding. Note that the placing of the foreleg on the feeder is always prolonged in positive trials; this is due to the fact that the dog keeps his leg on the feeder during the act of eating and puts it down only after the portion of food is consumed. (After Brutkowski *et al.,* 1956.) Reprinted by permission of Polish Scientific Publishers, Warsaw.

In order to see whether the disinhibitory syndrome appears selectively after prefrontal ablations, a parietal area of the same size was removed. The animal's instrumental responding was completely normal after the lesion, and no disinhibition was ever observed.

The next task was to see whether the prefrontal cortex is "equipotential" with regard to the Pavlovian R—no R differentiation, or whether there are some crucial areas responsible for the performance of this task. Experiments performed by Szwejkowska, Kreiner, and Sychowa (1963) and Brutkowski and Dabrowska (1963, 1966) have shown that lesions limited to the medial part of the prefrontal area (pregenual area and medial precruciate area, Fig. 4) give rise to the clear disinhibitory syndrome. On the other hand, lesions sustained in the dorsal part (proreal area) or the lateral part (so-called orbital area, not to be confused with orbital area in monkeys) failed to produce this syndrome, provided that the intertrial intervals are about 1 min or more. Lesions sustained in the subproreal area situated in the basal part of the prefrontal region also fail to produce disinhibition (Szwejkowska, Stepien, and Kreiner, 1965). Finally, it should be mentioned that when the intertrial intervals are shortened to 15 sec, disinhibition of inhibitory responses is also obtained after dorsal prefrontal lesions (Brutkowski and Dabrowska, 1963, 1966). This fact will be commented upon further in the text.

Now we should turn to the problem of whether there are other regions in the brain where damage produces a disinhibitory syndrome. First, as found by Brutkowski and Mempel (1961), the genual portion of the anterior cingulate gyrus (but not the posterior cingulate gyrus) also produces disinhibition of inhibitory responses in R—no R differentiation. This shows that the medial frontal lesion producing that syndrome is larger than originally suggested, a fact which may partially account for restoration of inhibitory CRs during post-operative training.

Second, the lesions in subcortical structures related to inhibition of hunger drive—lateral amygdala (Fonberg, 1969) and ventromedial hypothalamus (Rozkowska and Fonberg, 1971)—also produce the disinhibitory syndrome closely connected with increase of hunger drive. Interestingly enough, after ventromedial hypothalamic lesions, the intertrial responses were noticed, but the no-response to the CS— was not affected.

Finally, Dabrowska (unpublished experiments) performed an extensive study on R—no R Pavlovian differentiation after hippocampal lesions. She found that these lesions produce in many dogs (but not in all of them) a severe, disinhibitory syndrome. This finding would support Kimble's (1968) thesis claiming an important role of the hippocampus in "internal inhibition." It remains to be elucidated whether hippocampal lesions affect the same or different aspects of the inhibitory mechanism than that affected by prefrontal lesions.

Investigations on R—no R Pavlovian differentiation in monkeys are less numerous. In experiments carried out in the Wisconsin General Test Apparatus, Brutkowski, Mishkin, and Rosvold (1963) have shown that after orbitofrontal lesions R—no R differentiation to visual stimuli is strongly impaired. Dorsal ablations involving principal sulcus and surrounding area, including the anterior bank of the arcuate sulcus, fail to produce these effects. In a modified Wisconsin General Test Apparatus (no screen between the animal's cage and the food well, with manipulandum permanently available to animals) Lawicka, Mishkin, and Rosvold (1966, 1972) performed experiments with auditory stimuli analogous to those carried out in dogs. It has been found that orbital ablations in monkeys produce almost exactly the same impairment of R—no R Pavlovian differen-tiation as that obtained in dogs after medial ablations (or complete prefrontal lobectomies). The intertrial responses became very abundant and the animals vigorously responded to the CS—. After a lapse of time the correct CR performance was restored, but the number of errors on the negative trials in postoperative retraining was much higher than it was preoperatively. On the contrary, dorsolateral lesions failed to produce this effect.

To sum up, we see that after removal of a definite part of the prefrontal region there occurs a dramatic impairment of alimentary (but not defensive, see Soltysik and Jaworska, 1967) inhibitory CRs. The problem arises as to what is the mechanism of this phenomenon. In my recent book (Konorski, 1970, Chapters 7 and 10) it was postulated that besides the hunger drive system responsible for alimentary instrumental CRs, there is a higher order "antihunger center" whose role is to suppress the hunger drive in those situations in which food is not available. This "antihunger center" may be considered an extension of the limbic system, serving for the most delicate adaptation of alimentary behavior to the environment.

When at the start of the Pavlovian differentiation training a stimulus similar to the CS+ was presented without reinforcement, its center was already connected with the hunger drive center, owing to generalization. This is why the new stimulus elicits the instrumental response. During differentiation training, however, apart from these connections, which remain intact, new connections are formed between the new CS center and the antidrive center; these connections are responsible for the suppression of the instrumental response to this CS [Fig. 6(A)].

The mechanism of conditioned inhibition is a little more complicated. The CI, being dissimilar to any of the CSs used and never being reinforced by food, forms no connections with the hunger drive center (cf. the notion of the "primary inhibitory stimulus", Konorski and Szwejkowska, 1952), but it forms connections exclusively with the antihunger center [Fig. 6(A)]. The fact that the instrumental response to the CS+ which shortly followed the CI is suppressed, is primarily due to the inhibitory aftereffect which the CI exerted upon this response (the slight contamination of the CS itself by inhibitory properties is here neglected).

Now, the fact that lesions sustained in the mediofrontal area in dogs, or in the orbitofrontal area in monkeys, produce disinhibition of inhibitory CRs indicates that the postulated higher order antihunger drive center is localized precisely in this part of the prefrontal cortex. Accordingly, removal of this area [Fig. 6(B)]

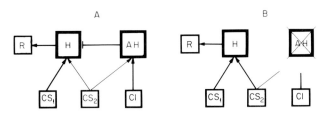

Fig. 6. Block model of the mechanism of inhibitory instrumental CRs (A), and their impairment after medial prefrontal (in dogs) or orbitofrontal (in monkeys) lesions (B). CS_1, positive CS center; CS_2, negative CS center; CI, conditioned inhibitor center; H, hunger system; AH, antihunger center situated in the prefrontal extension of the limbic system; R, instrumental response center. Arrows, excitatory connections; stopped lines, inhibitory connections. Thin lines denote weak connections. For simplicity, the direct connections between CSs and R are not drawn.

will not affect the excitatory CRs, but will impair those inhibitory CRs which have a mixed excitatory-inhibitory character. Thus the animal will perform the intertrial responses, because the experimental environment *was* originally a CS+ (see preceding section), and will also perform the responses to negatively differentiated CSs. As far as the CI is concerned it will not produce the instrumental response, because it has never been linked with the hunger center. However, since the antidrive center with which the CI center was connected has been destroyed, CI will no longer exert any inhibitory influence upon the CS+ following it; in effect, the inhibitory CR to the CI-CS compound will be dramatically disinhibited.

Since the prefrontal antihunger center is considered the rostral extension of the limbic system, it is clear that it is connected functionally with both the lateral amygdalar nucleus and the ventromedial hypothalamic nucleus. Accordingly, the disinhibitory syndrome is produced after lesions in these structures, although its symptomatology is not quite the same.

As noted before, lesions in the dorsolateral prefrontal area in dogs produced disinhibition in R–no R differentiation when the intertrial intervals were very short (15 sec instead of 1 min) (Brutkowski and Dabrowska, 1963, 1966). Although this disinhibition is quite significant, it differs from that produced by medial lesions in that during the intertrial intervals the dogs are quiet and fail to perform instrumental responses. Since these dogs fail also to display any increase of the hunger drive manifested by searching and sniffing movements, disinhibition of their instrumental responses to the CS– cannot be attributed to impairment of drive inhibition. It may be supposed that their defect is due to an inability to switch rapidly from excitatory to inhibitory responses, a capacity required in rapid succession of positive and negative CSs.

IV. R–no R Both Reinforced Differentiation

The effects of prefrontal lesions upon the performance of this test were recently studied in dogs (Dabrowska, 1971) in the following way. First, the dog was trained to lift his right foreleg to a 1000 cps tone and to place it on the feeder situated before him. Each such trial was reinforced. Thereafter, a 700 cps tone was presented in random order with the 1000 cps tone. At first, the animal performed the trained movement in response to the 700 cps tone, but since no food reinforcement followed, after a number of sessions he stopped doing so. If during 5 sec of the 700 cps tone no trained movement occurred, food was offered. This led to restoration of response to the 700 cps tone, until after several successions differentiation was achieved: the dog performed the trained movement to the 1000 cps tone, while during the operation of the 700 cps tone he clearly refrained from doing so.

After the animals reached criterion they were operated upon: in one group ablations included the medial part of the prefrontal area, in the other group the dorsolateral part was removed. The results of these lesions were exactly opposite those obtained by Brutkowski and Dabrowska (1966) with Pavlovian differentiation: medial lesions which were detrimental for Pavlovian differentiation produced only a slight effect, while the dorsolateral lesions produced total and irreversible disorder of symmetrical differentiation: the animals either performed the trained movement to both CSs, or refrained from performing that movement to either one. A comparison of data obtained in experiments on R–no R Pavlovian differentiation and in studies on R–no R both reinforced differentiation is presented in Fig. 7.

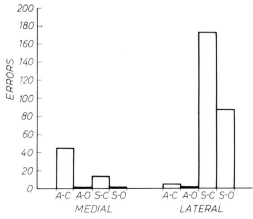

Fig. 7. Commission and omission errors in dogs in Pavlovian and both-reinforced R–no R differentiation after medial and lateral lesions. A–C, commission errors in Pavlovian differentiation; A–O, omission errors in Pavlovian differentiation; S–C, commission errors in both-reinforced differentiation; S–O, omission errors in both-reinforced differentiation. (After Brutkowski and Dabrowska, 1963, 1966; Dabrowska, 1971.)

Further experiments by Dabrowska (1971) have shown that whereas selective dorsal ablations, involving the proreal gyrus only, are not harmful for the performance of the R–no R both reinforced task, lateral ablations involving the orbital gyrus produced the same effect as dorsolateral lesions. Thus, the lateral and not the dorsal prefrontal area has appeared to be responsible for the integrity of an R–no R both reinforced differentiation.

Analogous experiments were performed much earlier on monkeys by Weiskrantz and Mishkin (1958), Gross and Weiskrantz (1962) and Gross (1963). In these experiments, too, auditory CSs were used to demonstrate that removal of the dorsolateral prefrontal cortex produced severe impairment of an R–no R both reinforced differentiation. It should be noted that in Gross and Weiskrantz's experiments (not supported by those of Gross, 1963) only ablations of cortex surrounding the principal sulcus but not its depth were responsible for this impairment.

How should we explain the fact that in spite of a seemingly small difference between two procedures of R–no R differentiation, the areas responsible for these two programs are different. This fact implies that the mechanisms underlying these programs should also be distinct.

In view of our concept of Pavlovian differentiation, the difference between the two programs is quite understandable. In the Pavlovian R–no R program, hunger drive is the essential link for occurrence of differentiation. The animal stops performing the instrumental response to the CS– because this stimulus becomes a signal of antihunger, or to speak freely, the animal does not expect food in its presence. On the contrary, in learning that no–R to CS_2 is reinforced, the animal must decide whether the R response or the no–R response should be performed to a given stimulus.

V. $R_1 - R_2$ Differentiation

The program of this task consists in the formation of two instrumental responses: $CS_1 - R_1$ and $CS_2 - R_2$. In our own experimental practice we used two methods. In Lawicka's experiments the left feeder and the right feeder in the setup presented in Fig. 2 were used, and two auditory stimuli served as cues which evoked locomotor responses to each of them respectively. In Dobrzecka's experiments the animal was required to place either the right or the left foreleg on the feeder (Fig. 1) in response to one or the other auditory CS, respectively. Before discussing $R_1 - R_2$ differentiation, it should be noted that we shall deal here exclusively with the situation where both CSs are noncontiguous to the feeders. When, in locomotor $R_1 - R_2$ differentiation, the cues are contiguous with the goals (e.g., buzzers are placed on the respective feeders), then practically no training is necessary and the animals make no errors even if a triple choice is presented; the CS simply "pulls" the animal to the corresponding feeder (Konorski and Lawicka, 1959). The situation is, however, quite different when the CSs are not contiguous to the feeders. In that case the task requires a more or less prolonged discriminatory training before the animal learns which CS signals which feeder.

An important rule should be followed in this training, originally discovered by Lawicka (1964, 1969a) for locomotor CRs, and later confirmed by Dobrzecka and Konorski (1967, 1968) for manipulatory CRs. If the two CSs differ only in quality but operate from the same place (e.g., two tones emitted from the same loudspeaker), the task is very difficult and requires prolonged training. If, however, the CSs differ in location, e.g., the source of one sound is above the source of the other (Lawicka's experiments), or one source is in front and the other behind the animal (Dobrzecka and Konorski's experiments), then the task does not present serious difficulties to the subject. Incidentally, the same rule appears to be valid not only for dogs but also for monkeys (Lawicka *et al.*, 1966, 1972). Konorski (1970, Chapter 10) explains this phenomenon by assuming that the quality of a sound is an inadequate cue for establishing direct CS–R connections because potential connections linking auditory and kinesthetic gnostic units are poorly developed. Consequently, the CS–R connections are mediated by kinesthesis produced by orienting responses to the CSs; the greater the difference between the kinesthetic feedback of those responses (as is the case when the CSs operate from different places), the easier is the discriminatory training.

Let us now analyze in more detail the formation of the R_1–R_2 differentiation to two auditory CSs, with the help of the block model presented in Fig. 8. Since in the experimental situation the animal has learned to perform both instrumental responses, the situation itself becomes a subthreshold CS, producing readiness for response occurrence. Releasing stimuli are provided by both CSs, due to the fact that they increase excitation of the hunger drive center and thus elicit both responses.

Since "direct" connections between auditory stimuli centers and centers of particular movements are poor, the instrumental responses to both CSs are indiscriminate, unless the CSs differ also in eliciting two distinct orienting responses. Orienting responses can easily establish connections with corresponding instrumental movements (e.g., look up–go right, look down–go left), and these connections determine which movement is performed to which stimulus.

Returning now to the problem of prefrontal representation of a R_1–R_2 differentiation, it should be noticed that when the CSs are contiguous with the appropriate feeders, even complete frontal lobectomies fail to impair the locomotor R_1–R_2 differentiation (Lawicka and Konorski, 1959).

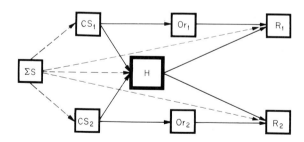

Fig. 8. Block model of R_1-R_2 differentiation to CSs noncontiguous with the place of feeding. CS_1, CS_2, centers of CSs; Σ S, experimental situation center. H, hunger system; Or_1, Or_2, centers of orienting reactions to CS_1 and CS_2; R_1, R_2, centers of instrumental responses. Arrows, excitatory connections; interrupted lines, facilitatory connections. $Or_1 \rightarrow R_1$ and $O_2 \rightarrow R_2$ are supposed to be situated in the prefrontal extension of the kinesthetic analyser.

The situation is, however, different when the CSs are not contiguous to the feeding places. As shown in some preliminary experiments, complete prefrontal lobectomies do impair locomotor (Lawicka, unpublished) and manipulatory (Dobrzecka *et al.*, unpublished) R_1-R_2 differentiation; however, the effects of partial prefrontal lesions have not yet been fully investigated. Recently Lawicka (1969b) reported that ablations of the proreal gyrus failed to impair this task (see Fig. 10). Let us recall that the same negative effect was obtained after this lesion with regard to R—no R where both were symmetrically reinforced (Dabrowska, 1971).

The study of this problem is more advanced in monkeys. In recent experiments by Lawicka *et al.* (1966, 1972) dorsolateral prefrontal lesions, including the rostral bank of arcuate sulcus, impair considerably the R_1-R_2 differentiation to CSs, differing from each other either in direction (up versus down) or in quality (frequency of tones). Remember (Section III) that R—no R Pavlovian differentiation in monkeys was not impaired after dorsolateral lesions. On the other hand, orbitofrontal lesions, which strongly impaired the R—no R Pavlovian differentiation, failed to affect seriously R_1-R_2 differentiation, at least to directional cues (up—down). The R_1-R_2 differentiation established to frequency cues, being an exceedingly difficult task for normal monkeys, *is* impaired also after ventral lesions—a fact which is elaborated upon elsewhere (cf. Lawicka *et al.*, 1972).

In this connection a recent study by Goldman and Rosvold (1970) should be cited, because they clearly demarcate the extent of lesions producing impairment of R_1-R_2 differentiation to directional auditory CSs (up—down). They have shown that the optimal lesions are those affecting the arcuate sulcus. Dorsolateral lesions around the principal sulcus produce a less severe effect, while those involving the principal sulcus alone are virtually without effect.

Similar results were obtained by Stepien and Stamm (1970a). These authors trained monkeys in the R_1-R_2 test with cues spatially opposed to the feeders—the cue near the left feeder signaled "go right," and that near the right feeder signaled "go left." They found that dorsolateral prefrontal lesions, surrounding the principal sulcus and involving the arcuate sulcus, severely impaired this test. On the other side, lesions inside the principal gyrus were almost ineffective. Lesions sustained in the premotor and the orbitofrontal areas produced a very insignificant deficit.

To sum up, we see that, as far as dogs are concerned, total prefrontal lobectomy does impair the R_1-R_2 differentiation, but the area specifically concerned with this test has not so far been demarcated. In monkeys the R_1-R_2 differentiation is impaired after lesions located in the dorsolateral area excluding the principal sulcus. The crucial area for this test lies in the arcuate sulcus.

In order to explain these findings we should recall that the R_1-R_2 differentiation to cues noncontiguous to the place of feeding is mediated by the orienting responses elicited by these cues (Fig. 8). Since the dorsolateral area of the prefrontal cortex including the arcuate sulcus may be regarded as a gnostic extension of the kinesthetic cortical region (Konorski, 1970), it may be supposed that precisely in this area associations are formed between kinesthetic patterns, representing particular behavioral acts, for instance, between patterns generated by orienting responses and those patterns generated by particular instrumental movements. When this area is removed, these associations are broken, and the animal is no longer capable of responding selectively to the corresponding cues. However, the more general connections, which link *both* CS centers with *both* instrumental movement centers via the hunger drive center, are fully preserved. Therefore the animal performs these movements indiscriminately, depending on the instantaneous higher excitability of a given motor center.

The fact that the R_1-R_2 test is *not* impaired when the animal is required to approach the feeder signaled by the contiguous CS is understandable; this response is based on a much more primitive mechanism previously discussed in Section II.

To end these considerations, we should ask the question whether the R_1-R_2 differentiation is fully equivalent to R–no R both reinforced differentiation. In experiments on monkeys the areas responsible for both tasks are, in fact, overlapping, but the crucial experiment, testing whether the arcuate sulcus, responsible for R_1-R_2 differentiation (Goldman and Rosvold, 1970), is also responsible for R–no R both reinforced differentiation has not yet been performed. In dogs the area responsible for R_1-R_2 differentiation is still unknown.

The difference between the two tasks is that one of them involves reciprocally related movements of one leg only (flexion–extension), while the other task involves two symmetrical movements (turn right–turn left, or lifting the right foreleg–lifting the left foreleg). As stated before, the R_1-R_2 task is acquired by the mediation of orienting responses; whether the same is true of an R–no R task, we do not know. Therefore, the problem of whether the two tasks are identical or different must still await its solution.[1]

VI. Delayed Responses

The program of delayed responses derives from the R_1-R_2 differentiation program, except that the animal is not allowed to display the instrumental

---

[1] Addendum in proof: Recent experiments of Dabrowska (*Acta Neurobiol. Exp.*, 1972, 32) and Stepien and Stepien (*ibid.*) have shown that R_1-R_2 differentiation and R–no R both reinforced differentiation depend on two different mechanisms since they are impaired after different prefrontal lesions. Probably the main difference between the two tests consists in that the first test involved only locomotor responses whereas the other one is based on two manipulatory responses, namely flexion of the fore leg versus its extension.

response in the presence of the corresponding CS but only to its trace. Since, however, in the majority of studies using this task the CSs were contiguous with food wells and the responses consisted of running toward them, or reaching for food by hand, the complexity of the R_1-R_2 programs with noncontiguous cues was omitted. Consequently, delayed response tests are typically concerned with the problem of mere delay, without being contaminated with the problem of making a learned choice. This is the advantage of using a procedure with cues contiguous to the feeders.

From the early 1930's, when Jacobsen (1936) performed his famous experiments showing impairment of delayed responses after prefrontal ablations in monkeys, studies on this problem were very numerous and the essential fact discovered by Jacobsen was fully confirmed. Most authors, however, did not agree with the original explanation, namely his attributing the delayed response deficit after prefrontal lesions to an impairment of short-term memory.

Since the experimental paradigm for the delayed response tasks with monkeys is well known to American readers, I shall describe here only the method used in our laboratory with dogs (Lawicka, 1959). Figure 2 illustrates the experimental setting. The buzzers are placed on each feeder. Before every trial the dog was attached by a leash to the starting platform, and in several seconds one of the buzzers operated for 3 sec; after various delay periods (usually 15 and 60 sec), the animal was released and allowed to approach the feeder. When he reached the correct feeder, a bowl of food was placed into position. An important factor introduced in these experiments was the application of trials with distractions during the delay period, the usual distractor consisting of a small portion of food being placed on the starting platform before the animal was released. This measure prevented the animal from preserving a directional posture toward the signaled feeder during the delay period. In this way pseudodelayed responses produced by the animal's maintaining his orientation posture to the buzzer were avoided.

Having established that delayed responses were dramatically impaired in dogs following prefrontal lobectomies (Lawicka and Konorski, 1959), the next aim was to isolate which part of this region was responsible for this deficit. In experiments by Lawicka et al. (1966) it was found that the dorsomedial part of the prefrontal area (proreal gyrus, Fig. 4) was crucial for this test, whereas lesions sustained in the lateral area (orbital gyrus and presylvian sulcus) did not produce any deficit (Fig. 9). On the other hand, pure proreal lesions which severely impaired the delayed response test failed to affect the R_1-R_2 differentiation (Konorski and Lawicka, 1964; Lawicka, 1969b) (Fig. 10).

As far as monkeys are concerned, many investigations have shown that the area necessary for successful performance on the delayed response task (including the spatial delayed alternation) lies in the depths of the principal sulcus (Blum, 1952; Mishkin, 1957; Gross and Weiskrantz, 1964; Goldman and Rosvold, 1970).

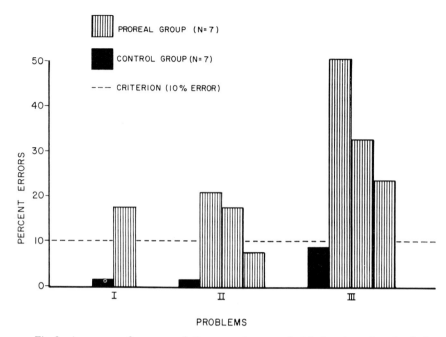

Fig. 9. Average performance of the proreal group (hatched columns) and of the combined orbital and presylvian group (black columns) for blocks of 60 trials on the three delayed response problems: I, 15-sec delay; II, 60-sec delay; III, 60-sec delay with intradelay feeding (Lawicka et al., 1966).

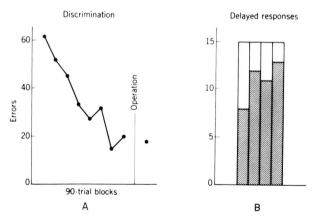

Fig. 10. Comparison of the effect of proreal lesions on R_1 - R_2 differentiation and triple choice delayed responses. (A) Training of differentiation before operation, and its full preservation after operation. (B) Number of errors (hatched parts of the columns) in delayed responses with distractions; performance on the chance level (66.6% of errors). (From Konorski and Lawicka, 1964.) Reprinted by permission of McGraw-Hill, New York.

Now we proceed to the main problem of our discussion, namely the role of the prefrontal area in delayed response performance. Perhaps the best evidence to demonstrate that the deficit caused by a prefrontal lesion is not due to the abolition of short-term memory has been provided in experiments on cats in a three-choice situation (Lawicka and Konorski, 1961). These animals, although severely impaired after prefrontal ablation, behaved regularly in the following way; when released from the starting platform after the delay period, they approached the feeder from which they had received food on the preceding trial; not finding food in this feeder, they would turn immediately to the *correct* one. This means that they did remember the signaled feeder, but simply could not suppress the perseverative (or rather one-trial learning) tendency to perform that locomotor response which was just reinforced. The same results were obtained on dogs, although corrections were less frequent (Fig. 11).

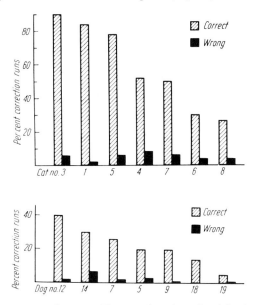

Fig. 11. The percentage of errors with corrections in prefrontal cats (upper graph) and dogs (lower graph). Each hatched column denotes the percentage of errors with "correct" corrections; each black column denotes the percentage of errors with wrong corrections (Lawicka, 1969b). Reprinted by permission of Polish Scientific Publishers, Warsaw.

Another important fact relevant for our discussion was recently obtained by Lawicka (1969b) on dogs. This author introduced a procedure described by her as the sham-trial method. It consisted of releasing the animal from the starting platform without a signaling stimulus. Normal animals, after being released in sham-trials remain, as a rule, on the platform or may slowly visit one of the feeders (Lawicka, 1969b). In contrast, the dorsofrontal animals, when released without a signaling stimulus, rush quickly to one of the feeders, and repeat these responses over a long series of sham-trials. When, however, they finally stop doing so, and a true trial follows, the delayed response is correct. Moreover, with increasing delayed response impairment, the responses in sham-trials following each correct true trial become more numerous.

All these data indicate that the deficit in delayed response after proreal lesions in dogs does not consist in abolition of short-term memory of directional cues, but in the vulnerability of the response system controlled by this memory. Accordingly, dominance of the proper delayed response over various concomitant instrumental reflexes, such as reacting to the unleashing procedure itself, or repeating the last reinforced run, is now overthrown. To restore this dominance we must extinguish these concomitant reflexes in order to give way to the operation of the delayed response.

One can argue whether this overthrow of delayed response dominance results from an increase in conditionability of actual stimuli, which may be related to an increase of orientation reactions to exteroceptive agents (Lawicka, 1969b), or is it due to a weakening of the memory traces of locomotor kinesthetic cues. We have some evidence to believe that these cues are primarily affected. According to data collected by Mishkin, Vest, Waxler, and Rosvold (1969) after lesions in the dorsolateral area including principal sulcus, delayed spatial alternation (go left—go right) is much more severely impaired than object alternation. In fact, in the former test, in order to react correctly the animal must remember the last direction of run, whereas in the latter test he must remember the visual cue. This finding is in good agreement with the fact that the dorsolateral frontal cortex may be considered a rostral extension of the kinesthetic analyzer, being the gnostic representation of kinesthetic directional cues.

VII. General Discussion

The main set of findings described in this paper is that different "parallel" types of programs of animal motor behavior, each involving two or more motor tasks in response to various stimuli, are represented by different parts of the prefrontal cortex. These programs are: R—no R Pavlovian differentiation, R—no R both reinforced differentiation, R_1—R_2 differentiation, and R_1—R_2 delayed responses. It has been shown that these programs are, in fact, different as far as their operations are concerned and therefore it was only to be expected that their central representations should be different.

The important problem arises as to whether all other programs of complex motor behavior can be reduced to these four models. It should be realized that the tasks with which we have dealt in the present article are only a small part of all tasks of motor behavior used in experimental practice. Here belong: (1) drive reversal, (2) response reversal, (3) delayed spatial alternations, (4) delayed object alternations, (5) delayed responses to cues not contiguous to the feeders, (6) delayed Pavlovian alternation, and many others. Furthermore, there are sequential types of programs such as locomotor maze habits on the one hand and chains of manipulatory movements on the other. The reason we are not concerned with these other programs in the present survey is simply because we do not have enough experimental documentation for both dogs and monkeys.

Let us try to analyze the enumerated programs in order to see whether they can or cannot be reduced to those described above.

Drive reversal consists in changing the signaling role of the CS with regard to *drive*. The simplest reversal of this kind is represented by extinction, in which the CS is no longer reinforced by food, and in consequence the instrumental response is inhibited. What is the role of the prefrontal cortex (or its parts) in this task? We have not studied this problem with dogs because we considered it to be identical with R—no R Pavlovian differentiation. Indeed, extinction is based on the formation of the connections between the CS center and the antihunger center (Fig. 6), exactly as is the case with a differentiated negative CS. Therefore the normal course of extinction should depend on the integrity of the same area as Pavlovian differentiation. In fact, as found by Butter, Mishkin, and Rosvold (1963) on monkeys, resistance to extinction after orbitofrontal lesions is much stronger than after dorsolateral lesions or in control animals.

Response reversal consists in changing the signaling role of the CS with regard to the instrumental response. The usual way of experimenting on this task is to confront the animal with two food wells and teach him, first, to approach one well in response to a given CS, and then to switch his response to the other one. This procedure is usually repeated many times in succession, and animals with various cortical lesions are compared.

In Lawicka's experiments (unpublished) performed on dogs, it has been established that proreal lesions fail to affect this test, at least when reversals begin after the animal has reached criterion in the preceding response.

An illustrative example of response reversal in monkeys has been provided by Mishkin (1964), who performed a number of successive reversals in two tests—spatial reversal and object reversal—after ablations sustained in the laterofrontal area, the orbitofrontal area, and inferotemporal area. His results are shown in a modified version (Fig. 12) presenting only the optimal case in which differences between the groups were most conspicuous; this took place when the task was neither too easy nor too difficult.

Notice that in spatial reversals orbital and lateral monkeys were equally impaired, while the temporal monkeys were not impaired. On the contrary, in object reversals orbital monkeys were as impaired as in spatial reversals, lateral monkeys were almost normal, and temporal monkeys were impaired.

These informative data have shown that: (1) the inferotemporal area plays the same role with respect to object reversal as does the laterofrontal area with

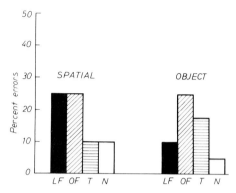

Fig. 12. Mean percentage of errors on object- and place-differentiation reversal in monkeys after lateral prefrontal lesions (LF), orbital prefrontal lesion (OF), inferotemporal lesion (T), and in normals (N). On the basis of Mishkin's data (1964), four reversals per day, each reversal includes eight trials.

regard to spatial reversals, and (2) both reversals are equally impaired after orbital lesions.

Thus the specific program concerning spatial reversal in monkeys depends on the integrity of the dorsolateral prefrontal area whereas the specific program concerning object reversal depends on the integrity of the inferotemporal area.

An unspecific role in response reversals (both spatial and object) is played by the orbitofrontal area. This role is easy to conceive if one takes into account that response reversal necessarily involves extinction of the instrumental response leading to food, whether it is a spatially guided response (where to go) or a visually guided response (to which object to go).

Thus we see that response reversal is a complex task involving either spatial or visual gnosis secured by the laterofrontal or inferotemporal cortex respectively, *and* the normal ability to extinguish instrumental responses secured by the orbitofrontal cortex.[2]

Delayed spatial alternation again combines two mechanisms: one functions to remember what was the last response (left or right), the faculty depending in monkeys on the integrity of the principal sulcus (Mishkin, 1957; and others); the other mechanism functions to easily "extinguish" the preceding response in order to alternate, the faculty depending on the orbitofrontal area. Consequently lesions in both areas impair this test.

---

[2] Recent experiments by Butter (1969) seem to indicate that lesions in the lateral orbital area produce an impairment of reversal learning, while lesions in the posteromedial orbital area affect mainly extinction. This result suggests that there might be a difference between simple extinction and response reversal training. This problem requires more detailed investigation.

On the other hand, delayed object alternation is obviously impaired for the same reason after orbital lesion, but it is not (or at least less) impaired after lateral lesions (Mishkin *et al.*, 1969).

Tests on delayed responses to cues noncontiguous to the feeders were performed in monkeys by Stepien and Stamm (1970b). Cues were spatially opposed to the signaled feeders so this test combined two programs: delayed responses and $R_1 - R_2$ differentiation. Therefore it should be impaired both after dorsolateral and principal sulcus lesions. As seen in Fig. 13, this is precisely what occurred. After dorsolateral nonprincipal lesions, $R_1 - R_2$ differentiation with and without delay was severely impaired. Note that initially the no-delay task was even more "impaired" (errors much above chance), because of the magneto-reaction. The delay task begins with chance level responding and remains at this level throughout the experiment, even when the no-delay responses become normal—demonstrating that $R_1 - R_2$ differentiation with delay is even more difficult than it is without delay. On the other hand, lesions in the principal sulcus destroyed irreversibly the delayed response, while the no-delay differentiation was only insignificantly impaired. After total dorsolateral lesions,

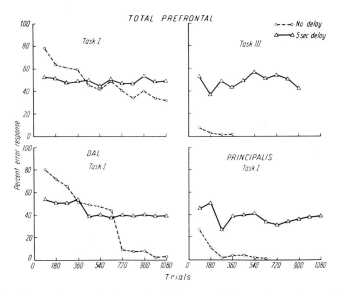

Fig. 13. Means of errors (two monkeys per group) for postoperative testing under no-delay and delayed response conditions. Task I, spatial opposition of CSs; Task III, spatial contiguity between CSs and food locations. Total prefrontal means dorsolateral cortex; "DAL" means cortex surrounding principal sulcus. In task I: total dorsolateral lesions produce severe impairment (chance level) on both no-delay test and 5-sec delay test, DAL lesions produce the same effect, principalis lesions produce impairment in only 5-sec delay test; on task III: total dorsolateral lesions produce impairment in 5-sec delay test, but not in no delay test (Stepien and Stamm, 1970b). Reprinted by permission of Polish Scientific Publishers, Warsaw.

R_1-R_2 differentiation was equally impaired with and without delay, but in the task with spatial contiguity between the cue and the feeder (task III in Fig. 13) only the delayed response was impaired.

Delayed Pavlovian alternation occurs when the same CS is reinforced every second time. These experiments were performed on dogs with 1-min intertrial intervals, which means presentation of food every 2 min (Szwejkowska, Lawicka, and Konorski, 1964). When the task was mastered, it turned out that the animal did not solve the problem according to the alternation program; instead, the act of eating on reinforced trials became a conditioned inhibitor with regard to the next CS, with the inhibitory aftereffect of about 1 min. This was proved by the following facts: (1) when food was given "gratis" without the CS, the dog never performed the trained movement on the next trial; (2) when CSs were presented twice or thrice during the inhibitory aftereffect (about 90 sec) the animal did not perform the trained movement, and (3) when the intertrial interval amounted to 2 min, that is, the negative trial was lacking, the animal did perform the trained movement, as if the negative CS were interspersed. Thus we have here a good example of a situation in which the program established by the experimenter and that adopted by the animals were quite different (cf. Section I).

In order to eliminate this pseudoalternation and teach the animal to perform true alternation, the intertrial intervals varied from half a minute to 2 min, and eventually, after long training the animals succeeded in solving the task (Szwejkowska, 1965a). Animals trained by a fixed or variable intertrial interval sustained prefrontal ablations either medial or dorsal (Szwejkowska, 1965b). The effects of these lesions are represented in Fig. 14. It may be seen that in the group with fixed intertrial intervals (which reacted according to the R—no R Pavlovian differentiation program) medial lesions produced a clear disinhibitory syndrome, whereas dorsal lesions failed to do so. However, in the group with variable intervals, the impairment was much more severe and concerned animals with both dorsal and medial lesions. This suggests that the true Pavlovian delayed alternation test is rather complex and involves both drive inhibition and some delay component. In fact the animal *must* now remember at each trial whether the preceding trial was negative or positive.

As far as sequential types of programs are concerned, we do know from experiments on rats (Dabrowska, 1964, locomotor sequences) and primates (Jacobsen, 1934, manipulatory sequences) that prefrontal lesions are detrimental for these tasks. We do not know, however, which particular anatomical areas are crucial.

To summarize all the programs discussed in this section, we may observe that in all probability they *can* be reduced to those dealt with in our previous sections. The only exception is object alternation and object reversal. They are essentially visual tasks controlled by inferotemporal cortex; however, the orbitofrontal cortex largely contributes to their proper performance.

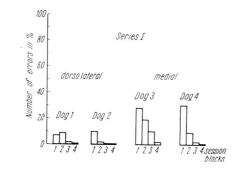

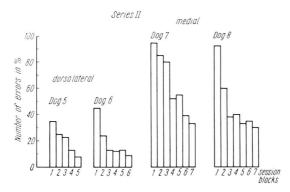

Fig. 14. The effects of prefrontal lesions on Pavlovian R—no R alternation. Series I: fixed intertrial intervals of the 1-min duration; Series II: varying intertrial intervals from ½ min to 2 min. Each column denotes 10-session block (80 inhibitory trials). (From Szewjkowska, 1965b.)

VIII. Summary

Acquired behavioral acts denoted as instrumental conditioned reflexes may be divided into two categories differing in their central mechanisms. To the first category belong simple instrumental responses to appropriate conditioned stimuli, according to the paradigm CS—R, where CS stands for the conditioned stimulus and R stands for the instrumental response. In the second category belong discriminative responses: a subject must select a particular instrumental response among two or more responses which are likely to occur in the given situation. In contradistinction to the first category, the second category demands that the animal make a decision what response should be performed in order to achieve the goal. The general paradigm for this category is: CS_1-R_1, CS_2-R_2, etc., and the corresponding training consists in learning which response is correct and which is wrong in the presence of a given conditioned stimulus. This paper was concerned mainly with the second category of instrumental responding.

In experimental practice we may discern the following tasks in which decision making is necessary; for the sake of simplicity, only instrumental responses based on food reinforcement are taken into consideration.

1. The subject must learn that in the presence of a given stimulus he should perform a given movement in order to receive food, but in response to a similar stimulus he should not, because this stimulus is never followed by food. The appropriate paradigm is: $CS_1 - R_1 \to$ Food, $CS_2 -$ no R $\to$ no Food.

2. The subject learns a similar task, but whereas CS_1 is reinforced when R is executed, CS_2 is reinforced when R is *not* executed. The paradigm of this procedure is: $CS_1 - R \to$ Food, $CS_2 -$ no R $\to$ Food.

3. The subject learns to perform R_1 in response to CS_1, and R_2 in response to CS_2, both these responses, when performed to the proper stimulus, being reinforced by food. The corresponding paradigm is

$$CS_1 - R_1 \to \text{Food}, CS_2 - R_2 \to \text{Food}.$$

4. The subject first learns the task specified in the preceding paragraph, but thereafter performance of the response is allowed by the experimenter to occur only to the trace of the CS (the so-called delayed response). The corresponding paradigm is

$$\text{tr } CS_1 - R_1 \to \text{Food, tr } CS_2 - R_2 \to \text{Food}$$

where "tr" stands for "short-term memory trace of."

In experiments performed on dogs and monkeys it has been shown that correct performance of these tasks depends on the integrity of the prefrontal region of the cerebral cortex, but for a given species each task requires the integrity of a specific part of this region. Thus the first task is impaired after ablation of the medial part of the prefrontal region in dogs and the ventral part in monkeys; the second task is impaired after ablation of the lateral prefrontal region in dogs and dorsolateral part (excluding the principal sulcus) in monkeys; the third task is impaired in monkeys after ablation of the arcuate sulcus; the fourth task is impaired after ablation of the dorsal prefrontal area in dogs and the principal sulcus in monkeys.

This functional compartmentalization of the prefrontal cortex is understandable if we take into account that in these experiments we have to deal with at least three different physiological mechanisms: task one is based on drive inhibition, tasks two and three are based on discriminative connections between stimuli and responses, while task four is based on short-term memory of the decisions made in advance. The problem remains whether or not other tasks requiring the integrity of the prefrontal cortex are reducible to these three mechanisms.

Acknowledgments

The author is greatly indebted to Dr. Waclawa Lawicka for many valuable comments and constructive criticism during the writing of this paper.

Most investigations performed on dogs were partly supported by Foreign Research Agreement No. 05-275-2 of U.S. Department of Health, Education and Welfare under PL 480.

Chapter 7

The Development of Operant Responses by Noradrenergic Activation and Cholinergic Suppression of Movements

D. L. MARGULES AND ADRIENNE S. MARGULES

DEPARTMENT OF PSYCHOLOGY
TEMPLE UNIVERSITY

I. Introduction

The brief presentation of a motivationally significant stimulus to an organism results in the activation of a broad spectrum of exploratory movements. These movements have consequences that exert powerful effects on the future movements of the organism. Some of these movements may be unsuccessful in producing the reoccurrence of the motivationally significant stimulus, whereas others may produce harmful consequences. Gradually, these unsuccessful or harmful movements are suppressed. When a successful movement occurs, an active organism will refine this movement by the suppression of unsuccessful variations. In this way, the movements of the organism are narrowed down and shaped into one discrete, purposeful, and highly predictable operant response. Often we ignore the long-lasting, tedious process of the suppression of unsuccessful or risky movements in the development of an operant response and overemphasize the final refinements of the response. Obviously, the operant response of pressing a bar could never have developed if the organism had failed to suppress his tendencies to wander away from it.

Two complementary processes seem to be necessary for the development of an operant response. One is the general activation of the organism's repertoire of exploratory movements upon the presentation of a motivationally significant stimulus. This could be accomplished by a neural system that carries a message of activation from the brainstem, where motivationally significant sensations are registered, to a number of motor command systems in the diencephalon and telencephalon. We propose that the norepinephrine-containing neurons in the brain mediate the general activation of a broad sequence of exploratory movements.

This theory is a version of Stein's noradrenergic theory of reward (Stein, 1969) with several important modifications.

The second process necessary for the formation of an operant response is the suppression of movements that are inefficient, ineffective, risky, or otherwise unsuccessful. This could be accomplished by a neural system that carries a message of suppression from the brainstem, where sensations of pain and frustration are registered, to the noradrenergic terminals in the diencephalon and telencephalon that initiated the movement. This process would eliminate a large number of unsuccessful movements and eventually result in the differentiation of a distinct operant response. We propose that cholinergic neurons in the brain participate in the differentiation and refinement of a specific operant response from the activated pool of exploratory movements by a continuous process of suppressing unsuccessful and risky movements. Eventually this process would reduce the pool of activated movements to those movements that appear to exert control over the motivationally significant stimulus. This theory is in agreement with the pioneering theory of Carlton (1963, 1969) on the cholinergic basis of nonreinforcement and inhibition. Carlton's theory (1963) suggests that portions of the cholinergic systems mediate the suppression of operant behavior associated with nonreinforcement (extinction). Evidence presented by Margules and Stein (1967) and Carlton (1969) extended the function of the cholinergic systems to the suppression of operant behavior associated with punishment and other inhibitory conditions.

An organism equipped with a noradrenergic activation system and a cholinergic suppression system would produce operant responses appropriate to his homeostatic needs and in harmony with his environment. He would not, however, have any way to discontinue successful operant responses. Such an organism would be trapped forever by the first motivationally significant stimulus he encountered.

Three known processes deactivate successful operant behavior. The first produces a relatively short-term deactivation known as satiety. The second produces a long-term deactivation known as sleep. The third produces a short-term deactivation associated with intense fear and freezing behavior. Recent evidence (Robichaud and Sledge, 1969) suggests that these reactions may be mediated, in part, by serotonergic neurons. Elsewhere (Margules, 1969b, 1970a, b), we present evidence that satiety for food may be mediated, in part, by high levels of norepinephrine in the hypothalamus. Sleep we believe, is mediated, in part, by an increase of serotonin levels in the brain (Jouvet, 1967; Koella and Czicman, 1966). The serotonergic deactivation system would function on a daily basis to disengage the organism from his operant endeavors. This would allow him to begin each new day at a relatively low level of activation. In effect, the serotonergic deactivation system provides a time-out period that would partially reset both cholinergic and noradrenergic activity. Systems for the deactivation of operant behavior are indispensable for a comprehensive theory of behavior. Unfortunately, we cannot deal extensively with the noradrenergic satiety, the serotonergic deactivation, or the serotonergic freezing systems in the present paper.

Movements with large respondent components such as chewing and swallowing of food are excluded from the present theory. Many theories of behavior assume that respondent and operant responses have the same motivational substrate. Thus, the rate of food-rewarded operant responses has been used as a measure of the strength of the tendency to engage in feeding responses. This assumption may be valid under certain experimental conditions; however, it is invalid during starvation, and during systemic administration of drugs such as d-amphetamine, physostigmine, and estrogen (Hamilton, 1969; Coons cited in Miller, 1960; Stark et al., 1968; Hoebel, 1969). These treatments have opposite effects on feeding responses and food-rewarded operant responses. Such dissociations indicate that the brain mechanisms that mediate feeding responses may be separate from those that control food-rewarded operant responses. In another paper (Margules and Margules, in preparation) we consider the properties of brain systems that mediate feeding responses and satiety.

The neuroanatomical circuitry of noradrenergic and cholinergic brain systems imposes constraints on theoretical interpretations of their functions. This chapter focuses on these constraints. We have given high priority to experiments based on direct chemical intervention in local brain areas. This technique can help to reveal the particular role of various brain areas in the noradrenergic activation and cholinergic suppression processes.

In order to test the noradrenergic-activation, cholinergic-suppression theory, it is necessary to quantify the process of suppression of unsuccessful or risky voluntary movements. We start with a milk-reinforced bar press response that has a stable frequency of occurrence. An organism will learn to suppress this response if it no longer produces the milk (extinction) or if it causes a painful shock to the paws (punishment). The suppression of operant responses produced by punishment can be adjusted to produce a fixed level of suppression without significant reductions of nonpunished milk-rewarded responses (Geller and Seifter, 1960). Furthermore, it is possible to alternate punished periods with periods of nonpunished voluntary responses. This provides a control baseline that is helpful in the interpretation of drug treatments that affect punished responses. The experimental technique of punishment is used extensively in this chapter. We focus on the effects of drugs placed directly in various brain areas concerned with the activation and suppression of voluntary movements.

For many years, operant behavior in mammals was believed to mediated, for the most part, by the pyramidal system. Recently, Towe (1971) has pointed out that the evidence for this assertion is at best, marginal. Towe suggests that it may be necessary to revise classical concepts of motor organization, with a shift in emphasis to subcortical mediation. The limbic system contains a number of structures known to be important in the activation and suppression of voluntary movements. The work of McCleary established the location of anatomically discrete movement-activation and movement-suppressant areas in the telecephalic portions of the limbic system. McCleary's work emphasizes the septal area, cingulate gyrus, amygdala, and hippocampus (McCleary, 1961, 1966).

The posterior diencephalic portion of the limbic system also participates in the initiation and control of voluntary movements (Hess, 1957). Electrical stimulation anywhere within Hess's dynamogenic zone (posterior hypothalamus and anterior midbrain) causes a general activation of exploratory movements. This includes a heightening of motor excitability accompanied by a discharge of the sympathetic nervous system. The overall effect prepares the organism for strenuous muscular exertion. Electrical stimulation of the medial forebrain bundle (MFB), a main pathway in the dynamogenic zone, increases locomotor exploration (Christopher and Butter, 1968), and reinforces operant responses that produce such stimulation (Olds and Milner, 1954). Finally, cuts that isolate the neural influence of the hypothalamus from the rest of the brain abolish operant responses (such as approach responses to food) without affecting consummatory feeding responses (such as swallowing) (Ellison, Sorenson, and Jacobs, 1970). The MFB may contain pathways for the activation of a broad spectrum of exploratory and operant responses.

In contrast to the broad spectrum of effects produced by electrical stimulation of the dynamogenic zone, such stimulation in a widespread anterior diencephalic region (anterior hypothalamus, supraoptic and preoptic areas, septum and inferior lateral thalamus) produces specific parasympathetic reactions that suppress motor excitability in individual organs (Hess, 1957). The particular reaction varies with the site of stimulation. Each of these reactions is antagonistic to that of the dynamogenic zone. These reactions are protective and conservative in their overall effects. The individual and site-specific organization of the parasympathetic suppressant reactions in the diencephalon contrasts sharply with the relatively diffuse organization of sympathetic activation reactions within the dynamogenic zone.

These antagonistic brain systems appear to be extensions of the autonomic nervous system postulated by Cannon (1929). Synaptic transmitter substances utilized in the periphery often are employed in the brain. For example, norepinephrine, a synaptic transmitter substance of the sympathetic nervous system in the periphery, is present in the brain (Fuxe, 1965) in dorsal and ventral pathways of the MFB (Fig. 1). Stein's theory (1969) suggests that the noradrenergic components of the MFB participate in the selection and strengthening of a specific voluntary movement by reinforcement.

The neuroanatomy of Fuxe's dorsal and ventral noradrenergic systems is not consistent with Stein's theory of the selection and strengthening of a specific response. First, Fuxe's systems consist of monosynaptic connections between

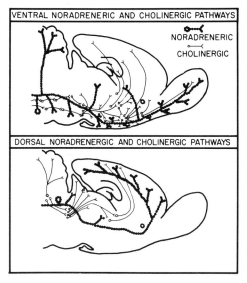

Fig. 1. The dorsal and ventral noradrenergic and cholinergic ascending neural pathways. Note that the noradrenergic pathways are monosynaptic and contain many collaterals. Activation of these pathways would release norepinephrine massively at many brain levels. In contrast, the cholinergic systems are multisynaptic chains of individual neurons. These could release acetylcholine selectively at certain brain levels and not at others (From Fuxe, Hökfett, and Ungerstedt, 1970).

the brainstem and forebrain. Monosynaptic systems are closed to a large portion of synaptic input from other brain areas. They lack the multiple sensory input necessary for a selective process. Second, Fuxe's systems have massive numbers of collaterals. Collaterals of the same neuron would release the same synaptic transmitter substance at all their synaptic terminals. Therefore, activation of dorsal or ventral noradrenergic pathways would cause a massive release of norepinephrine in many forebrain structures, simultaneously. This massive release of norepinephrine argues against the selective activation of a particular response. The "zeroing in" on a particular response may depend on a nonnoradrenergic system that can release its transmitter selectively in individual forebrain areas.

The specific function of norepinephrine in each forebrain area is not known, but self-stimulation studies indicate that electrical excitation of both dorsal (Margules, 1969a) and ventral (Dresse, 1966) noradrenergic pathways produce high rates of response. It is interesting to note that the most consistent response elicited by electrical stimulation of self-stimulation sites is increased locomotor exploration (Christopher and Butter, 1968). If we assume that all collaterals of the same axon mediate effects that are physiologically and behaviorally related, then the function of norepinephrine in forebrain structures must be consistent with an increase in positive reinforcement and locomotion. The activation of an organism's repertoire of exploratory movements is consistent with such increases. This activation of movements would provide the organism with an adaptive mechanism in new and potentially rewarding situations.

The trained organism has developed an effective response, appropriate to the experimental situation. He no longer makes movements that delay or interfere with successful responding. It would appear that the trained organism has inhibited unsuccessful movements. In trained organisms, experimental manipulations that release norepinephrine in the brain (such as self-stimulation) cause increases in a trained movement but very little general activation of movements. For example, electrical stimulation of self-stimulation sites during a Sidman avoidance test increases relevant operant responses much more than irrelevant lever responses that have no programmed consequences (Margules and Stein, 1968). Perhaps, during the training of animals, strong suppressant influences develop that prevent or counteract the release of norepinephrine in those forebrain areas not concerned with the trained response. The suppressant influences that develop during training may originate from cholinergic systems in the brain (Carlton, 1963).

A system that suppresses maladaptive movements must be strongly attuned to many aspects of the environment. Information about the environment is represented in multiple sensory systems that provide input to many brain areas, including the reticular formation of the brainstem. This area contains polysynaptic chains of neurons that are open to afferent input of an extremely divergent nature (Ramón-Moliner and Nauta, 1966). Moreover, the long dendrites of reticular formation neurons and hypothalamic neurons overlap extensively and may form dendrodendritic synapses (Millhouse, 1969). These may provide a mechanism for gradients of lateral inhibition, which would sharpen sensory discriminations (Rall and Shepherd, 1968). A system that is armed with accurate and current sensory information would be well equipped to select behaviors to be suppressed.

Acetylcholine, the synaptic transmitter substance of the peripheral parasympathetic nervous system, is present in the reticular formation in two multisynaptic chains of cholinesterase-containing neurons; the ascending dorsal tegmental pathway, and the ascending ventral tegmental pathway (Fig. 1) (Shute and Lewis, 1967; Lewis and Shute, 1970). According to Shute and Lewis, there are no descending cholinergic pathways. The ascending cholinergic pathways that arise from the reticular formation appear to have many of the anatomical requirements necessary for the suppression of an operant response. These multisynaptic pathways are open to a variety of synaptic inputs that can promptly modify their activity. Moreover, these systems contain multiple independent pathways between the reticular formation and the forebrain. This arrangement allows acetylcholine to be released discretely in an individual forebrain area. Such a release would suppress a particular movement without affecting other movement tendencies. The location and arrangement of the cholinergic pathways is ideally suited to convey inhibitory feedback from unsuccessful movements to the forebrain. The release of acetylcholine in the forebrain could prevent the reoccurrence of specific unsuccessful movements. Cholinergic systems may allow the organism to profit from past experiences by the feedback of corrective information concerning maladaptive movements. In the present studies, norepinephrine, a noradrenergic synaptic transmitter, and atropine, a cholinergic receptor blocker were bilaterally applied directly to specific brain areas by means of chronically implanted cannulae of variable depth (Morris, Walker, and Margules, 1970).

II. The Suppression of Operant Behavior Associated with Punishment

A multiple schedule of reinforcement developed by Geller (Geller and Seifter, 1960), provides a sensitive measure of the effects of drugs that intensify or abolish the suppression of operant behavior. Subjects maintained at a body weight of 300 gm perform operant responses for a 0.2 ml sweet milk reward in a Skinner box. They work for 72 min on a VI-2 schedule of reinforcement, a schedule relatively sparse in reward density. This schedule generates a slow, steady rate of nonpunished responding.

At fixed intervals during a 72-min session, a tone comes on for a 3-min period, which indicates a change in the reinforcement schedule. During tone periods, milk is available on every lever press, a schedule of optimal reward density. Each response, however, also produces a ¼-sec electrical shock to the paws. The intensity of this shock is adjusted in gradual steps during tone periods until operant responses are almost completely suppressed. Operant responses during the VI-2 periods remain at relatively high rates, indicating that the punished behavior is under good stimulus control. Patterns of responses are stable with this procedure for many months of testing.

In the Geller reward-punishment test, systemic administration of antifear agents such as meprobamate (Geller and Seifter, 1960) and oxazepam (Margules and Stein, 1967) disinhibit suppressed operant responses. The reward-punishment test also is sensitive to the effect of elimination of punishment when the foot shock is reduced to zero (Margules and Stein, 1967). If the decrease of pain can cause a release of suppressed voluntary behavior, then the increase of pain and/or the expectation of increased pain (fear) should intensify the suppression of operant behavior associated with punishment. In order to determine the effects of increased pain, a partially suppressed (low shock) reward-punishment baseline was established. The fifth cranial nerve, which carries sensations of pain on the face, was stimulated for .15 sec every second, in rats. The parameters of electrical stimulation are reported elsewhere (Margules, 1969a). Such stimulation was presented 3 min before punishment periods, during punishment periods, and 3 min after punishment periods.

Repeated stimulation of the fifth cranial nerve significantly suppressed responses during the tone periods, but did not suppress the response rate during nonpunishment periods (Fig. 2, panels A and B). Apparently, a summation of peripheral and central pain inputs occurred during the punishment periods. The suppressant effects of this stimulation also were observed on the day after the experiment (Fig. 2, panel C). This experiment demonstrates that a centrally applied painful stimulus can selectively intensify the suppression of operant movements associated with peripherally applied pain.

The initial stimulation of the fifth cranial nerve during the prepunishment period, caused a decrease in responses (Fig. 2, panel B 25 ua), but subsequent stimulation periods at higher intensities showed normal and moderately increased rates of nonpunished responses (particularly in the pretone periods). The centrally induced pain appeared to have a response-increasing effect during nonpunishment periods. Both punishment and nonpunished responses returned to their respective prestimulation control baselines, from 2 to 5 days after stimulation of the fifth cranial nerve (Fig. 2, panel D).

III. Evidence for a Cholinergic Punishment System in the Periventricular Hypothalamus (PVS)

The hypothalamic portion of the system, which participates in the suppression of feeding behavior by satiety (Anand and Brobeck, 1951) also participates

EFFECTS OF ELECTRICAL STIMULATION OF Ⅴ™ NERVE ON THE
REWARD - PUNISHMENT TEST

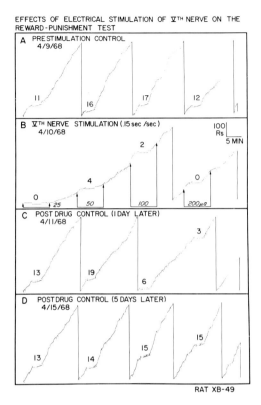

RAT XB-49

Fig. 2. Cumulative records of operant responses in the reward-punishment test before, during, and after painful stimulation of the fifth cranial nerve. Each response makes the pen move upward a constant step. Downgoing slashes represent milk-reward responses during the nonpunished (VI-2) schedule of reinforcement. The punishment periods are represented by the offset position of the stepper pen with upgoing slashes indicating punished operant responses. The numbers above the punishment periods indicate the total number of punished responses. The stepper pen resets every 500 responses. In panel B, stimulation of the fifth cranial nerve occurred continuously (0.15 sec every second) during the time indicated by each set of connected arrows. The current level is indicated in microámps for each set of arrows.

in the suppression of operant behavior associated with punishment. Damage to the PVS by bilateral insertion of cannulae (Margules and Stein, 1969b) or by electrolytic lesions (Kaada, Rasmusssen and Kveim, 1962; Sclafani and Grossman, 1971) substantially reduces the suppression of operant behavior associated with punishment (i.e., produced a passive-avoidance deficit). Conversely, electrical stimulation of the PVS intensifies the suppression of operant movements (Delgado, Roberts, and Miller, 1954; Fernandez de Molina and Hunsberger, 1959; Hess, 1957; Krasne, 1962).

A number of drugs that influence cholinergic synaptic transmission have effects in the PVS consistent with the theory that the suppression of voluntary behavior associated with punishment is mediated by acetylcholine, acting as a synaptic transmitter substance. Carbachol, a cholinomimetic agent that is impervious to enzymic degradation, completely suppresses punished and nonpunished responses both in the reward-punishment test (Margules and Stein, 1967) and in a modified version of the reward-punishment test (Sepinwall and Grodsky, 1969). Neostigmine, an anticholinesterase agent with cholinomimetic properties, has a similar effect that lasts several days (Margules and Stein, 1969b). Physostigmine, an anticholinesterase agent that increases endogenous acetylcholine, has a smaller suppressant effect, but again, both punished and nonpunished responses are affected (Margules and Stein, 1967, 1969b; Sepinwall and Grodsky, 1969). These results may be due to a drug-induced intensification of suppression and its generalization to the nonpunished responses, or they may be the result of a general incapacitation. As a test of these alternatives, physostigmine hydrochloride was bilaterally applied to the PVS (at a dose of $10\mu g$) under two experimental variations of the reward-punishment test, low shock and no shock. In the first test, the intensity of the punishing foot shock was low during tone periods and, as a result, responses during punishment periods were only partially suppressed (Fig. 3, panel A). In the second test, the intensity of the foot shock was reduced to zero for several weeks. There was a full release of responses during tone periods, before drug treatments were begun (Fig. 3, panel C). If physostigmine hydrochloride has a general depressant action, responses during both experimental procedures should be suppressed. If, however, the presence of punishment is necessary for physostigmine to suppress responses, this treatment should fail to suppress responses during the zero shock test, but would suppress responses during the low shock situation. This is exactly what occurred as shown in panel D of Fig. 2. A dose of physostigmine that had a substantial suppressant effect on punished as well as nonpunished responses in the low shock test (Fig. 3, panel B), did not suppress significantly total responses in the zero shock test. Similar results were obtained in two other rats (Margules, 1971a).

These results can be explained by the known mechanism of action of physostigmine. This drug acts by poisoning the endogenous enzyme, cholinesterase, which is responsible for the degradation of acetylcholine in the synaptic cleft. Without this enzyme, acetylcholine released from presynaptic terminals accumulates in extra quantities and exerts an intensified effect on the postsynaptic receptor site. This suggests that physostigmine intensifies the suppressant effects of punishment by increasing the accumulation of endogenous acetylcholine in the synaptic cleft. When punishment is absent (zero shock), no acetylcholine would be released and therefore, no acetylcholine could accumulate when cholinesterase is poisoned by physostigmine. A cholinergic system that

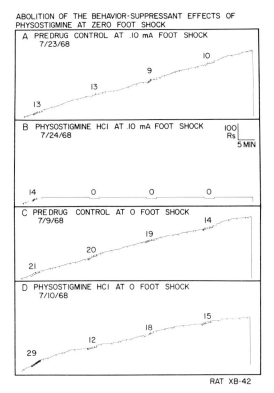

ABOLITION OF THE BEHAVIOR-SUPPRESSANT EFFECTS OF
PHYSOSTIGMINE AT ZERO FOOT SHOCK

RAT XB-42

Fig. 3. The influence of direct bilateral placement of physostigmine HCL in the PVS on punished and nonpunished operant responses. When foot shock was low, physostigmine suppressed both punished and nonpunished responses (panels A and B). When foot shock was eliminated and abolition of punishment had occurred, the same treatment with physostigmine failed to suppress either total punished or total nonpunished responses (panels C and D). A detailed analysis of panel D indicates a biphasic effect of physostigmine treatment. Early in the test physostigmine has the opposite effect, as indicated by the small increase of punished responses during the first punishment period (panel D). Note the similarity in time of onset of the physostigmine action in panels B and D (about 6 min into the test). Later in the test physostigmine has a small suppressant effect as indicated by the decreased response rate before, during, and after the second tone period (panel D). The details on the generation of these cumulative records are given in the caption for Fig. 2.

has access to sensory information could respond promptly to the absence of foot shock. When punishment is absent, no acetylcholine need be released, whereas a mildly painful shock would require small amounts of acetylcholine to control behavior. A large release of acetylcholine might accompany highly painful shock, and behavior would be severely curtailed.

Consistent with the proposal that cholinergic synapses in the PVS suppress operant behavior associated with punishment, bilateral placement of atropine methyl nitrate, a cholinergic blocker of muscarinic receptors, disinhibits punished behavior (Margules and Stein, 1967, 1969a, b; Sepinwall and Grodsky, 1969).

Punished responses are not the only responses disinhibited by direct bilateral application of atropine methyl nitrate to the PVS (Margules, 1967; Margules and Stein, 1969a). This treatment also disinhibits a general assortment of irrelevant movements; exploratory locomotion, head-bobbing, etc. The overall effect is to make the organism less effective by the reintroduction of this assortment of unsuccessful or risky movements. The release of these behaviors by cholinergic blockade strongly suggests that the cholinergic system of the PVS normally maintains inhibitory control over such movements.

This release of assorted suppressed behaviors caused by atropine suggests that the suppression of behavior is mediated by the occupation of the muscarinic type of cholinergic receptor in the PVS. Here, we assume that atropine prevents endogenously released acetylcholine from occupation of muscarinic receptor sites. To test this hypothesis we must determine if blockade of muscarinic receptors by atropine methyl nitrate could reverse a physostigmine-induced intensification of punishment. First, it is clear that atropine methyl nitrate administered bilaterally to the PVS at a 20-μg dose reduced the suppressant effects of punishment (Fig. 4, panels A and B). Such treatment with physostigmine hydrochloride strongly suppressed both punished and nonpunished responses (Fig. 4, panel C). When atropine was administered after a physostigmine-induced suppression was fully established, both punished and nonpunished responses returned to previous atropine-induced levels (Fig. 4, panels B, C, and D). The blockade of muscarinic receptors by atropine apparently prevents their occupation by the physostigmine-induced accumulation of endogenous acetylcholine. This supports the theory that endogenous acetylcholine in the PVS mediates the suppression of voluntary behavior associated with punishment, by occupation of muscarinic receptors. Thus, the suppression of a learned operant response associated with punishment may be mediated in part by a release of endogenous acetylcholine in PVS.

In order for acetylcholine to be released at the appropriate point in time, the cholinergic system must have access sensory representations of the foot shock and the bar-pressing response. It also must have access to the motor system. Finally, it must have access to some representation of the results of past bar-pressing responses. The cholinergic response suppression system must have a memory mechanism.

IV. A Glycinergic Influence of Long-Lasting Duration in the Periventricular Hypothalamus

Glycine has been put forth as a candidate for a synaptic transmitter substance in the central system (Curtis *et al.*, 1968; Werman, Davidoff, and Aprison,

REVERSAL OF PHYSOSTIGMINE INDUCED SUPPRESSION OF BEHAVIOR
BY METHYL ATROPINE

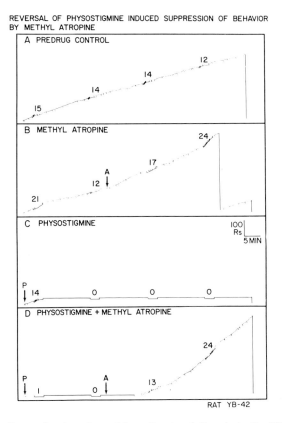

RAT YB-42

Fig. 4. The effects of various drugs, bilaterally placed directly in the PVS, on punished and nonpunished operant responses in the reward-punishment test. Note that the effects of a dose of physostigmine that completely suppresses both punished and nonpunished responses (panel C) are reversed by the direct bilateral application of methyl atropine nitrate (panel D). The details on the generation of these cumulative records are given in Fig. 2.

1968). Glycine meets many of the requirements for transmitter identity. First, it is present in the central nervous system (Aprison, Shank, and Davidoff, 1969). The application of glycine to the spinal cord (Werman *et al.,* 1968) and medulla (Hösli, Tebecis, and Filias, 1969) hyperpolarizes neurons with greater potency than gamma-aminobutyric acid (GABA), another potential synaptic transmitter substance. This depressant action of glycine is blocked by strychnine, a selective blocker of postsynaptic inhibition that fails to block the depressant action of GABA. Glycine and other amino acids are released from brain slices during electrical stimulation (Katz, Chase, and Kopin, 1969). These data have been interpreted as evidence that glycine is a major synaptic transmitter substance (Werman *et al.,* 1968; Curtis *et al.,* 1968). The interpretation that glycine serves as a neuroregulator rather than a neurotransmitter also has been suggested (Katz *et al.,* 1969).

In the reward-punishment test, glycine (bilaterally applied at a dose of 20 μg) has a weak suppressant effect at sites in the PVS where atropine causes a large disinhibition of suppressed behavior. Such treatment reduced punished responses from the predrug control of 5 to 2 ($P < .05$), and nonpunished responses from the predrug control of 4567 to 3497 ($P < .05$). On the day after this treatment, punished responses (5) and nonpunished responses (4739) returned to predrug control levels. Essentially the same results were obtained with a group of four rats. A typical record is shown in Fig. 6, panels A and B.

Pretreatment of PVS sites with strychnine sulfate (bilaterally applied at a dose of 20 μg) abolishes the weak suppressant effect of glycine on punished as well as nonpunished responses. The reversal was complete on the day of the treatment, with no effects (such as rebounds or undershots) on the day after the treatment. This result was obtained in three of four rats tested. Strychnine is known to block the electrophysiological effect induced by glycine. This block is selective; other stimulants such as picrotoxin fail to antagonize glycine-induced hyperpolarizations. This has led to the proposal of a specific strychnine-sensitive glycine receptor (Curtis, Duggan, and Johnston, 1969). According to these authors, the reversal of a glycine-induced suppression of behavior by strychnine would constitute strong evidence for glycinergic receptor sites. Glycinergic receptor sites may participate in the suppression of operant behavior.

To further investigate the weak suppressant properties of glycine, this drug was administered bilaterally in the PVS, 5 min before bilateral treatment with atropine methyl nitrate. In a control test, the atropine treatment was shown to have a large disinhibitory effect on suppressed responses (Fig. 5, panels A and B). The pretreatment with glycine substantially reduced the disinhibitory action of atropine (Fig. 5, panel C). The animal no longer showed high rates of punished responding. This effect was long lasting. Bilateral treatment with atropine alone, 1 week later, did not produce the large release of behavior typical of atropine treatment. That is, 1 week after the glycine pretreatment, the antisuppressant action of atropine methyl nitrate was still substantially reduced (Fig. 5, panel D). The following week, atropine was again applied to the PVS. In this second week, after glycine pretreatment, the antisuppressant action of atropine was still not completely restored. Total punished and nonpunished responses were still slightly below preglycine control (compare panels E and B, Fig. 5). These findings indicate that glycine exerts a strong and long-lasting interference with the antisuppressant action of atropine. Long-lasting chemically induced changes in behavior are of particular interest in relation to the neurochemical basis of memory. Glycine acting as a neurotransmitter or as a neuroregulator in the PVS may be part of a memory circuit that provides a storage mechanism for cholinergically suppressed information.

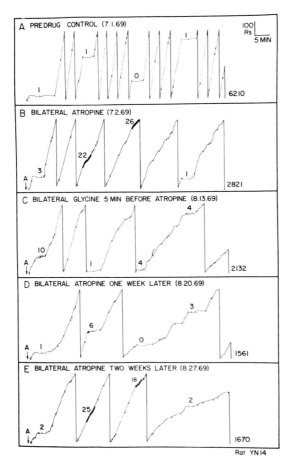

Fig. 5. The effects of various drugs, bilaterally placed directly in the PVS on punished and nonpunished operant responses in the reward-punishment test. Pretreatment with glycine 5 min before methyl atropine reduces methyl atropine's antipunishment properties (panels B and C). One week later bilateral application of atropine has a very weak antipunishment effect (panels D and B). Two weeks later bilateral application of atropine produces an antipunishment effect (panel E) almost back to control (panel B). The details on the generation of these cumulative records are given in Fig. 2.

In summary, bilateral application of glycine to the PVS produces a small decrease in responses when punishment is intense. Although glycine shows only a weak suppressant effect, it is a powerful antagonist of the strong suppressant effect of atropine for periods as long as 2 weeks.

The weak suppressant effect of glycine may be antagonized by systemic administration of the "antifear" agent oxazepam. It has been shown that the systemic administration of oxazepam effectively antagonizes the intense suppression of voluntary behavior caused by direct bilateral placement of carbachol into the PVS (Margules and Stein, 1967).

In the present study, systemically administered oxazepam failed to reverse the weak suppressant effect of glycine bilaterally placed in the PVS, but effectively reversed the strong suppressant effect of carbachol bilaterally placed at this same site (Fig. 6, panel D). At this site in the PVS, the weak suppressant effect of glycine apparently cannot be reversed by systemic administration of oxazepam at a dose that reverses the strong suppressant effects of carbachol.

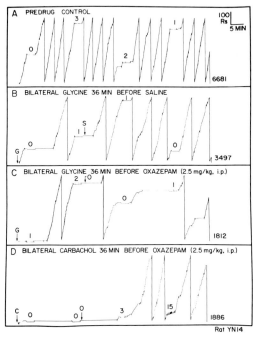

Fig. 6. Comparisons of effects of systemic administration of oxazepam (2.5 mg/kg, i.p) on the glycine- and carbachol-induced suppressions of punished and nonpunished responses in the reward-punishment test. Note that the oxazepam treatment easily reverses the intense suppression produced by direct bilateral placement of carbachol into the PVS (panel D). Note also that the same oxazepam treatment fails to reverse the weak suppression produced by direct bilateral placement of glycine into the PVS (panel C). Oxazepam appears to intensify the suppression of nonpunished responses produced by glycine (panels B and C). The details on the generation of these cumulative records are given in Fig. 2.

V. Atropine Disinhibits Suppressed Behaviors at Sites Where Norepinephrine Is Ineffective

Direct bilateral placement of atropine in the PVS caused a large disinhibition of suppressed behavior. Norepinephrine failed to elicit such effects at these same sites (Margules and Stein, 1969b). Atropine also has large antisuppression effects at bilateral sites in the dorsal and ventral hippocampal gyrus (see Fig. 7) (Margules and Lowes, in preparation), and in the entopeduncular nucleus (Margules, 1971b). Norepinephrine was relatively ineffective in these areas.

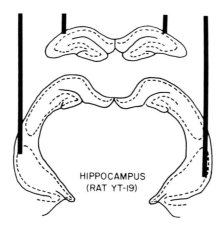

Fig. 7. The location of cannulas in the dorsal and ventral hippocampal gyri of a typical rat used to generate the results in Fig. 8.

Figure 8 shows that bilateral placement of atropine in the dorsal and ventral hippocampal gyrus produced a much larger disinhibition of punished operant responses in the reward-punishment test than such treatment with *dl*-norepinephrine. Direct treatment of the hippocampal gyrus with atropine also reduced nonpunished operant responses in this test (from the mean predrug control of 2482 to 1015). The PVS, hippocampal gyrus, and entopeduncular nucleus appear to contain a cholinergic system or systems for the suppression of operant behavior associated with punishment. They do not appear to contain major elements of the noradrenergic-activation system. Verification of the presence of cholinergic synaptic terminals in the entopeduncular nucleus, hippocampus, and periventricular system has been provided by the work of Shute and Lewis (1967).

VI. Separation of Brain Systems for Operant and Consummatory Responses

For several years evidence has been accumulating that indicates that separation exists in the brain between those systems concerned with operant responses and those concerned with consummatory responses. This mounting evidence appears to contradict several theoretical explanations of food-motivated behavior outlined in Hoebel's comprehensive review (1971). These theories make the assumption that operant response rates can be used as an

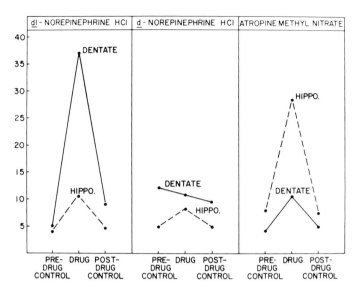

Fig. 8. The effects of various bilateral drug treatments placed directly in the dorsal and ventral hippocampal gyrus are compared to such treatments placed directly in the dorsal and ventral dentate gyrus on punished responses in the reward-punishment test. Numbers along the ordinate represent mean punished responses.

accurate index of the reward value of food in the hungry organism. This basic assumption is firmly embedded in the literature of physiological psychology and is worth reexamination.

Consummatory and operant responses usually employ different muscles in their execution. There must be separation of the central motor neurons that mediate these responses. The crucial question is whether or not separation exists in the central nervous system at levels concerned with the activation and the suppression of movements.

A. Dissociation of Activation Systems for Operant and Consummatory Responses

A number of pharmacological treatments have opposite effects on operant and consummatory responses. Systemic administration of *d*-amphetamine, an agent that causes the release of norepinephrine in the brain (Stein and Wise, 1969), lowers self-stimulation thresholds, but raises thresholds of electrically elicited feeding obtained from the same brain site (Coons, cited in Miller, 1960; Stark and Totty, 1967). This treatment also increases operant responses for food without increasing food consumption (Weissman, 1962). Amphetamine is not the only treatment that produces dissociations between food-reward operant responses and consummatory behavior. Systemic administration of drugs that decrease general movements, such as chlorpromazine, decreases food-rewarded operant responses, but increases feeding responses (Stolerman, 1967; Margules and Stein, 1967). Systemic administration of physostigmine increases thresholds for self-stimulation responses but decreases thresholds for stimulus-bound feeding at the same site (Stark *et al.*, 1968). Systemic administration of estrogen increases rates of self-stimulation from the lateral hypothalamic sites but decreases feeding responses (Hoebel, 1969). Pfaffmann also has emphasized the dissociation between consummatory and operant responses. In the same animal, two different sugars elicited equal rates of consummatory responses but unequal rates of operant responses (Pfaffmann, 1969). It is difficult to reconcile this large body of experiments with a theory that the same noradrenergic cells that are responsible for the activation of food-rewarded operant responses also activate feeding responses (Berger, Wise, and Stein, 1971).

B. Dissociation of Suppression Systems for Operant and Consummatory Responses

Blockade of cholinergic synapses in the PVS by direct bilateral application of atropine methyl nitrate disinhibits operant responses for a milk reward suppressed by satiety or by punishment, but suppresses milk licking responses (Margules, 1967; Margules and Stein, 1969a). Rats under this treatment increase operant responses for milk but fail to consume the milk they earn. Recently this paradoxical result has been confirmed by Miczac and Grossman (personal communication). Apparently, the cholinergic system that suppresses operant behavior does not suppress feeding behavior. In their analysis of this result, Margules and Stein (1969a) postulated that neurons in the PVS that suppress feeding responses (Anand and Pillai, 1967), either fail to form synaptic terminals in the hypothalamus or form noncholinergic synaptic terminals there. Recent evidence favors the latter alternative and suggests that the noncholinergic synapses in the hypothalamus for the suppression of feeding by satiety may be noradrenergic (Margules, 1969b, 1970a,b).

The atropine-induced dissociation of food-rewarded operant responses and feeding responses constitutes a pharmacological dissection of an operant response suppression system from its underlying consummatory response suppression system. In the preceding section, we reviewed evidence that suggests a similar separation exists between the activation systems for operant and consummatory responses. The same concept is used by Vanderwolf, Bland, and Whishaw in their analysis of hippocampal mechanisms in the control of movements (Chapter 8). At the present time, the neurochemical basis for the consummatory activation system is unknown. Preliminary evidence exists for two candidates, norepinephrine (Grossman, 1962) and acetylcholine (Stark *et al.*, 1968). If the candidacy of acetylcholine receives additional experimental support, there would be perfect symmetry between the systems for the activation and suppression of operant and consummatory responses. Norepinephrine appears to activate operant responses and to suppress consummatory responses. Acetylcholine appears to suppress operant responses and may activate consummatory responses.

VII. Selectivity of Action of the Cholinergic Suppression System in the Septal Area

Recent evidence indicates that a deficit in striatal dopamine may be responsible for the adipsia associated with the lateral hypothalamic syndrome. This suggests that striatal dopamine may participate in the initiation of thirst.

The cholinergic system in the hypothalamus that suppresses operant movements does not appear to participate in the suppression of consummatory responses. Further evidence for specificity of function of the cholinergic system has been obtained in the septal area (Hamilton, McCleary, and Grossman, 1968). These authors found that blockade of cholinergic synapses in the septal area by atropine caused a punishment deficit, and a deficit in extinction, but failed to affect performance of a position-habit reversal problem, or the acquisition of a one-way avoidance problem. Lesions of the septal area caused deficits on all four problems. This indicates that use of a battery of tests will be most likely to identify further specificities of function in cholinergic suppression systems (McCleary, personal communication).

VIII. Functions of the Noradrenergic Neurons in the Amygdala

On the basis of the neuroanatomy of the noradrenergic system of collaterals, any stimulus that activates this system would cause a release of norepinephrine in many diencephalic and telencephalic brain areas simultaneously. The neuroanatomy of this system does not permit a discrete release of norepinephrine in a single brain area. It is of considerable interest therefore that direct placement of exogenous norepinephrine and epinephrine, but not dopamine, dopa, or serotonin, into one highly localized region of the amygdala has a large antipunishment action (Fig. 9) (Margules, 1968, 1972). It is of further interest that this treatment is highly specific; it increases punished operant responses for food without increasing nonpunished operant responses for food. An increase such as this may be due to an increase in reward or it may be the result of a decrease in the suppressant effects of punishment. If placement of norepinephrine in the amygdala increased reward, nonpunished as well as punished responses should increase. The failure of this increase to occur suggests that the effects of punishment have been decreased. Thus, the increase in punished responses caused by such treatment appears to be a disinhibitory effect.

The disinhibition of punished responses induced by placement of norepinephrine in the amygdala is much more specific than the disinhibitions induced by

EFFECTS OF DIRECT APPLICATION OF DRUGS TO THE AMYGDALA ON PUNISHED BEHAVIOR

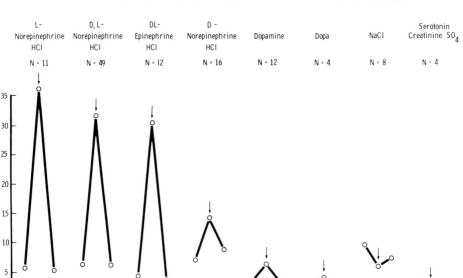

Fig. 9. Effects of direct bilateral application of various drugs to the amygdala on punished responses in the reward-punishment test. Arrows indicate the day of bilateral application of the drugs.

placement of atropine in the hypothalamus. Atropine-induced disinhibitions of punished responses are accompanied by disinhibitions of exploratory behaviors and repetitive movements such as head-bobbing. A disinhibition of operant responses for food that is dissociated from consummatory feeding responses occurs also (Margules, 1967; Margules and Stein, 1969a). The overall effect of placement of the anticholinergic drug, atropine, in the hypothalamus is similar to the activation of the broad spectrum of behaviours produced by systemic administration of amphetamine. This sympathomimetic agent causes a massive release of norepinephrine (and other biogenic amines) in many brain areas. Placement of atropine in the hypothalamus may allow norepinephrine to predominate in many brain areas by blockade of the cholinergic suppressant systems. The cholinergic suppressant systems have been described as a multisynaptic set of series circuits between the brainstem and the forebrain. Multisynaptic systems that form series circuits become nonfunctional at all sites at and above a blockade. Therefore, the cholinergic block induced by placement of atropine in the hypothalamus may remove all cholinergic suppressant influences at sites in and above the hypothalamus.

Direct bilateral placement of norepinephrine in the amygdala affects only a small fraction of the total number of noradrenergic collaterals. More precisely, it affects one branch of a parallel circuit. Activation of a branch of such a circuit would not influence other parallel branches, nor would it influence series circuits attached to these branches.

The noradrenergic terminals in the amygdala may increase punished responses by a direct effect on motor command cells in the amygdala or they may have an indirect influence by an effect on cholinergic systems in other brain areas. The theories of Stein (1969) and Carlton (1969) assume that noradrenergic terminals on forebrain cells in amygdala, hippocampus, and other brain areas increase punished behavior by an inhibitory action on descending cholinergic neurons that activate the PVS suppression system. At the present time there is no anatomical support for such descending cholinergic connections (Lewis and Shute, 1970). It is possible that the noradrenergic activation system may gain inhibitory control over specific cholinergic suppressant systems by way of descending noncholinergic connections from the forebrain. This would provide a means of removal of suppressant influences that no longer provide adaptive movements. It is also possible that the amygdala contains motor command cells that receive both direct noradrenergic messages of activation and direct cholinergic messages of suppression. Finally, it is possible that the noradrenergic terminals form synapses directly on motor command cells in the amygdala and other forebrain structures, and that the cholinergic terminals act indirectly by presynaptic inhibition of these nordrenergic terminals. According to this view, cholinergic influences would act as governors of operant behavior. A recent experiment provides support for this theory (Margules and Margules, submitted). The suppression of operant behavior produced in the initial segments of a fixed-interval schedule of reinforcement was shown to be uninfluenced by cholinergic stimulation or blockade of the PVS. In contrast, these treatments produced large effects on operant behavior produced in the terminal segments of the fixed-interval schedule at the time of maximal noradrenergic activation of behavior. These results suggest that noradrenergic cells must be active in order for the cholinergic and anticholinergic drugs to exert their effects. Once noradrenergic cells are active, cholinergic presynaptic influences would increase and begin to regulate the noradrenergic activity. Cholinergic suppressant influences could not build up until the noradrenergic facilitation system is activated. It should be possible, however, for an animal to suppress behavior even though he is not particularly aroused or activated. Recently, other suppression systems have been identified that may mediate this function. These systems release the synaptic transmitter substance known as serotonin and have a monosynaptic pathway that parallels the noradrenergic system (Fuxe, 1965). We assume that these systems suppress behavior by a direct action on motor command cells in the forebrain. Thus, the serotonergic freezing system and the serotonergic sleep system (Robichaud and Sledge, 1969) may provide the necessary link to deactivate operant behavior directly without prior noradrenergic activation.

It has been possible to localize the precise region of the amygdala responsible for the increase in punished responses caused by norepinephrine. This appears to be the dorsal portion of the corticomedial division of the amygdala (Margules, 1971b). The nucleus amygdaloideus centralis seems to be the most likely site in this region for norepinephrine's action.

It also has been possible to specify the adrenergic receptor site in the amygdala where norepinephrine causes its effect. This appears to be an alpha-adrenergic receptor site. Direct bilateral pretreatment of the amygdala with alpha, but not a beta-adrenergic receptor blocker, reduces the disinhibitory action of norepinephrine. Moreover, direct bilateral treatment of the amygdala with a beta-adrenergic stimulant, isoproterenol, has the opposite effect: it intensifies the suppressant effects of punishment (Margules, 1972). This finding suggests that beta-adrenergic receptors in the amygdala antagonize the effects of alpha receptors. In summary, the amygdala is differentiated from medial hypothalamus, the hippocampus, and the entopeduncular nucleus by a double pharmacological dissociation. These three brain areas appear to contain components of cholinergic systems that mediate the suppression of operant movements by punishment and other suppressant influences. The amygdala appears to contain a noradrenergic system that facilitates voluntary behavioral movements by a direct action on motor command cells in the limbic system and forebrain. This system is controlled by a cholinergic governor that appears to act by presynaptic inhibition. Finally, the noradrenergic system appears to be directly antagonized, at the level of the motor command cells, by serotonergic systems that deactivate operant movements. The noradrenergic and serotonergic systems have anatomical features indicative of nonspecific behavioral reactions (general activation and deactivation of a broad sequence of exploratory movements respectively). The cholinergic system has an anatomical arrangement that allows specificity and selection of behavioral responses by a process of elimination of noradrenergically activated movements that have been unsuccessful or risky.

IX. Norepinephrine Has an Antipunishment Action in the Dentate Gyrus

The dentate gyrus contains a high density of noradrenergic synaptic terminals in the zone just below the granular layer (Fuxe, 1965). These terminals disappear ipsilaterally, after lesions of A-10, a region rich in noradrenergic cell bodies. Prolonged self-stimulation causes a reversible decrease in the fluorescence of these terminals, an indication of exhaustion of norepinephrine reserves. These findings were interpreted as support for the proposal that the noradrenergic neurons of A-10 provide the anatomical substrate for self-stimulation (Dresse, 1966). This suggests that the release of norepinephrine in the dentate gyrus would have behavioral effects consistent with reward. In order to test this proposal, crystalline *dl*-norepinephrine hydrochloride was applied bilaterally to the dorsal and ventral portions of the dentate gyrus in three rats. Typical sites are shown in Fig. 10. Treatments with *dl*-norepinephrine HCl but not atropine methyl nitrate, produced a large increase in punished operant responses in the reward-punishment test as shown in Fig. 7. Such treatment with *d*-norepinephrine failed to have this effect. Nonpunished responses were also increased by treatment with *dl*-norepinephrine hydrochloride (from a mean predrug control level of 2300 to 3076) but not by the other drug treatments. The increases in nonpunished as well as punished responses suggests that the function of norepinephrine in the dentate gyrus is to increase the reinforcing effects of reward.

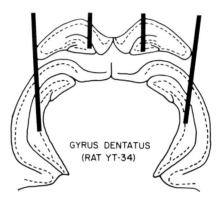

GYRUS DENTATUS
(RAT YT-34)

Fig. 10. The location of cannulas in the dorsal and ventral dentate gyrus of a typical rat used to generate the results in Fig. 8.

Olds (1969) suggests that the dentate gyrus may be part of a computerlike biological memory mechanism. Highly rewarded events are easily retained in memory and events that have little motivational significance are quickly forgotten. The function of noradrenergic synaptic terminals in the dentate gyrus may be to activate a storage mechanism, or to inhibit a forgetting mechanism. In either case, noradrenergic messages of reward that reach the dentate gyrus could ensure that a highly rewarding event becomes a memorable one.

The hippocampal gyrus also has been implicated in the formation of memories (Olds, 1969). Here direct bilateral placement of atropine methyl nitrate increased responses during the punishment periods (Fig. 7) and decreased responses during the nonpunished periods (from the mean predrug control of 2482 to 1015). This same pattern of responses occurs when the suppressant effects of punishment are abolished by reduction of foot shock to zero. At zero shock, the continuous reinforcement schedule (CRF) produces much greater incentive for responses than the VI-2 schedule. As a result of this, VI-2 responses decline as responses during CRF increase. During atropine treatment, this same pattern occurs and this suggests that the atropine treatment has reduced the suppressant effects of punishment. This could be the result, at least in part, of an atropine-induced selective amnesia for painful events. The hippocampal gyrus may contain part of a cholinergic system for the suppression of movements associated with painful memories. We would like to tentatively suggest that cholinergic messages of pain and frustration that reach the hippocampal gyrus activate a memory mechanism which preserves painful events. These could be used on future occasions to help prevent the reoccurrence of maladaptive movements.

X. Summary

Evidence is presented in this chapter for a reevaluation of traditional concepts of somatosensory integration of voluntary movements. The output of the pyramidal system is deemphasized as the main determinant of movements. Instead, emphasis is placed on multiple motor outputs from structures in the limbic system.

Motor mechanisms in the limbic system appear to be concerned with operant movements (such as pressing a lever for a milk reward) and not with respondent movements (such as swallowing the milk). These operant movement neurons are postulated to receive three main inputs: one is an excitatory noradrenergic input from cells in the brainstem where motivationally significant sensations are registered and expectations are formed of the reoccurrence of those sensations. Another is an inhibitory cholinergic input from other cells in the brainstem where stimuli associated with recently made unsuccessful and risky movements are registered. The noradrenergic input appears to be governed presynaptically by the cholinergic suppression system. The third input consists of direct serotonergic connections with operant movement neurons, which cause a general deactivation of behavior.

The known neuroanatomy of ascending noradrenergic, serotonergic and cholinergic neurons imposes several constraints on the functions of these systems. The noradrenergic and serotonergic systems are monosynaptic (closed) sets of multiple collaterals. These collaterals release norepinephrine or serotonin massively in many forebrain structures, simultaneously. We propose that the function of the noradrenergic neurons is to activate the organism's repertoire of previously successful instrumental behaviors (including exploratory movements). These behaviors are viewed as attempts to gain operant control over the expected reoccurrence of motivationally significant stimuli. In other words, we propose that the noradrenergic system deals with the organism's expectations of future active movements. The serotonergic systems deactivate movement tendencies tonically. This occurs during freezing behavior, intense fear (such as that generated by the conditioned emotional response paradigm) and during sleep. This system appears to be capable of the immediate deactivation of movements regardless of the intensity of the noradrenergic urge to respond.

The cholinergic system is a polysynaptic chain of neurons. It is open to diverse sensory input and has the capacity to release acetylcholine selectively in one forebrain area at a time. Its function is to eliminate unsuccessful or harmful specific movements that have been already activated. We propose that cholinergic systems utilize feedback from unsuccessful movements to govern the reoccurrence of those movements. This continual process of monitoring and suppressing movements is necessary for the development and refinement of an operant response. In agreement with Carlton (1963), we assume that learning involves the joint participation of both cholinergic and noradrenergic systems. Accordingly, the trained organism would have many more cholinergically suppressed movements and less noradrenergically activated movements, than the naive organism. The suppression generated by the cholinergic system appears to be directly proportional to the intensity of the noradrenergic urge to respond.

The anatomical arrangement in the cholinergic suppression system resembles a series circuit. A block in this circuit would remove all cholinergic suppressant influences at and above the level of the block. Our experimental evidence indicates that direct cholinergic blockade in the hypothalamus by atropine produces a general disinhibition of movements. In contrast, the anatomical arrangement in the noradrenergic activation and serotonergic suppression systems resembles a parallel circuit. Manipulation of one branch of a parallel circuit would be expected to have limited influences. Our experimental evidence shows that noradrenergic activation in the amygdala by norepinephrine produces a very specific disinhibitory action on punished responses.

Finally, preliminary evidence is presented in this chapter for neurochemical memory mechanisms in the brain. Glycine, acting in the PVS as a neurotransmitter, or as a neuroregulator, exerts a long-lasting suppressant effect that reduces the antipunishment action of atropine for several weeks. In addition, evidence has been presented that suggests (1) noradrenergic synapses in the dentate gyrus may participate in the storage of rewarding events in memory, and (2) cholinergic synapses in the hippocampal gyrus may participate in the storage of punishing events in memory.

Chapter 8

Diencephalic, Hippocampal, and Neocortical Mechanisms in Voluntary Movement[1]

C. H. VANDERWOLF, B. H. BLAND[2] AND I. Q. WHISHAW[3]

DEPARTMENTS OF PSYCHOLOGY AND PHYSIOLOGY
UNIVERSITY OF WESTERN ONTARIO

I. Introduction

A number of years ago P. D. MacLean reported that regular electrical activity appeared in the hippocampus of a freely moving rat when the animal "seemed to focus its attention or was exploring, and disappeared when it was eating or drinking" (MacLean, 1957). The fact that hippocampal activity is related to behavior in some way has been confirmed repeatedly, but different observers have interpreted the relation in various ways, usually in terms of inferred processes such as attention, stimulus processing, learning, memory, motivation,

[1] This research was supported by a grant from the National Research Council (APB-118). Drugs used in some experiments were contributed free of charge by: Poulenc Ltd., Montreal; Schering Corp. Ltd., Montreal; and Smith, Kline and French, Corp., Montreal.

[2] Now at Institute of Neurophysiology, University of Oslo, Oslo, Norway.

[3] Now at Department of Psychology, University of Lethbridge, Lethbridge, Alberta.

etc. Other studies, to be summarized here (see also Black, 1971; Black, Young, and Batenchuk, 1970; Bland and Vanderwolf, 1971a, b; Dalton and Black, 1968; Sainsbury, 1970; Vanderwolf, 1969, 1971; Whishaw, 1971; Whishaw and Vanderwolf, 1971) have shown that hippocampal electrical activity is closely related to the actual movements made by an animal and cannot easily be interpreted in terms of traditional psychological concepts.

In these experiments, recordings have been derived from bipolar electrodes chronically implanted in the hippocampus, neocortex, or various brainstem structures. Slow electrical activity has been recorded using an inkwriting polygraph or an oscilloscope and camera. Behavior has been recorded simultaneously with the EEG record by means of manually operated signal markers attached to the polygraph. In experiments in which a precise indication of the instant of occurrence of a given behavior was required, an accelerometer or an electronic movement sensor of the type described by Griffiths, Chapman, and Campbell (1967) was used and the type of behavior performed was indicated, as before, by the signal markers and by written notes. In some experiments the hypothalamus or hippocampal formation was electrically stimulated, using trains of rectangular pulses and a stimulus isolation unit.

In some experiments rats were trained to avoid shock by jumping out of a plywood box whick measured 30.5 x 30.5 x 30.5 cm, and was mounted on foam rubber blocks. A grid floor, placed 28 cm below the top, could be electrified by an inductorium. A plywood shelf, 6.4 cm wide, ran around the outside of the box 1.3 cm below the upper edge. Thus, a rat could jump out of the box, catch the raised edge with its forepaws, and pull itself up on to the outside shelf. Movements of the box were recorded by the movement sensor placed beneath a metal plate fixed to the outside, a system which produced an almost instantaneous response.

Recordings of brain electrical activity were analyzed by inspection and counting. Measurements of the frequency and amplitude of hippocampal rhythmical slow activity (RSA) were made on the polygraph records, using a transparent plastic ruler.

II. Relation of Hippocampal and Neocortical EEG to Behavior

It is useful to classify the EEG derived from the hippocampal pyramidal cells in the waking rat, gerbil, or guinea pig into three main types, as was done previously by Stumpf (1965a) in the rabbit. Rhythmical slow activity (RSA) consists of trains of nearly sinusoidal waves of a frequency varying from about 6 to 12 Hz. Amplitude varies widely depending on the exact location and orientation of the electrode tips with respect to the dipole of the pyramidal cell, as shown by Green, Maxwell, Schindler, and Stumpf (1960). At a given electrode site, both amplitude and frequency of RSA vary in relation to the behavior of the animal.

Large amplitude irregular activity (LIA) is a second waveform which differs from RSA in that it has a component of very slow waves and lacks the rhythmical character of RSA. The LIA pattern is sometimes accompanied by irregularly occurring spikes with a duration of about 50–100 msec and a large amplitude (2–5 times the amplitude of the background activity).

A third waveform is small amplitude irregular activity (SIA) which appears as a sudden reduction of the amplitude of hippocampal activity and ordinarily lasts only 1–2 sec, in contrast to the two preceding types which may continue steadily for many minutes.

All three of the foregoing patterns will occur at a single placement in the hippocampus of an alert rat, guinea pig, or Mongolian gerbil. The particular pattern exhibited depends on the behavior of the animal. Recordings are particularly clear and free of artifact when taken using a difference amplifier connected to an electrode pair placed with one tip above the pyramidal cell layer, and the other below it (see Freeman, 1963; Matthews, 1934). In this way, potentials of 2 mV or more can be obtained in the hippocampus, using gross electrodes.

A basic finding has been that in a normal freely moving animal, RSA accompanies voluntary types of movement, including walking, running or galloping straight ahead, turning, backing up, rearing up on the hind legs, climbing, mounting (prior to copulation), swimming, jumping, struggling when held, head movements, postural changes, manipulation of objects, digging with the forepaws, and isolated movements of the limbs, such as a phasic retraction of one forepaw.

LIA usually occurs in the hippocampus (SIA is also observed, but less frequently) during behavioral immobility and during the performance of automatic or reflexive types of behavior, including licking (during drinking, grooming, or sexual activity); chewing food, gnawing wood, biting the fur during grooming; chattering the teeth (part of agonistic behavior in the rat and guinea pig); piloerection, shivering, urination, defecation; pelvic thrusting and ejaculation during coitus; face-washing, scratching the fur with one hind foot; and vocalization (such as fear-induced squealing). Trains of RSA may occur during automatic types of movement if the animal makes a voluntary type of movement at the same time. For example, RSA appears when a rat moves a paw slightly while drinking.

These EEG-behavior relations persist under a great variety of motivational or stimulus conditions, including deprivation of food or water, sexual arousal, exposure to extreme temperatures, electric shock, immersion in water, different types of apparatus, presence of other animals, etc. Thus, hippocampal activity is related to what an animal *does* in response to sensory stimulation rather than to the stimulation itself.

Clear EEG-behavior relations can be observed consistently in the hippocampus only if the recording electrodes are placed in relation to the pyramidal cells in such a way that clear large amplitude RSA can be recorded. Electrodes placed in the dentate gyrus or subiculum yield a good deal of fast activity with an amplitude up to 1 mV (see Fig. 1). Electrodes placed at random in the hippocampal formation are likely to pick up mixtures of RSA and fast activity, and the presence of RSA may pass undetected, especially when its amplitude is low.

Electrical activity in the neocortex may be related to behavior in much the same way as it is in the hippocampus. This can be demonstrated clearly

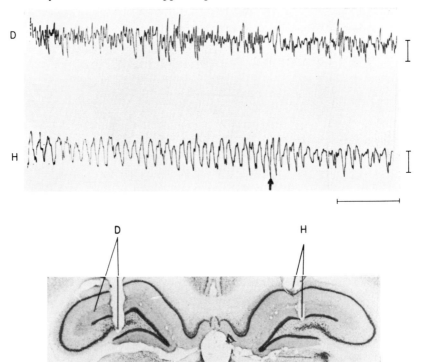

Fig. 1. Simultaneous recordings of activity at two sites in the hippocampal formation of a rat performing an avoidance response. The arrow indicates the point of initiation of a vertical jump of 28 cm. Note: fast activity recorded from an electrode pair placed on either side of the granule cell layer of the dentate gyrus (one of the wire tips was rostral to the plane of the section shown); rhythmical slow activity (RSA) from a similar electrode pair placed on either side of the pyramidal cell layer of the hippocampus. RSA tends to increase in frequency as the jump occurs. Cal: 1 sec, 500 μV.

following large doses of atropine or scopolamine. In the rat, atropine produces slow activity in the cortex when given in doses above about 6 mg/kg (i.p.) (Burešova, Bureš, Bohdanecký, and Weiss, 1964). We have confirmed this, and found that larger doses produce increasing effects up to about 25 mg/kg, with little further change up to 150 mg/kg. During RSA-related behavior (walking, running, jumping, struggling, head movement) in a heavily atropinized rat, low amplitude slow waves (3–10 Hz) can be recorded continuously from frontal, parietal, or occipital neocortex. This rhythm does not resemble anything seen in the cortex of a normal rat during the same behavior. If the rat engages in an LIA-related behavior (standing or lying motionless, washing the face, chattering the teeth, gnawing on wood, or scratching itself) cortical activity consists of irregular spindles and large amplitude slow waves, a pattern almost identical to the waveforms seen in normal deep slow wave sleep in the same rat. Thus, in a heavily atropinized rat, cortical activity has a more "activated" or "aroused" appearance during RSA-related behavior than during LIA-related behavior (see Fig. 2).

It is a traditional belief that cortical activation is correlated with sensory stimulation; possible detailed relations to motor activity have received less attention. However, the cortical EEG in an atropinized rat is closely related to actual movement; sensory stimuli have an effect only to the extent that they modify behavior. Thus, if a drugged rat is walking about and arousing stimuli are presented (hand claps, whistles, pure tones, touching, etc.) little effect is seen as long as the rat continues to walk or move its head. On occasions when it responds to such stimulation by an arrest of movement (freezing), slow large amplitude spindles appear in widespread cortical areas after a latency of not more than 1–3 sec. This also happens when movement stops spontaneously without any obvious eliciting stimulus (Fig. 3). Sensory stimuli applied during behavioral immobility have little effect on the ongoing large amplitude slow activity unless they elicit head movement or locomotion as well.

In summary, it may be said that atropine abolishes a rat's normal ability to maintain an activated cortical EEG while standing motionless or performing an automatic behavior. A clear, though incomplete, activating effect is associated with walking, head movements, etc., and can be recorded from a widespread cortical area including frontal (sensorimotor) cortex as well as parietal and occipital cortex.

Large doses of atropine or scopolamine seem to have an effect on the hippocampus which is analogous to the effect on the neocortex. The drugs alter the normal activation pattern (RSA), but do not abolish it altogether, even following extremely large doses. Thus, RSA is less regular than normal, but there is always a clear increase in regularity when a drugged rat changes from a state of immobility to active locomotion (Fig. 3).

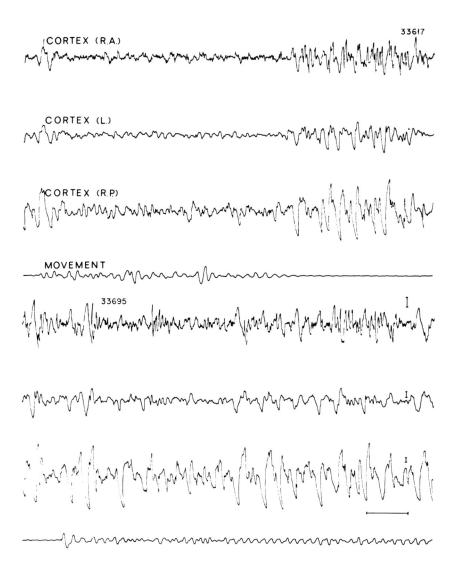

Fig. 2. Motor activity and neocortical electrical activity following atropine SO$_4$ (25 mg/kg i.p.). Cortical recording sites: R.A., right anterior; L., left parietal; R. P., right posterior. Upper four tracings: head movements and stepping followed by immobility; lower four tracings: face washing. Note large-amplitude slow waves during immobility and face washing and smaller, faster waves during head movements and stepping. Cal. 1 sec, 50 μV.

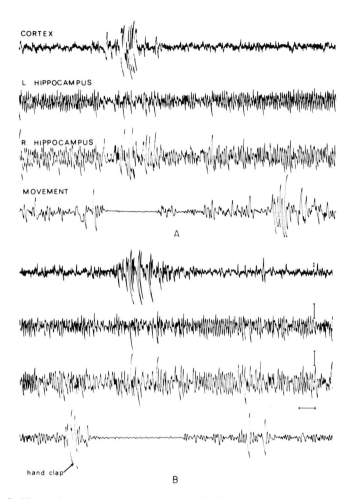

Fig. 3. Neocortical (sensorimotor cortex) and hippocampal activity in relation to behavior following scopolamine HBr (10 mg/kg). Top four tracings: Note RSA in the hippocampus during walking and head movement, and almost immediate development of large amplitude slow waves and spindles when movement stops momentarily. Lower four tracings: Comparable effect produced by a hand-clap, which produced an "arrest" of movement. Cal. 1 sec; hippocampus, 500 μV; neocortex, 50 μV.

The physiological basis of these effects is unknown. Studies in acute preparations have shown that in atropinized cats large amplitude waves can be suppressed by stimulation of the thalamus or mesencephalic reticular formation but that lower amplitude slow waves persist (Loeb, Magni, and Rossi, 1960). This is similar to the effect observed here during behavior. A possible hypothesis is that there are multiple ascending activating systems to the cortex and that one, responsible for cortical activation during immobility and the performance of automatic behavior, contains muscarinic synapses. A second activating system, related to the production of voluntary movement, would be less readily affected by atropine. Additional factors might also be involved since cortical activity is never entirely normal following atropinization. Atropine exerts widespread effects on the forebrain both directly on the neocortex and subcortically (see Dudar and Szerb, 1969; White and Rudolph, 1968).

Although extensive evidence is lacking, neocortical electrical activity appears to be related to ongoing movement in normal animals as well as in those that have been atropinized. Clemente, Sterman, and Wyrwicka (1964) and Roth, Sterman, and Clemente (1967) have reported that slow waves and spindles appear in the neocortex of a cat drinking milk or grooming, but do not occur during walking. We have observed these waveforms in the neocortex during chewing, facewashing, scratching, shivering, or immobility but not during the performance of behavior associated with hippocampal RSA. Thus, these observations are consistent with the general rule that hippocampal RSA is associated with low voltage fast activity in the neocortex, while irregular hippocampal activity *may* be accompanied by slow waves and spindling (Green and Arduini, 1954). That is, there are many occasions when the cortical EEG appears fully activated during immobility or automatic types of behavior (e.g., facewashing, shivering) even though RSA may be absent from the hippocampus.

The foregoing results indicate that the performance of a voluntary type of movement is associated with increased activation of the cerebral cortex as compared with the performance of more automatic movements or behavioral immobility. The effect is clearest in the hippocampus but apparently occurs in the neocortex as well. It is well known that the cerebral cortex can be activated by electrical stimulation of ascending pathways from the brainstem nonspecific system (Green and Arduini, 1954; Moruzzi and Magoun, 1949). This suggests that during behaviors such as walking or the manipulation of an object, cortical mechanisms, driven from below, play a role in the control of the ongoing movement. This control must be of a generalized type, involving wide areas of the cerebral mantle. Automatic or reflexive types of movement, such as shivering or emotional expression, need not be associated with such activation, suggesting that cortical structures play a lesser role in their performance.

This interpretation assumes that low voltage fast activity in the neocortex and RSA in the hippocampus are associated with an active functional state of those structures. Such an assumption has sometimes been questioned, especially in the case of the hippocampus; RSA is sometimes regarded as an indication of inhibition (Grastýan et al., 1959).

The following experiments on the effects of hippocampal stimulation on electrical activity and behavior support the hypothesis that the hippocampus plays an important role in RSA-related behaviors and a lesser role in the control of LIA-related behaviors.

III. Effects of Electrical Stimulation of the Hippocampal Formation

Different effects on voluntary RSA-related behavior and more automatic LIA-related behavior were observed in experiments in which the dentate-gyrus-CA4 area was stimulated while recording hippocampal EEG in freely moving rats (Bland and Vanderwolf, 1972a). Low voltage unilateral stimulation (0.1 msec pulse duration) at sites in the dentate gyrus produced a bilateral evoked potential in the pyramidal cell layer, as shown in Fig. 4. Response latencies, measured from the stimulus artifact to the onset of the evoked waveform, varied from 2.5 to 7 msec, and were usually about 5 msec for ipsilateral responses, and 4 msec for contralateral responses, a result which may be related to the relatively extensive myelinization of the commissural pathway. Repetitive stimulation at low frequencies produced a steady driving of hippocampal activity, but at frequencies of 40 Hz or more it resulted in a rapid diminution of the amplitude of the evoked potentials during a 1–2-sec train.

The pathways producing these effects could not be positively identified, but probably involve activation of the mossy fiber projections to CA2 and CA3. The best effects were obtained from electrodes placed in the hilus of the dentate gyrus and the evoked potentials themselves were quite similar in latency and

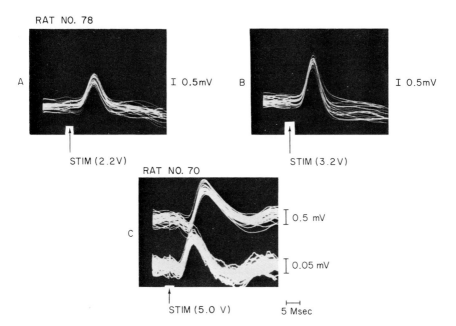

Fig. 4. Evoked responses in the hippocampus during dentate-CA4 stimulation. A and B, responses recorded contralateral to the stimulating electrode; C, upper beam illustrates an ipsilateral response, lower beam illustrates a contralateral response. Each record consists of about 25 superimposed sweeps. (From Bland and Vanderwolf, 1971a.)

duration to those observed by Gloor, Vera, and Sperti (1963) who stimulated the mossy fiber system in the cat while recording from pyramidal cells.

Dentate gyrus stimulation at the intensities employed here had no observable behavioral effect in a motionless rat. Posture was unaffected. Neither was there any change in respiration or heart rate. However, if the animal was engaged in an RSA-related movement, stimulation of 10 Hz or more produced an immediate arrest of movement (accompanied by hippocampal driving) which continued for the duration of the stimulus train. Shortly after stimulus offset, the spontaneous hippocampal EEG was restored, RSA returned, and the rat would continue moving as before. This effect was observed during spontaneous walking, swimming, or climbing behavior, during shock avoidance behavior (jumping out of a box), during struggling movements produced by manual restraint and during bar-pressing behavior in a Skinner box. The effect was demonstrated quantitatively using the jump avoidance procedure described above. Rats were trained to jump out of the box in 1 sec or less when placed inside. Stimulation of the dentate gyrus (100 Hz, 0.1 msec pulse duration, 1.4–5 V, 2 sec train duration) suppressed jumping behavior, increasing response latency up to an average of 3–7 sec (Bland and Vanderwolf, 1971a).

Behavioral arrest did not occur with stimulation of 1–5 Hz but became obvious at 8–10 Hz or more. Figure 5 suggests that this is due to a progressive invasion of the RSA wave cycle by the electrically produced waveform. At 5 Hz RSA waves still appear between successive evoked potentials and the rat is able to struggle (attempting to escape the experimenter's hand). At 10 Hz or more the RSA waveform (which has a maximum frequency of about 12 Hz) is obliterated and the rat can no longer perform the type of movement which is normally accompanied by RSA.

It was suggested earlier that the presence of LIA in the hippocampus during a given motor pattern in a normal animal is an indication that the hippocampus does not play an essential role in the performance of that motor pattern. The effects of stimulation of the dentate gyrus support this idea. Figure 6 shows that stimulation of the dentate gyrus need have no effect on the lapping movements of the tongue in a rat drinking water. Similarly, in another series of experiments, it was found that dentate gyrus stimulation had no visible effect on shivering (recorded by needle electrodes inserted subdermally in the hip) in a slightly cooled rat, although it suppressed voluntary types of movement.

A control series of experiments showed that stimulation of the pyramidal cell layer (loci yielding good RSA) did not produce widespread evoked potential activity in the hippocampal formation or any obvious behavioral effect. Jumping behavior, for example, was unaffected. However, stimulation of the pyramidal cell layer produced seizure discharges very easily, and if the discharges became self-propagating, hippocampal activity was subsequently depressed for several minutes. These abnormal electrical patterns were associated with a complex

RAT NO. 78

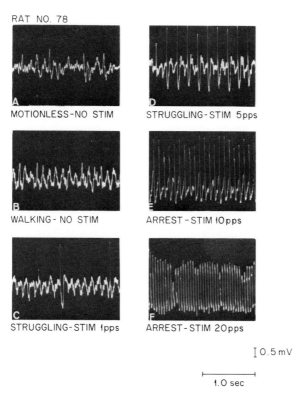

A. MOTIONLESS-NO STIM

B. WALKING-NO STIM

C. STRUGGLING-STIM 1pps

D. STRUGGLING-STIM 5pps

E. ARREST-STIM 10pps

F. ARREST-STIM 20pps

$\mathbb{I}$ 0.5 mV

$\longmapsto$ 1.0 sec

Fig. 5. Effects of the evoked response produced by dentate-CA4 stimulation on rhythmical slow activity in the dorsal hippocampus. A. Irregular activity present while the animal was motionless. B. RSA during walking. C. Animal struggling while receiving dentate-CA4 stimulation at 1 Hz. D. Animal struggling while receiving stimulation at 5 Hz. E. Effect of stimulation at a frequency of 10 Hz. The struggling was arrested at 10 Hz and also at 20 Hz as illustrated in (F). Stimulus intensity was 2 V throughout. (From Bland and Vanderwolf, 1972a.)

series of behavioral effects including grooming, feeding, and increased spontaneous locomotion, together with defective jump avoidance performance (Bland, Wishart, Altman, Whishaw and Vanderwolf, unpublished observations).

The actual mechanism of the inhibition of voluntary movement produced by dentate stimulation requires further investigation. According to Fox *et al.* (1967) evoked potentials can be recorded in the anterior cerebellum following hippocampal stimulation. We have confirmed this in two rats and have also observed very clear evoked activity in the hypothalamus during dentate gyrus stimulation. It is conceivable that these effects, rather than the evoked activity in the hippocampus, are responsible for the behavioral arrest which is observed. RSA can be recorded in some parts of the medial thalamus and hypothalamus

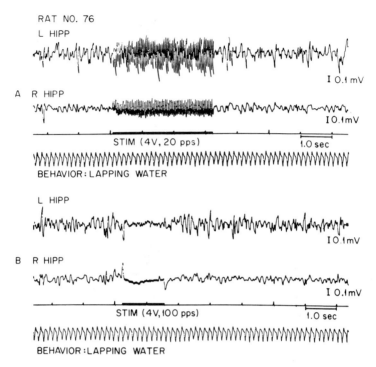

Fig. 6. Effect of dentate-CA4 area stimulation on hippocampal electrical activity and on drinking behavior. Licking movements continue undisturbed during hippocampal driving. (From Bland and Vanderwolf, 1972a.)

and this waveform has the same basic relation to movement as it does in the hippocampus. Thus, the interference postulated above might occur subcortically as well as in the hippocampus itself.

High frequency (100 Hz) stimulation of the dentate gyrus reduces the amplitude of ongoing hippocampal activity in a manner which bears some resemblance to the naturally occurring SIA wave pattern. This may be more than a coincidence since the occurrence of SIA is associated with an abrupt arrest of ongoing voluntary movement. If the same waveform occurs during scratching the fur, sniffing or pelvic thrusting, however, the ongoing movement may continue unaffected (Whishaw, 1971).

In summary, electrical stimulation of the dentate gyrus produces evoked potentials bilaterally in the hippocampus. At stimulation frequencies above about 10 Hz, these induced waveforms supplant the naturally occurring rhythms, and are associated with suppression of voluntary movement, whereas normal posture and certain automatic motor activities (licking, shivering) appear unaffected. Together with the data on the relation between behavior and the spontaneous rhythms of the hippocampus and neocortex, the findings suggest that there are special cerebral mechanisms required for the performance of voluntary movements which are not necessary for the maintainance of a fixed posture or the performance of automatic movements.

IV. RSA Amplitude and Frequency in Relation to Behavior

Correlation of the amplitude and period of individual waves in a train of RSA shows that these parameters are not closely related even when samples are taken during a wide range of behaviors, possibly suggesting that they are independently regulated to some extent. It is also possible to manipulate RSA amplitude and period independently by different experimental procedures (Whishaw, 1971). If rats are cooled by immersion in ice water or heated with a lamp, RSA amplitude remains fairly constant between core temperatures of 26–40°C, but frequency varies with temperature. Thus, mean RSA frequency accompanying walking can vary from 3 to 10 Hz in a rat at different core temperatures. Following seizure activity produced by direct electrical stimulation, hippocampal electrical activity is temporarily depressed. If a rat walks about during this postictal state, RSA may be present at normal frequency but with an attenuated amplitude (see Fig. 7). Thus, the amplitude and frequency of the RSA waveform can be made to vary independently. A simple hypothesis might be that amplitude is related to the number of neurons participating in the rhythm while frequency is related to the intensity of the afferent bombardment (see below).

However, during most behaviors there is an overall correlation of amplitude and frequency. For example, the RSA accompanying an isolated head movement (the rest of the body remaining motionless) is, on the average, about half the amplitude of the RSA accompanying walking.[4] Correspondingly, the mean RSA frequency (averaged over 1–2 sec or more) is about 7 Hz during head movement and about 8 Hz during a brief episode of walking. (For reasons discussed below, mean RSA frequency is usually less than 8 Hz during steady walking after the behavior has been in progress for several seconds.)

It is common for a series of RSA waves accompanying a given act to have a uniform amplitude although the period of individual waves within such a train can vary considerably. Thus, it appears that although some behaviors are accompanied by large amplitude RSA with a high mean frequency and others by small amplitude RSA with a lower mean frequency, on a wave-to-wave basis, amplitude and frequency are poorly correlated. Our impression is that RSA

---

[4] It is interesting that the small amplitude low mean frequency RSA accompanying slight movements is not due to low "motivation" as has sometimes been thought. A rat attempting to remove a bulldog clamp from its vibrissae by pulling with its forepaws will exhibit an RSA pattern appropriate to slight paw movements even though it may squeal with pain as it pulls.

RAT 183

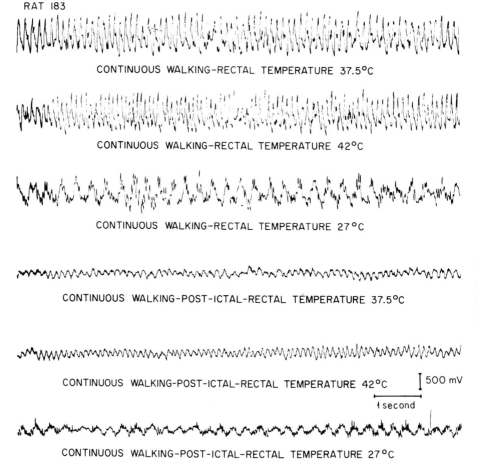

CONTINUOUS WALKING-RECTAL TEMPERATURE 37.5°C

CONTINUOUS WALKING-RECTAL TEMPERATURE 42°C

CONTINUOUS WALKING-RECTAL TEMPERATURE 27°C

CONTINUOUS WALKING-POST-ICTAL-RECTAL TEMPERATURE 37.5°C

CONTINUOUS WALKING-POST-ICTAL-RECTAL TEMPERATURE 42°C   500 mV

1 second

CONTINUOUS WALKING-POST-ICTAL-RECTAL TEMPERATURE 27°C

Fig. 7. The effect of changed core temperature and electrically induced hippocampal seizure activity on hippocampal RSA. RSA frequency varies with core temperature independent of wave amplitude; amplitude is reduced following a hippocampal seizure, independent of frequency. Cal. 1 sec, 500 μV. (From Whishaw, 1971.)

amplitude is related particularly to the extent of the muscular field activated during a movement and that frequency increases are related to the initiation of movement. The latter point can be demonstrated in the shock avoidance task described above (rats are required to jump out of a box). This task has several advantages: (1) the moment of initiation of muscular activity can be defined accurately using the movement sensor, (2) a large movement is required, ensuring large amplitude RSA, and (3) the use of shock reinforcement suppresses irrelevant spontaneous motor activity, permitting the observation of a sudden transition from immobility to vigorous movement. Using well-trained rats which exhibit a minimum of irrelevant motor activity immediately preceding the jump response, it can be shown that RSA with a frequency of 6–7 Hz precedes the jump by several seconds (Figs. 8, 9, and 16). Between 1 and 2 sec before the jump, the frequency rises, reaching a peak value, varying from 8 to 12 Hz, near the time that overt motor activity begins. Similar frequency shifts accompany

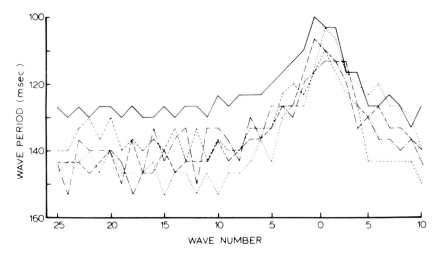

Fig. 8. Changes in frequency of RSA associated with performance of jump response in avoidance task. Jump occurs at "O." Points shown are means of 24–143 waves in each of five rats. Rats remained motionless prior to the jump, aside from a slight tensing, and did not take a step or move their heads.

the initiation of running, whether it occurs as an avoidance response, or spontaneously, or in a motor-driven wheel (Whishaw, 1971). However, it should be emphasized that long periods of low frequency RSA appearing in advance of overt movement are unusual in the spontaneous behavior of rats, guinea pigs, or Mongolian gerbils. So far, this has been observed consistently only in situations involving painful electric shock. Normally, movement occurs almost simultaneously with the onset of RSA and it may be that aversive situations (and their elicitation of freezing behavior) prolong a process which is normally completed in a fraction of a second.

In attempts to discover factors producing variations in RSA frequency during the initiation of various movements, it was found (Whishaw, 1971) that RSA frequency is regularly about 2 Hz faster (up to 12 Hz) when a rat must jump 56 cm to avoid shock than when it jumps 28 cm (Fig. 9). This may be related to the greater acceleration required for the higher jump since we have also found

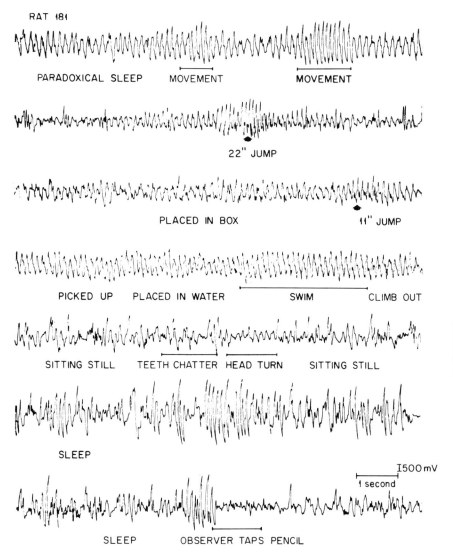

Fig. 9. Electrical activity at a single hippocampal site during sleep and various behaviors in a rat. Note: RSA during paradoxical sleep, jumping, struggling when held in the hand, swimming, and head movement; LIA during sitting while alert and while chattering the teeth; irregular slow activity and "spindling" during slow wave sleep; SIA when the rat was awakened but did not move about. Note also: Increased RSA frequency and amplitude associated with twitching during paradoxical sleep and with jumping in avoidance tasks; different frequencies and amplitudes of RSA associated with head movement, swimming, jumping 11 in (28 cm) and jumping 22 in (56 cm). Cal. 1 sec, 500 μV. (From Whishaw, 1971.)

that the initiation of fast running is associated with higher frequency RSA than the initiation of slower running. Preliminary results from work now in progress suggest that increasing a rat's total mass (by means of a pack saddle loaded with up to 125 gm of lead shot) has less effect on RSA frequency, producing an increase of 1 Hz or less.

RSA amplitude usually rises as the frequency increases during the initiation of movement, but there are also occasions when the amplitude remains unchanged or even falls as the frequency rises. RSA amplitude is also greater during a 56-cm jump than during a 28-cm jump (see Fig. 9).

Whishaw (1971) has investigated the relation between speed of running and RSA frequency in rats and gerbils trained to run at different speeds in a wheel measuring about 61 cm in diameter and 20 cm in width (i.e., width of the running surface). Animals could be placed inside and EEG recordings taken while the wheel was turned at different speeds by an electric motor and set of pulleys. The data shown in Fig. 10 are based on recordings taken when the animals were walking or running steadily (without pausing) at speeds ranging from 33 to 144 ft/min (10–44 m/min). There is no consistent relation between RSA frequency and running speed.

RSA frequency also remains constant if running continues at the same speed for prolonged periods. After a training period, rats were able to run for 8 hr at 33 ft/min (10 m/min) without stopping. RSA frequency remained at about 8 Hz throughout. A similar experiment was performed on two cats which walked continuously for 8 hr in a treadmill. RSA was continuously present and maintained a constant frequency of about 5 Hz.

In summary, if a motionless rat or gerbil begins to run, let us say, and continues steadily for some time, low frequency RSA (6–7 Hz) may precede the actual movement by several seconds. More commonly, the onset of movement is almost simultaneous with the onset of RSA. Frequency rises to a peak at the

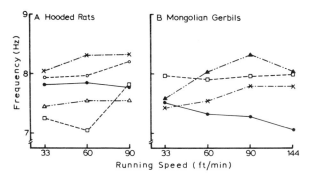

Fig. 10. The relation between running speed in a motor-driven wheel and RSA frequency in five rats and four gerbils. Each point represents the mean frequency of RSA during a 2-min period of steady running. (From Whishaw, 1971.)

moment that actual movement begins, then falls off to a stable level (7–8 Hz) as running continues. The height of the frequency peak (up to 12 Hz) is related to the speed with which running is initiated, but the final stable frequency is not closely related to running speed.

These results can be related to previous electrophysiological and behavioral findings. It is well established that the reticular formation exerts an ascending influence on the hippocampus via the diencephalon and a relay in the septal nuclei. Electrical stimulation of the reticular formation or medial diencephalon produces RSA in the hippocampus. Certain septal neurons fire in phase with hippocampal RSA and are thought to act as pacemakers for this rhythm. If the reticular formation of hypothalamus is stimulated at different intensities, RSA frequency is initially higher (i.e., at stimulus onset) when stronger stimuli are employed, possibly reflecting an increased excitatory bombardment of the septal pacemaker cells. RSA frequency is always highest at the onset of stimulation, and declines as stimulation is continued (see Stumpf, 1965b).

On this basis, one might imagine that the initiation of voluntary movement in a freely moving animal is associated with an intensification of ascending unspecific activity to the hippocampus, succeeded by a steady upward discharge as movement continues. The more intense the initial burst, the higher the RSA frequency will be and the faster the movement will be initiated. One may think of the ascending activity as a nonspecific trigger or initiator of movement, since similar frequency shifts accompany a number of quite distinct motor patterns such as running, jumping, or swimming.

Study of animals with chronic lesions of the diencephalon has also suggested the existence of a mechanism for the triggering of voluntary movement (Vanderwolf, 1962, 1971). Rats with large lesions of the medial thalamus are unable to avoid electric shock by running or jumping promptly (within 5 sec) away from the place where it is administered. (Normal rats do this after 2–12 shock reinforcements.) The animals are not paralyzed in the ordinary sense, and control experiments indicate that they are able to learn what to do and are motivated to avoid electric shock. Thus, they are able to solve a three-choice brightness discrimination problem with escape from shock as a reinforcement almost as well as normal, and are well able to avoid shock passively by refraining from movement. During active avoidance training they exhibit many of the automatic behaviors characteristic of fear in a normal rat (vocalization, piloerection, chattering the teeth, defecation, etc.) even though they remain absolutely motionless when placed on the grid where shock is to be presented. Vocalization may occur as a conditioned response in anticipation of shock. The failure to avoid is dependent to some extent on the time allowed for the initiation of flight; many rats with medial thalamic lesions can avoid fairly well if given a longer time to perform. They are able to initiate running or jumping only after a considerable delay.

It has been suggested that failure to avoid shock following medial thalamic damage is due primarily to an impaired ability to initiate voluntary motor activity, an effect which might result, in part, from interruption of ascending pathways to the hippocampus. The main ascending pathway appears to run through the hypothalamus, but a part is also present in the medial thalamus, and the hippocampus would be deprived of part of its unspecific input by a large lesion placed there (Eidelberg, White, and Brazier, 1959; Kawamura, Nakamura, and Tokizane, 1961; Kawamura and Domino, 1968). Thus, the process associated with production of RSA and increases in its frequency might be defective in a rat with a medial thalamic lesion and the animal would be unable to initiate running or jumping in a shock avoidance test.

This idea has been tested in rats with lesions in the medial thalamus and with recording electrodes implanted in the hippocampal formation. Medial thalamic lesions, even when very extensive (including the habenula and the intralaminar, medial, and midline nuclei), do not permanently abolish hippocampal RSA and do not change its main relations to motor activity. Thus, apparently normal RSA accompanies walking, struggling, jumping, etc. During avoidance testing, two main patterns of electrical activity occur on trials when the rats fail to avoid (Fig. 11). The most common pattern is irregular, resembling normal LIA.

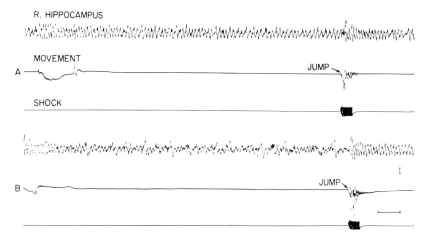

Fig. 11. Hippocampal electrical activity during shock avoidance testing in a rat with medial thalamic damage. At left the rat is placed in a grid box. Shock is presented about 15 sec later, but can be avoided by a vertical jump of 28 cm. Note that prior to shock the hippocampal record may consist of low frequency (6 Hz) RSA (upper three tracings) or of irregular activity (lower three tracings). In either case the rat remains motionless, failing to avoid. Shock elicits a short latency startle response followed by development of RSA of 8–10 Hz and a quick scramble out of the box. Jumping out of the box occurs only when RSA is present and reaches a frequency of about 8 Hz or more.

However, on some trials a clear RSA pattern appears, but no visible movement occurs unless the frequency rises above 6–7 Hz. Presentation of shock elicits a short latency startle response followed by the development of higher frequency RSA (8–10 Hz) and jumping out of the box. On those occasions when a medial thalamus-damaged rat avoids shock successfully, RSA appears in the hippocampus prior to the initiation of movement and rises in frequency as motor activity begins, much as in a normal rat. Therefore, a medial thalamic lesion apparently does reduce unspecific input to the hippocampus during a behavioral test. This results in: (1) failure to develop RSA in response to the conditioned stimuli, or (2) development of RSA but of a frequency too low to trigger motor activity. On some trials RSA development is minimal, suggesting a graded transition from irregular to regular activity. The results support the conclusions drawn from the earlier ablation studies: medial thalamic lesions block shock avoidance behavior by impairing the operation of a movement-triggering mechanism.

According to the view presented here, different frequencies of RSA are related to varying degrees of activation of a movement triggering system. It is uncertain whether this hypothesis can account for all the relations between RSA frequency and behavior which have been observed so far. Figure 12 illustrates frequency histograms of RSA during various behaviors (see also Vanderwolf, 1969, Fig. 3). Walking, rearing, swimming, or running in a motor-driven wheel are associated with RSA with a mode of 7.5 Hz and a mean of 7.1 to 8.3 Hz in different rats. There are no significant differences in RSA frequency among these behaviors, but the RSA associated with isolated movements of the head, the manipulation of a food pellet, or lever pressing in a Skinner box has a lower mean frequency, resulting from an increase in 6 Hz activity and a decline of 9–10 Hz activity. Conceivably, this low frequency activity is a consequence of slow initiation and frequent pausing during the latter types of behavior, but there is no direct evidence bearing on this point as yet.

The lower left corner of Fig. 12 illustrates a frequency histogram of RSA in rats in a type of classical conditioning situation. Using a delay conditioning procedure with a 5-sec CS-US interval, a tone was paired with an inescapable electric shock delivered to the grid floor of the experimental chamber (Whishaw, 1971). After 20 paired presentations or more, the tone would produce a train of regular 5–6 Hz waves in the hippocampus when the rat remained absolutely motionless throughout the trial, except for changes in respiration. (A similar effect may have occurred in an experiment by Bremner, 1968, but movement was not looked for.) Movements of the head, or locomotion, were associated with higher frequency RSA, as they normally are. Thus, during classical aversive conditioning, long trains of low frequency RSA (about 6 Hz) can occur in a normal rat while it remains absolutely motionless. It is our hypothesis that this activity is related to low-level activation of a central movement controlling

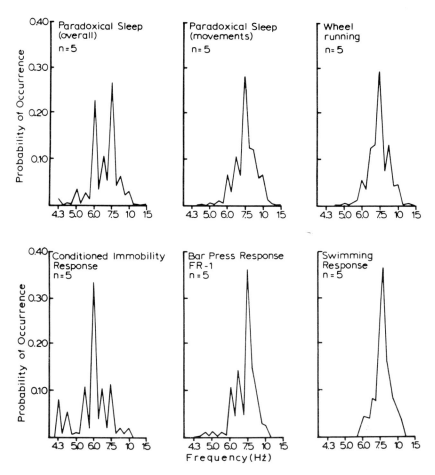

Fig. 12. Frequency distributions of hippocampal RSA during six different behaviors. Mean frequencies are: paradoxical sleep (over all), 6.7 Hz; paradoxical sleep (movements), 7.6 Hz; wheel running, 7.7 Hz; swimming, 7.6 Hz; conditioned immobility, 5.9 Hz; bar-pressing, 7.2 Hz. Measurements based on 27,978 waves obtained from five rats in each case. (From Whishaw, 1971.)

mechanism, even though no movement is observed. That is, some sort of voluntary movement is "planned" but is not actually triggered. Evidence supporting this view is indirect at present, but the following points may be cited. (1) During shock avoidance testing, trains of 6–7 Hz RSA may precede the movements of running or jumping (as the rat "prepares" to respond) but movement occurs only when the frequency rises to 8 Hz or more. (2) Rats with medial thalamic lesions may develop RSA in the hippocampus during avoidance testing but unless the frequency rises to about 8 Hz the avoidance response fails to occur. Previous behavioral work had indicated that medial thalamic lesions block avoidance performance by an effect on the initiation of movement rather than an impairment of learning ability or fear. (3) Evidence presented below shows that phenothiazines affect avoidance behavior and concurrent hippocampal activity in much the same way as medial thalamic lesions do. Therefore, in several situations in which low frequency RSA is observed, independent behavioral evidence suggests that preparation for movement is occurring even though actual movement is absent.

Paradoxical sleep is another instance in which hippocampal RSA occurs in the absence of extensive motor activity. During this stage of sleep RSA is present almost continually and there is also a remarkable reduction of tone throughout the somatic musculature. Despite this there are frequent small movements or twitches of the limbs, back, head, or vibrissae. At such times the ongoing RSA rhythm increases in frequency and in amplitude. Figures 9 and 12 show that the RSA accompanying movements during paradoxical sleep has a frequency much like the RSA occurring during running or swimming. Amplitude is as large or larger than it is during very violent movements in the waking state. Between movements, the RSA rhythm decelerates and a strong 6-Hz component appears.

According to Pompeiano (1967) there is increased activity in descending pathways (including the pyramidal tract and rubrospinal tract) during the twitching of paradoxical sleep but movement is largely prevented by descending postsynaptic and presynaptic inhibitory influences which are simultaneously present. The results of hippocampal recording are consistent with this in showing that there is a great deal of central motor activity during paradoxical sleep, but that such activity is largely prevented from reaching the muscles.

Related explanations may be invoked to account for the fact that RSA can occur during animal hypnosis even though the animal is completely immobilized. (1) The RSA tends to have a low frequency, insufficient to trigger vigorous voluntary movement, and (2) monosynaptic and polysynaptic spinal reflexes and midbrain reflexes are depressed (Carli, 1969; Harper, 1968; Klemm, 1966, 1969; McBride and Klemm, 1969). Therefore, overt muscular activity is unlikely even though central movement—controlling systems are active.

V. Hypothalamic-Hippocampal Relations and Behavior

There is a great deal of evidence that electrical stimulation of the hypothalamus has potent effects on behavior and also on hippocampal electrical activity. Initial attempts to relate the behavioral and bioelectrical effects of such stimulation led to the hypothesis that RSA is related to approach behavior (Grastyán, Karmos, Vereczkey, and Kellényi, 1966) but this has not been confirmed (Ito, 1966; Pond and Schwartzbaum, 1970; Routtenberg and Kramis,

1968; Routtenberg, 1970) and it is unlikely that hippocampal RSA bears any relation to positive or negative reinforcement.

We have attempted to study the relations between hippocampal activity and the pattern of movements made by an animal during hypothalamic stimulation (Bland and Vanderwolf, 1972b; Whishaw, Bland, and Vanderwolf, 1972). Preliminary experiments in rats anesthetized with chloral hydrate (300 mg/kg) showed that electrical stimulation of the dorsomedial posterior hypothalamus was especially effective in producing RSA in the hippocampus. Later, chronically prepared rats were tested in a large open field in which food, water, sawdust (for digging), pieces of wood (for gnawing), and, occasionally, other rats, were available. Stimulation (0.1 msec pulses, 100/sec, 1–15 V) of the dorsomedial posterior hypothalamus produced head movements, walking, rearing, or running, i.e., movements that are normally accompanied by RSA. Although stimulation above threshold (about 4.0 V) ensured that movements of this general type would occur, it did not dictate the exact pattern. Rats could turn to either side, avoid obstacles, etc., showing that the elicited pattern of movement was under environmental control. The thresholds for producing movement and RSA were generally identical; whenever a voluntary type of movement occurred, RSA was also present. Stimulation of the dorsomedial posterior hypothalamus never produced behavior of the type which is normally associated with LIA. Immobility, licking, chewing, etc., were not observed. In fact, if stimulation was presented while one of these behaviors was spontaneously in progress, it was interrupted and head movements or locomotion appeared instead.

Stimulation of hypothalamic sites outside the dorsomedial area usually failed to produce locomotor behavior reliably. Automatic behaviors, including chewing, licking, washing the face, and chattering the teeth (a component of agonistic behavior) often occurred, interspersed with periods of walking and head movement. Figure 13 illustrates hippocampal activity during spontaneous walking and drinking (induced by water deprivation) together with activity at the same hippocampal site accompanying walking and drinking occurring during stimulation of the lateral hypothalamus, at a point just lateral and dorsal to the fornix.[5] In this experiment, the rat could stimulate its own hypothalamus by pressing a bar, initiating a 10-sec train of stimulation. At intensities just above threshold, stimulation resulted in walking to the water spout, head movement and lapping, the total performance resembling normal behavior very closely. Hippocampal activity also appeared very similar to the normal pattern, becoming very regular during walking and rather irregular during the lapping movements. With more intense hypothalamic stimulation, drinking behavior persisted but the

[5] Stimulation of this site produces maximal increases in drinking behavior (Mogenson, 1969).

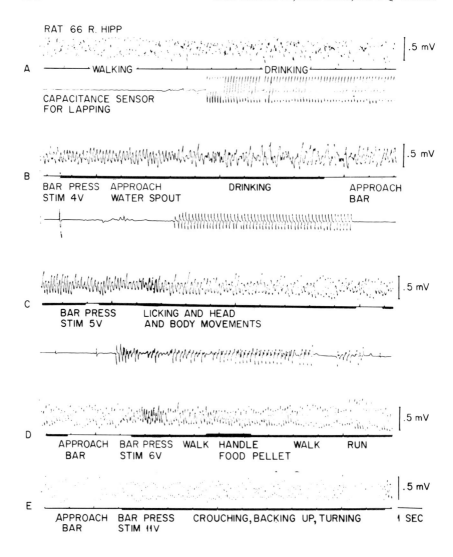

Fig. 13. Hippocampal activity accompanying "spontaneous" behavior or behavior resulting from self-administered stimulation of the lateral hypothalamus. A. Approach to water and drinking following water deprivation. B-E. Drinking and other behavior during hypothalamic stimulation (indicated by downgoing black bar). Note irregular hippocampal activity during induced drinking at 4.0 V. At higher voltages drinking is accompanied by head and body movements and RSA appears in the hippocampus. Note increasing RSA frequency as the stimulus voltage is increased. (From Whishaw, Bland, and Vanderwolf, 1972.) Reprinted by permission of the American Psychological Association, Washington, D.C.

rat was no longer motionless for long periods during lapping. Small movements of the head, limbs, and trunk occurred almost continuously and, correspondingly, hippocampal activity consisted of low-frequency RSA. As stimulation intensity was increased still further, RSA frequency rose as locomotor activity became more and more common. Simultaneously, the bouts of drinking became progressively shorter and water intake declined. Self-stimulation behavior continued at a high rate, however (Whishaw, Bland, and Vanderwolf, 1972).

Analogous effects occurred during eating elicited by hypothalamic stimulation. At low stimulation intensities, walking and picking up and manipulating a food pellet were associated with regular hippocampal activity while chewing was associated with more irregular hippocampal activity, just as these activities are during normal spontaneous behavior. The elicited behavior also resembled spontaneous behavior quite closely. However, stronger stimulation produced almost continuous "fidgeting" during chewing, and a corresponding increase in the regularity of the hippocampal record. At the highest voltages tested, both behavior and hippocampal electrical activity became unlike anything seen during spontaneous activity. Figure 13 shows that 11 V stimulation of the lateral hypothalamus produced continuous RSA at a mean frequency of 10 Hz or more, associated with crouching and slow backing up. This behavior pattern does not occur naturally and correspondingly, RSA is not maintained at frequencies above 10 Hz for more than about 1 sec during spontaneously occurring behavior (i.e., behavior occurring in the absence of brain stimulation).

In a further study, chronically prepared rats were placed in a light Plexiglas wheel (61 cm in diameter, with a running surface 7.6 cm wide) which turned on ball bearings. Struts, radiating out from the circumference at 20.3 cm intervals, activated a movement sensor to indicate running speed on the polygraph chart. Hippocampal recordings were taken while a 60-sec train of hypothalamic stimulation (100 Hz, 0.1 msec pulses) was administered to rats in this apparatus. One stimulation trial was given per day. Figure 14 illustrates RSA frequency over time during stimulation of the dorsomedial posterior hypothalamus at different intensities. Higher voltage stimulation produces higher frequency RSA at stimulus onset, but as stimulation continues, frequency declines to a stable level which has no consistent relation to stimulation intensity. Similar phenomena were reported by Stumpf (1965b) in acute preparations. It has also been shown that speed of running in a wheel is directly related to the intensity of hypothalamic stimulation (Gerben, 1968, 1969). The two types of experiment are here combined and the results are illustrated in Fig. 15. As stimulation of the dorsomedial hypothalamic area increases in intensity, RSA onset frequency rises in relation to running speed. A similar effect probably occurs in normal behavior. Whishaw (1971) showed that initial RSA frequency was consistently higher in two gerbils when the animals were initiating a run of

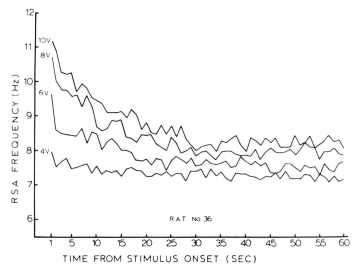

Fig. 14. Changes in RSA frequency in a rat during wheel running induced by various intensities of dorsomedial-posterior hypothalamic stimulation. Each curve represents data from one stimulation trial, frequencies being averaged over 1-sec intervals. (From Bland and Vanderwolf, 1972b.)

144 ft/min (44 m/min) in a motor-driven wheel than when they were initiating a run of 33 ft/min (10 m/min).

Stimulation of hypothalamic sites outside the dorsomedial posterior area did not produce reliable wheel running behavior. Such sites did not produce RSA in the hippocampus either, except on those occasions when the rats walked about, moved their heads, etc.

VI. Effect of Phenothiazines on Hippocampal Activity and on Behavior

Phenothiazine derivatives, such as chlorpromazine, have the property of suppressing conditioned avoidance behavior in experimental animals, but do not affect escape to the same extent. General CNS depressants, such as barbiturates, affect avoidance and escape behavior equally (see Herz, 1960). The phenothiazines also affect the electrical activity of the hippocampal formation (see Stumpf, 1965b) but the relation of this to behavior has not been well understood.

We have studied the effects of several phenothiazines on hippocampal and neocortical EEG in rats trained to jump out of a box to avoid shock. After 2 days of training the rats jumped out very consistently several seconds after being placed on the grid floor. On succeeding test days, drugs were dissolved in saline and given intraperitoneally in the following dosages: chlorpromazine,

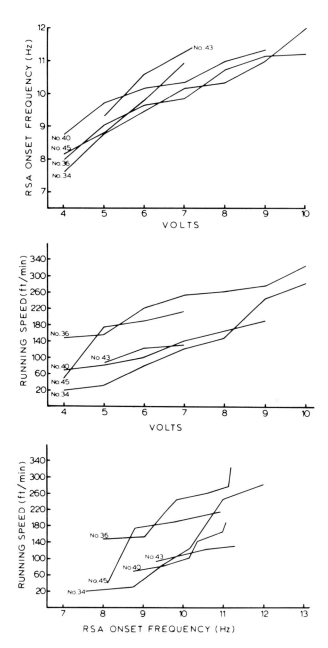

Fig. 15. Relations among intensity of dorsomedial-posterior hypothalamic stimulation, RSA onset frequency, and running speed. (From Bland and Vanderwolf, 1972b.)

5-15 mg/kg; trifluoperazine, 1 to 5 mg/kg. Perphenazine (2-5 mg/kg) was dissolved in polyethylene glycol 400. Control injections of saline and polyethylene glycol were also given. The testing procedure was first to give a rat several avoidance trials in the normal state while recording hippocampal and neocortical activity. Next, the drug or control solution was administered, and testing was continued immediately. The intertrial interval was about 60 sec.

As discussed above, RSA precedes the act of jumping, often by several sec, and rises in frequency just before the actual movement begins. All three of the phenothiazine derivatives tested have qualitatively similar effects on this process and on the accompanying avoidance behavior. Following the administration of a large dose of one of the drugs, the first change observed is a prolongation or blocking of the anticipatory RSA frequency shift. RSA appears, but the critical triggering frequency at which the jump is normally initiated is not reached in the time allowed (15 sec) and the rat receives a brief foot shock. This usually results in a rise in RSA frequency associated with jumping out of the apparatus ("escape"). Trials of this type are at first interspersed with trials in which RSA rises to the normal triggering frequency and a jump is initiated before shock is administered (avoidance). As avoidance performance deteriorates further, RSA ceases to appear prior to shock. Nonetheless, the animal may squeal in anticipation of shock (conditioned vocal response) (Fig. 16). If a brief foot shock is given at this time, sometimes only a startle response occurs, unaccompanied by any other visible movement. This consists of a sudden flexion of the neck and trunk which tends to drive the rat's snout between the bars of the grid. Such a movement, occurring in isolation, may not be accompanied by any visible change in the ongoing pattern of irregular hippocampal activity. Usually, however, the rat responds to shock by moving its head, stepping, walking, or jumping, and these behaviors are accompanied by RSA with a normal frequency and amplitude (Fig. 16). Normal RSA also accompanies the struggling movements produced when a drugged rat is picked up, although neither movement nor RSA occurs in response to many normally effective stimuli such as the sight of a novel object.

No obvious relation was found between depression of avoidance behavior and changes in neocortical electrical activity. Following trifluoperazine and perphenazine in particular, rats may exhibit good low voltage fast activity in the neocortex even though they fail to avoid and may even be in an obvious cataleptic state. Chlorpromazine tended to produce a great deal of spindling in the neocortex, and following large doses, such activity would appear even when a rat was placed on the grid (without shock) provided that it remained motionless. Spindling did not occur during walking or jumping but it was common during immobility or an automatic behavior, such as gnashing the teeth following shock. On some occasions neocortical spindling was observed while a rat was receiving shock and biting viciously at the grid floor (making a loud

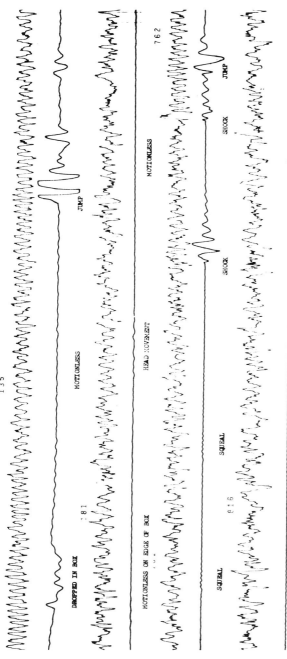

Fig. 16. Effects of chlorpromazine on hippocampal activity in a shock avoidance task. Lower tracing of each pair indicates the movements of the rat. A. Normal hippocampal activity (no drug) during a jump avoidance response. Note that the regular slow waves (RSA) increase in frequency immediately preceding the jump. B. Irregular hippocampal activity accompanying behavioral immobility during the intertrial interval. C. Following chlorpromazine HCl (10 mg/kg) rat fails to avoid but squeals (conditioned vocal response) prior to shock onset. RSA is not present. Note that the strong expiration activates the movement sensor. After two brief shocks, a normal RSA pattern appears, and the rat jumps. D. Irregular hippocampal activity accompanying behavioral immobility in rat following chlorpromazine. Cal. 1 sec, 500 µV.

grating noise), provided that head and limb movements were not made at the same time. Thus, these observations are consistent with those discussed previously; slow waves and spindling occur much more readily during immobility or automatic behavior than during a voluntary type of behavior.

There is evidence that phenothiazine derivatives inhibit avoidance performance by an effect on the control of movement. Large doses of the drugs produce symptoms of "extrapyramidal" disorders in man and cataleptic states in animals. Taeschler and Cerletti (1959) showed that the ability of different phenothiazines to produce catalepsy correlates with their efficacy as depressors of avoidance performance. Posluns (1962) showed that the effect of chlorpromazine on one-way avoidance is similar in many ways to the effect of medial thalamic lesions on this test. Conditioned vocal responses may occur when avoidance behavior is suppressed, suggesting that normal perception and fear can still occur. Failure to avoid seems primarily due to interference with the initiation of movement (running) since there is a strong correlation between "locomotor initiation latency" and impairment of avoidance behavior. In agreement with this, Irwin (1961) has demonstrated a correlation between depression of locomotion and depression of avoidance performance in a series of seven different phenothiazines.

In summary, phenothiazines appear to interfere with unspecific input to the hippocampus and with the production of the voluntary type of movement which is normally associated with it. Suppression of avoidance responding is associated with either a total failure of RSA development or with development of RSA of a frequency too low to trigger an avoidance response. In many ways, the effect resembles the impairment produced by medial thalamic damage. The hippocampus itself does not seem to be directly affected by the phenothiazines since strong stimuli (physical handling or electric shock) can produce normal RSA in association with voluntary movements. It may be that the drugs interfere with the ability of mild sensory stimuli to activate the subcortical mechanism which controls hippocampal RSA, and initiates voluntary movement. Nonetheless, such stimuli can still exert a behavioral effect, and behaviors such as conditioned vocal responses, which are not dependent on the RSA system, can still occur.

VII. Discussion

The data presented here show that certain aspects of the spontaneous electrical activity of the hippocampus are correlated with concurrent motor activity in a specific way. Rhythmical slow activity (RSA; hippocampal activation) normally occurs in the hippocampus during the performance of such motor acts as walking, swimming, manipulation etc. (voluntary movement) but need not occur during behavioral immobility or such motor acts as licking, chewing, shivering, etc. (automatic movement). Further, the frequency and amplitude of the RSA waveform is closely related to the time of initiation of a movement and to the extent of the muscular field activated.

Neocortical activity appears to be related to behavior in somewhat the same way as hippocampal activity; activated patterns (low-voltage fast activity; here assumed to be functionally analogous to hippocampal RSA) always occur during voluntary movement in a normal animal but need not be present during behavioral immobility or automatic movement. Relations between behavior and the electrical activity of the neocortex are especially clear in heavily atropinized rats. Large amplitude slow waves, indistinguishable from a sleep pattern, occur during immobility and automatic behavior. Smaller amplitude waves with a shorter period occur during voluntary movement.

It is often said that electrocortical activity is not consistently related to behavior since, for example, an atropinized animal may be very active at a time when slow waves are unusually prominent. This so-called "dissociation" of behavior and electrocortical activity is paradoxical only if it is insisted that slow waves and spindling are necessarily indicative of sleep. The abnormal electrocortical activity is, in fact, correlated with obvious behavioral deficits. Large doses of atropine produce a type of amnesia (state-dependent learning) in rats (Overton, 1966) and psychotic behavior and amnesia in man (Innes and Nickerson, 1965). We have found that atropinized rats are somewhat hyperactive (mostly movements of the head and forequarters), squeal when touched, and are very clumsy, often falling when placed on a narrow shelf. Escape behavior is intact, but one-way avoidance behavior is depressed in proportion to the $\log_{10}$ of the dose over the range of 5–150 mg/kg (unpublished observations).

A similar condition occurs during sleepwalking in man. Jacobson and Kales (1967) have shown that slow waves can occur in the EEG during actual walking and that, correspondingly, the movements made are repetitive and aimless, revealing a disturbance of higher level control of behavior. Further, the subjects subsequently do not remember the sleepwalking episode.

Therefore, gross electrical recordings probably provide a reasonably accurate index of the functional state of the neocortex. The presence of slow waves or spindles means that the cortex is incapable of normal control of any motor activity which may happen to be in progress at the time. This is not a disadvantage during normal sleep since motor activity is largely suspended.

The interpretation outlined here (also see Longo, 1966) is consistent with the results of experiments on the effect of cerebral lesions on behavior. A totally decorticated or even decerebrated rat (Woods, 1964) possesses reflexive licking and biting behavior and will lick at the spout of a water bottle or nibble bits of food when they are presented to the mouth. Such an animal is also able to walk and move its head about, but normal control of these movements is absent. Thus, a decerebrated rat does not make use of its reflexive feeding abilities by walking to a food pellet and placing its mouth in contact with it. It seems that licking and biting movements are still regulated (turned on or off, etc.) in a normal manner, but that the control systems for walking and head movement have been largely destroyed. Therefore, these behaviors are useless, making no contribution to survival.

Less extensive forebrain damage may have analogous effects. Localized destruction of the neocortex, dorsal medial (cingulate) cortex, or the hippo-campal formation does not abolish walking, running, jumping, etc., nor does it abolish licking, biting, holding objects lightly in the mouth, hovering, pelvic thrusting or ejaculation, but it does produce a disorganization of the total behavior patterns of which these behaviors form a part (feeding, food hoarding, nest-building, maternal care, sexual activity). In tests involving maze perfor-mance or care of the young, for example, rats with large cortical lesions often run about aimlessly, accomplishing little even though they may be very active (maternal behavior: Beach, 1937; Kimble, Rogers, and Hendrickson, 1967; Slotnick, 1967; maze performance: Hughes, 1965; Kaada, Rasmussen, and Kviem, 1961; Kimble, 1963; Lashley, 1929; Thomas and Otis, 1958; see also Teitelbaum and Milner, 1963). Male sexual behavior may also be abolished following cortical damage (Beach, 1940; Larsson, 1962, 1964).

Behavioral disorders of this type are often discussed in terms of inferred processes such as learning, attention, motivation, emotion, etc. Perhaps it would be advantageous to consider the problem from a more behavioristic point of view. The fact that a decorticate rat does not run through a maze accurately can be thought of as an indication of a deficit in learning, etc., but in a more descriptive sense it is a deficit in the control of locomotion. The rat still runs, but the movement is no longer biologically useful in that it does not carry the animal to the food in the goal box. Disorderly, uncontrolled running may also occur in situations where the role of special training is less obvious (e.g., pursuit of the female by the male, carrying of nesting material, carrying of the young by the female), suggesting that the deficits produced by decortication may not be crucially related to learning.

Regarded in this way, the neocortex and hippocampus play a very general role in the control of motor activity. Destruction of the cerebral cortex produces very little real paralysis in most mammals but does produce a severe behavioral disorder of a type which suggests that the destroyed tissue normally controls motor activity. Electrocortical recording in the intact brain confirms this. When a voluntary type of behavior is to be performed, brainstem structures call on (activate) the hippocampus and neocortex to select an appropriate course of action, guide movements in relation to sensory input, etc. If this process is interfered with in any way (by atropine, for example) movement may still occur, but cortical control of it is impaired.

According to the hypotheses advanced here, large lesions of the cerebral cortex should generally have less effect on the control of automatic types of movement than on the control of more voluntary movements. Unfortunately, only limited information is available on this point at the moment (see Vanderwolf, 1971; Whishaw and Vanderwolf, 1971). There is also very little systematic information available on the role of different types of cortex, or different neocortical areas, in the control of different patterns of movement. For example, maze performance and maternal behavior are seriously disturbed following extensive destruction of either the neocortex or the hippocampal formation. Are the effects really identical?

Electrical stimulation of the dentate gyrus illustrates that the hippocampal formation plays a greater role in the performance of voluntary movement than in the performance of certain automatic movements. Unilateral dentate gyrus stimulation at a frequency above 10 Hz appears to occlude, or otherwise interfere, with the RSA waveform. This interference is associated with an arrest of naturally occurring RSA-related behavior although LIA-related behaviors (licking, shivering) are not affected.

A major problem raised by the results is the manner in which cortical and subcortical structures collaborate in the control of movement. The basic circuitry for gross bilateral types of movement seems to lie in the brainstem. According to Bard and Macht (1958), chronically prepared cats in which the brainstem has been transected at a pontine level are not able to right themselves and walk about, but if the section is made through the mesencephalon the animals are able to do this. Rats which have been decerebrated at the level of the mesodiencephalic junction are able to walk, rear up on the hind legs, climb, bite, chew, lick, squeal, wash their faces, etc. (Woods, 1964).

The diencephalon apparently exerts a powerful facilitatory influence on lower level motor automatisms. Thalamic cats (tissue rostral to the diencephalon removed) are extremely active (Wang and Akert, 1962) whereas mesencephalic cats (tissue rostral to the mesencephalon removed) are rather inactive and may not walk at all except when strongly stimulated (Bard and Macht, 1958). (In Bard and Macht's experiments the mesencephalon itself was damaged to varying degrees.) Acute physiological experiments have shown that posterior hypothalamic stimulation facilitates spinal reflexes or movement produced by concurrent cortical stimulation (Murphy and Gellhorn, 1945; Peacock and Hodes, 1951) and increases the discharge rate of gamma motor neurons (Granit and Kaada, 1952). Also, as shown by Hess (Hess, 1957; also see Akert, 1961) and many subsequent researchers, localized electrical stimulation of different areas of the ventral diencephalon in conscious animals can produce virtually all the behavior patterns of which the animal is capable. On the other hand, large lesions of the posterior hypothalamic-subthalamic area produce akinesia (Ingram, Barris, Fisher, and Ranson, 1936; Magoun, 1950), a severe loss of spontaneous movement.

We have attempted to investigate hypothalamic control of movement and of hippocampal activity by stimulating the lateral or posterior hypothalamus while recording hippocampal slow waves and observing ongoing behavior. Lateral hypothalamic stimulation resulted in locomotion toward food or water, directed head movement, manipulation, etc., followed by licking, or biting and chewing. RSA occurred in the hippocampus during locomotion, head movement, manipulation, etc., but not during licking and chewing (when unaccompanied by voluntary movement). This suggests that the hippocampus took part in the first class of movements, guiding the rat toward food or water and bringing the lips and mouth into position for contact. At this point lower level reflex mechanisms were activated and the RSA system ceased to operate as the rat maintained a fixed posture, enabling reflex activity to continue. Such a result shows that lateral hypothalamic influences on the hippocampus must be quite complex; electrical stimulation does not activate a direct ascending anatomical pathway. Lateral hypothalamic stimulation can mimic closely the state produced by deprivation of food. A rat can walk in search of food, then stop to eat when it finds it. Stimulation of the posterior hypothalamus (or strong stimulation of the lateral hypothalamus) seems to have a more direct effect on hippocampal activity and on RSA-related movement. During stimulation RSA is continually present and the rat continually runs, jumps, moves its head, etc., the behavior bearing a close resemblance to normal movement as long as hippocampal activity retains a normal pattern.

Thus, it appears that the principal mechanisms of spontaneous movement in mammals are located in the upper brainstem. These mechanisms are capable of independent activity, being responsive to sensory stimulation in the absence of the cerebral cortex. However, in a normal animal, an ascending brainstem system can call on cortical mechanisms to select and direct motor activity, permitting a more adaptive control of behavior. In higher mammals, in particular, cortical neurons (e.g., pyramidal tract cells) achieve a relatively direct control of the motor neurons of the final common path, an evolutionary development that may reflect the survival value of increasingly detailed control of small body parts. However, such direct connections are apparently not essential for cortical participation in the control of movement. Hippocampal pyramidal cells do not project to the neurons of the final common path, yet (as shown here) the hippocampus does play an important role in the control of spontaneous motor activity.

Chapter 9

Intracranial Self-Stimulation Pathways as Substrate for Stimulus-Response Integration

ARYEH ROUTTENBERG

DEPARTMENT OF PSYCHOLOGY
NORTHWESTERN UNIVERSITY

I. Introduction

The attempt of this volume is to present a somewhat different picture of motor integration than one finds in recent edited volumes on the subject (Granit, 1966; Yahr and Purpura, 1967). The plan is to discuss some of the recent findings, particularly those gained from neurobehavioral studies, that demonstrate the need for a more expanded view of those systems which have been considered in the classical neuroanatomical and neurophysiological literature as important in motor integration. Recent research from our laboratory (Routtenberg and Malsbury, 1969) has suggested, for example, that certain brainstem extrapyramidal structures which have been related solely to motor coordination functions also appear to possess motivational components. Thus, animals with electrodes chronically implanted in the substantia nigra will press a bar to activate this region. This self-stimulation behavior, originally described in septal area and hypothalamus by Olds and Milner (1954) has until recently been related to limbic system structures. It appears now to be the case that some relation exists between the motor integration systems of extra-pyramidal structures and the motivational systems of limbic structures. The present chapter deals, in part, with this relationship.

From a theoretical point of view, Glickman and Schiff (1967) have recently emphasized the relation between the performance of species-typical motor patterns and the self-stimulation phenomenon. They note that "species-typical responses . . . are categorized as constituting approach to or withdrawal from a stimulus-object . . . and [such responses] demonstrate a relationship between these categories of behavior and the positive and negative rewarding effects of electrical stimulation, respectively" (p. 81). In more general terms, the central organization of particular motor patterns involved with approach or withdrawal behavior patterns forms the basis for positive and negative reinforcement, respectively.

At an intuitive level the Glickman-Schiff position appears reasonable. It would seem necessary, for example, that the motor nuclei involved with licking, chewing, and swallowing must be related to the physiological stimuli of hunger involved in initiating eating behavior. Or, as another example, the motor integration involved in sniffing, rearing, and perambulating through a new environment must be related to the capacity of novel stimuli to elicit such behavior. The present position differs from the Glickman-Schiff view by emphasizing the importance of both the motor system and the sensory system. They note, for example, that "reinforcement basically involves selective facilitation of motor patterns organized within brainstem" (p. 83). The present view emphasizes the contribution of both the stimulus and response mechanisms which form the substrate for behavior, placing a considerably greater emphasis on the stimulus-processing mechanism than do Glickman and Schiff (1967).

Other distinctions relate to the definition of reinforcement which I have discussed elsewhere (Routtenberg, 1968, pp. 73–74).

The present chapter describes, first, the anatomical organization of self-stimulation. Microelectrode data are next considered which delineate the response of single neurons to stimulation at hypothalamic self-stimulation sites. A third area of interest relates to hippocampal EEG activity as influenced by brain stimulation. This activity is compared to that recorded from freely behaving animals in an effort to consider the pathways of self-stimulation as substrate for observed behavioral activities. In a theoretical summary, these hippocampal patterns of activity are related to the anatomical pathways which mediate these electrophysiological responses in an effort to define the relationship between the organized motor patterns and the stimuli which guide these activities.

II. Demonstration of Self-Stimulation

Olds and Milner (1954), working at McGill, were interested in discovering those regions of the brain, particularly in the reticular formation, which would, when activated, produce an aversive effect. Reasoning from a model of optimal level of arousal (Hebb, 1955), they assumed that activation of the reticular formation would produce aversive effects as a consequence of stimulation. They set out to place electrodes in this region but due to a fortunate error, the electrode tip was placed several millimeters away in the septal region. They initially tested the animals for their distaste for the stimulation by applying brain stimulation to the animals in an open field (basically, it is a closed four-sided box; it is neither open, nor a field) and began looking for an aversive response to the stimulation. Presumably the animals would move away from that region of the box where they were stimulated. This the animals did not do. They seemed to be most interested, rather, in those regions of the open field where stimulation was applied. This result indicated to these researchers that the stimulation, far from being aversive, seemed to have a rewarding or pleasurable effect.

It is important to indicate, from a historical point of view, that the initial demonstration of the curious characteristics of brain stimulation was not obtained in a Skinner box, but was rather obtained in an open field in which the brain stimulation was applied when the animal was in a certain region of the field. The animal, then, seemed to be interested in the stimulation and would go to that area where the stimulation was presented. In this context one does not necessarily have to make use of the term reward in describing that stimulation. As history developed, however, this concept was impressively demonstrated by Olds and Milner (1954) who put the animals into a Skinner box to determine whether the animals would press a bar to activate their own brains. This is, indeed, what the animals did. An animal would continually and repeatedly press the bar and obtain stimulation. This demonstration was quite important and impressive from the point of view of indicating the quality of the stimulation. From the point of view of indicating the function of the fibers being stimulated, one cannot be so enthusiastic.

The highly repetitive, automatic form of the brain self-stimulation demonstration provoked a skeptical response from certain brain researchers. They considered the possibility that the stimulation was producing its intense repetitive behavior by provoking some form of abnormal seizure activity (Newman and Feldman, 1964). There now exists a literature concerning the relation of epileptiform activity to self-stimulation, indicating that while seizure activity can occur during self-stimulation, it is not necessary for its occurrence (e.g., Bogacz, St. Laurent, and Olds, 1965). Indeed, pharmacological agents which tend to reduce epileptiform activity tend to increase self-stimulation rate (Mogenson, 1964), indicating that seizure activity is an unlikely mechanism for the mediation of self-stimulation.

The use of operant conditioning for demonstrating intracranial self-stimulation also brought with it another series of experiments which determined whether this kind of stimulation had the characteristics of "real reward." Out of this view came a series of research endeavors in which various behavioral paradigms were employed involving both the straight-alley runway (Scott, 1967) and operant conditioning experiments in which delays were imposed between the time of pressing the bar and obtaining the stimulation (e.g., Pliskoff, Wright, and Hawkins, 1965). Other tests compared brain self-stimulation to sugar reward or a non nutritive saccharine reward (Gibson, Reid, Sakai, and Porter, 1965). The net result of such research (see Trowill, Pankseep, and Gandelman, 1969, for review) indicated that the use of operant conditioning procedures was not a necessary condition for demonstrating the approach-engendering character of the stimulation. When the highly repetitive behavior generated in the self-stimulation paradigm was altered, the performance of animals working for brain stimulation was similar in most details to the performance of animals working for conventional types of stimuli. The stimulation, in short, was "rewarding," and did not appear to differ, from a behavioral point of view, from conventional physiological incentives.

Another problem which has aroused considerable interest has been the anatomy of self-stimulation. Olds (1956) early recognized the importance of attempting to describe the anatomical systems which mediate self-stimulation. He assumed that one could delineate these systems by observing the pattern of points indicated by the deepest penetration of the electrode and determining whether this collection of points followed known fiber bundles. Olds and Olds (1963) demonstrated that self-stimulation placements did, in fact, appear to follow a particular fiber pathway, the medial forebrain bundle (MFB). Following Olds' discovery of the importance of MFB, and the suggestion that the lateral hypothalamus represented the "focus" of self-stimulation, one sees that localization of self-stimulation electrodes was subsequently based on the proximity of the electrode to this region (e.g., Routtenberg and Lindy, 1965), not its actual position. This indicates, I believe, that MFB was generally assumed to be the major fiber system involved with self-stimulation. If the electrode was near MFB this represented satisfactory anatomical localization. This view of the importance of MFB and particularly the importance of the so-called lateral hypothalamic focus of self-stimulation (Olds and Olds, 1964), has been questioned by several experiments (e.g., Valenstein and Campbell, 1964; Lorens, 1966). Valenstein and Campbell (1966) showed that self-stimulation in anterior telencephalic regions of the brain survived lesions which transected most of MFB, presumably cuttng the connection between the self-stimulation site and the MFB itself. This would not have been predicted by the view that MFB is critical for self-stimulation, and that the focus of the phenomenon, that is the cells which must be activated, is in the lateral hypothalamus (Olds and Olds, 1964). Indeed, the review of these difficulties *The Anatomical Locus of Reinforcement* by Valenstein (1966) would have been more accurately described had "Does Not Exist" been added to the title.

Given the difficulties created by the pathophysiological epileptiform activity generated by brain stimulation the abnormal behavioral activity generated, and the uncertain anatomical analyses of self-stimulation to this time, it is not surprising that the significance of self-stimulation itself remains to be established. In general, these difficulties, to be discussed below, relate to assumptions which were made but which were never established empirically. It seems necessary, therefore, in order to establish the functional significance of self-stimulation, to discuss these assumptions.

III. The Questioning of Basic Assumptions

A. THE BEHAVIOR ITSELF

It has been generally assumed that the behavior seen during the performance of self-stimulation is relevant to and, indeed, indicates the function of the fiber systems being stimulated by the animal. If the animal presses the bar to be stimulated in this area, the activation should be pleasurable. It would be expected, then, that the endogenous activity of this region should be related to the reward process. Although Olds (1967, 1969) has attempted such an approach, by recording unitary activity in freely moving animals, a convincing demonstration of reward-related activation of such neurons has not yet been made.

In addition to the lack of positive data to support the position that these fibers mediate reward, one can also consider certain logical arguments which weaken such a position. Thus, the understanding of the function of the fibers being stimulated does not necessarily have to relate *in any obvious fashion* to the behavior which immediately precedes or follows that stimulation. That is, the behavior itself may be far removed, in terms of causal steps, from the function of the stimulated fiber systems. Thus, fiber systems that support self-stimulation may be responsible for a particular function which cannot readily be appreciated by observing self-stimulation behavior.

This logical and conceptual difficulty may have been created by using the term rewarding and conceiving of the stimulation as having that particular function. In fact, making that assumption tends to preclude understanding of the detailed function of the fiber systems being stimulated. Nor does use of the term reinforcement, even when operationally defined, assist in resolving this issue. By having this convenient shorthand expression for describing the fact that the animal repeats certain acts, there exists an implicit explanation of why those acts were repeated. This is one difficulty with the Glickman-Schiff position which defines reinforcement essentially by itself. It is not surprising, then, that this phenomenon, which has elicited considerable interest from neuroscience disciplines, has not yet been firmly grounded in anatomical terms (Wetzel, 1968). I believe that part of the barrier to progress has been the focus on the definition of reward, rather than the description of the fiber pathways which mediate self-stimulation.

One might retrace history here. Consider, for example, the discovery of this system and the role of brain stimulation. It might have sufficed for early researchers to have indicated, making use of the Skinner box solely to automate the demonstration, that the animal had unfailing interest in the stimulus. They would have emphasized, then, that indicating that it was interesting would not explain why the animal paid attention to the stimulation, nor would it explain the actual function of the fiber systems being activated by the stimulation. Had such an approach been made, perhaps some of the characteristics of the fiber systems that support this particular phenomenon might be more adequately defined.

Historically, then, following the initial events leading to the discovery of self-stimulation, an assumption that the stimulation was rewarding was made. This was quite an inductive leap, and brilliant though that jump may have been, it also tended to obscure many of the steps that seem most critical in assessing the significance of the phenomenon. It would have been more helpful, rather than focus on the most general implications, had an attempt been made to direct more effort to the description of particular neuronal elements which contributed to that initial demonstration. This might have put the study of self-stimulation on a different course.

B. ANATOMY OF SELF-STIMULATION

In the past few years we have been studying the anatomical organization of self-stimulation, and have come to question another fundamental assumption: that the knowledge of the location of the tip of the electrode is of major significance and is sufficient for understanding the anatomical organization of self-stimulation. The knowledge of the location of the tip of the electrode is, of course, not unimportant, but it has become clear to us now that this represents only one piece of evidence in defining the self-stimulation system. This lesson has been learned as a consequence of the study of the anatomy of self-stimulation in the context of all fiber systems related to self-stimulation. Thus, a narrow view of a particular region of brain will not provide a clear indication of the neural elements that are involved. A broad but detailed analysis seems critical. Considerations presented in the next section will demonstrate why knowledge of the deepest penetration of the electrode tip is not adequate information for characterizing the anatomical organization of self-stimulation.

IV. Pathways of Self-Stimulation: Methodological Considerations

In order to delineate those regions from which self-stimulation could be obtained, it was necessary to make use of a set of simplifying procedures so that it would be possible to interpret our data in the least ambiguous fashion. It will be worthwhile, before describing our results, then, to describe the details and justification for procedures that we employed.

A. ONE ANIMAL—ONE ELECTRODE

Although it may have been of interest to compare self-stimulation from several sites in the same animal, it was clear that self-stimulation was not related only to the activation at the electrode site, but was, in fact, a product of the elaboration of activation throughout the nervous system. That being the case, the animal could possibly make comparisons between self-stimulation of two regions, one of which yielded self-stimulation, and the other which might not. This led us to presume that an animal might be influenced in his self-stimulation rate if a second electrode had a different motivational potency. We decided, therefore, to obtain more information by implanting fewer electrodes into each animal. Evidence reviewed by Robinson (1964), using multiple electrodes for brain stimulation, indicates that this choice was in fact a good one.

B. A SINGLE CURRENT LEVEL

We decided that to obtain a map of self-stimulation, it would be important to use a single current level, so that we might obtain a more uniform anatomical map of self-stimulation. Use of one current level had the following consequences.

1. Anatomical Considerations

Although the spread of current would be different, according to the electrical characteristics of the brain area in which the electrode tip was implanted, it could be assumed that the volume of tissue being stimulated was roughly similar in each case. Thus, every point could be compared with every other point, in the sense that it was activating the tissue having more or less the same field.

2. Contrast Effects

Using several current levels would have produced, in some sense, the same problem as using several electrodes. Thus, each current level would influence behavior at other current levels, so that the self-stimulation rate of a particular electrode would be influenced by the extent or range of current levels used (Valenstein, 1964). It was felt, therefore, that in order not to contend with interactions such as electrode placement by current level, a single current level would be used.

3. Consistency

We discovered another virtue when one employed a single current level. Since this procedure afforded a certain day-to-day consistency for the animal, it was clear that we were providing a stable condition under which self-stimulation rate would achieve a high degree of repeatability. To the extent that this rate did not vary could it be considered as a quantative index of the extent of involvement of the electrode in the fibers which mediate self-stimulation.

C. Fifteen Minutes/Day, 7 Days/Week

This procedure was also instituted primarily to provide a more stable environment in which to observe the self-stimulation behavior of these animals. It is clear that self-stimulation rates are different over a test session as a function of the placement of the electrode, as for example, in the septal area and hypothalamus (Routtenberg, 1968a). It was felt, therefore, that a single self-stimulation session of reasonably short duration would not yield preferential effects for a particular electrode placement. Our animals, in fact, self-stimulate at a similar rate throughout the entire session, and that rate seems to vary at different places; and the animals, once highly trained, maintain a stable rate across the 15-min test period.

D. Electrode Dimensions

In our initial studies using the above simplifying procedures, we used an 0.01-inch (254 μ) stainless steel wire in a bipolar configuration. We now use a smaller 0.0031-inch (78.7 μ) wire in a similar configuration because it is felt that a more restricted area of tissue can be activated. This restricted influence allowed the hope that the set of points gained by placing electrodes throughout the brain might yield a more readily interpretable pattern of points. With a smaller electrode and the consequent higher current density at the electrode tip, it was necessary to use a smaller current level. Thus, with the larger electrodes employed in the study of brainstem, a 25-μA, rms 60-Hz sine wave was used with the 254-μ wire, bipolar electrodes. In our forebrain experiments we used 15 μA, 60 Hz, sine wave stimulation, and in the study of hypothalamic self-stimulation we used 10 μA. In both experiments we used the 78.7-μ wire to make the bipolar electrode. We now routinely use the 10-μA current value, since this presumably gives us a more restricted volume of application of stimulation.

V. Pathways of Self-Stimulation: Results

For purposes of exposition, as well as for organizational purposes, I shall present three series of experiments. The first experiment was performed in the brainstem primarily concentrating on midbrain, pons, and medulla. The second series of experiments deals with self-stimulation in the hypothalamus and the pathways, primarily downstream, from such diencephalic regions. The third set of experiments focused on the forebrain telencephalon, particularly the frontal or pregenual cortex and septal area.

In considering the self-stimulation phenomenon in 1960, interest was generated in the relationship between the discovery of self-stimulation and the discovery of the reticular formation arousal system (Moruzzi and Magoun, 1949). It seemed quite reasonable to assume that some intimate relation did exist between these two systems. Indeed, the theoretical views of Hebb (1955) concerning an optimal level of arousal implied that an optimal level or change of reticular activity might be important for mediating self-stimulation. Both Glickman (1960) and Olds and Peretz (1960) reported, in fact, that reticular activation could support self-stimulation. This lent credence to the suggestion made earlier by Sharpless (1958) that some relationship did exist between reticular activation and self-stimulation.

Because Olds and Peretz were able to obtain self-stimulation from the ventral tegmental region, Ronald Kane and I (Routtenberg and Kane, 1966) compared self-stimulation effects from midbrain reticular formation, nucleus mesencephalicus profundus, and ventral tegmental area. We found that self-stimulation rate was, in fact, much higher in ventral tegmental area, as compared with the dorsal midbrain reticular formation. We also described behavioral effects of lesions at these sites which tended to confirm the importance of the fibers mediating self-stimulation for the maintenance of ongoing behavior. That is, lesions at self-stimulation sites in the ventral tegmentum had a more marked effect on the behavior of the animal, in terms of exploration and weight maintenance, than did lesions at sites in the reticular formation which did not support self-stimulation.

Since that study was a preliminary foray into understanding brainstem mechanisms of self-stimulation, we decided to repeat the experiment, and discovered that we could, indeed, obtain self-stimulation from dorsal regions of the brain (Routtenberg and Sugar, 1966). We were surprised, initially, because we had on the basis of the earlier study (Routtenberg and Kane, 1966) a considerably different effect from dorsal regions as compared to ventral ones. This forced a reassessment of the oversimplified distinction between the dorsal and ventral regions of the brainstem with regard to self-stimulation.

A. Brainstem Self-Stimulation

In order to clarify this ambiguity, Charles Malsbury and I (Routtenberg and Malsbury, 1969) decided to observe self-stimulation at brainstem sites. Initially, lesions were not made at these sites so that we could observe, without the uncertainty introduced by making a lesion, the deepest penetration of the electrode tip. Lesions were made subsequently to determine the pathways from self-stimulation sites. This series of experiments, then, was performed in two parts: mapping and degeneration.

1. Mapping

We placed a single electrode in 134 male albino rats and tested for self-stimulation as described earlier. The results obtained with that experiment analyzed placements of electrodes in the midbrain, pons, and anterior medulla. The most salient features of these results may be listed as follows: First, the highest rates of self-stimulation were obtained only from the anterior parts of the midbrain. As one moved to posterior regions such high rates were not observed. The second major feature of the results was that self-stimulation placements occurred in regions that were described as extrapyramidal. Thus, high rates of self-stimulation (>500 responses in 15 min) were observed in the ventral tegmental decussation, in the substantia nigra, and in the brachium conjunctivum.

We were surprised to find self-stimulation from these extrapyramidal structures. Perusal of the literature revealed, however, that earlier experiments indicated the involvement of these structures. Thus, Albino and Lucas (1962) reported self-stimulation from the substantia nigra and Spies (1965) reported self-stimulation from the brachium conjunctivum. Bogacz *et al.* (1965) reported self-stimulation from the ventral tegmental area, although the electrode placement was in the substantia nigra. Thus, self-stimulation obtained from the extrapyramidal system had been reported in earlier work, although such involvement was not emphasized.

A third point that needs emphasis was the lack of self-stimulation from placements in regions typically considered to be reticular formation. Although a placement in that region may yield self-stimulation, it may be related to fiber systems, not to reticular formation, traversing that region. This point will be discussed more fully in a later section of this paper. For the present, it is important to note that reticular formation may not be important in sustaining self-stimulation.

2. Degeneration Experiments

Although many placements in the mapping experiment indicated involvement of the extrapyramidal system, it seemed possible that fibers not related to this system were coursing through these brainstem regions mediating self-stimulation. Since we would not necessarily be able to observe such fibers with normal myelin-stained material, it was necessary to embark on a series of experiments that would answer this question.

For this purpose, then, we studied degeneration from self-stimulation sites. The general procedure of this approach was as follows: after testing the subject for self-stimulation until this behavior became stable, a lesion was made at the site of stimulation through the stimulating electrode. The animal was tested for self-stimulation for the next 5 days to determine whether the lesion eliminated self-stimulation Following preparation for either the Nauta technique (1957) or the Fink-Heimer modification (1967), pathways of degeneration were charted.

It was assumed that the pathways revealed by such degenerating fragments represented the pathways activated by the stimulation. There was no guarantee, however, that the stimulation field would not extend beyond the lesion, or that the lesion would not be larger than the stimulation field. The reduction of self-stimulation following the lesion, at the very least, would point to the fact that some fascicles related to self-stimulation had been destroyed.

Use of the Nauta (1957) or the Fink-Heimer (1967) technique along with the mapping procedure permitted certain important convergences. First, the pathways revealed by the Nauta technique could be referred to the mapping study to determine whether points along the pathway existed that supported self-stimulation. If it was so, the importance of the pathway for self-stimulation would be strongly suggested. If not, then this pathway would not be relevant. Second, the histology used in the mapping study does not always reveal the structure or pathway that is mediating self-stimulation. The typical fiber and cell stains, indeed, miss much of the structure of the nervous system. With the experimental anatomical technique, in addition to the mapping work, it is possible to reveal pathways related to self-stimulation that might, only with difficulty, be discerned with normal material. Thus, self-stimulation points revealed in the mapping study would be more clearly identified with regard to the neural pathways subserving self-stimulation after perusal of those pathways revealed by lesions at self-stimulation sites.

Using this approach, Routtenberg and Malsbury (1969) observed degeneration from self-stimulation sites in the posterior parts of the brainstem. In particular, we wished to determine whether the pathways revealed would overlap with those self-stimulation points which we observed in the mapping experiment. If such a relation would obtain, we could assume some relation among those self-stimulation sites. Thus, this convergent evidence would support the view that the self-stimulation sites observed in the mapping study were, in fact, related to the pathway of degeneration from a self-stimulation site in posterior parts of the brainstem. In general, then, it was hoped that this approach would allow us to replace the apparently infinite set of points with a numbered set of pathways.

What we observed (Routtenberg and Malsbury, 1969, Fig. 3) was demonstrated by a representative case of degeneration following a lesion made at a self-stimulation site in the posterior midbrain immediately ventrolateral to the central gray. Several features of these data should be pointed out. First, considering this case and others studied in the Routtenberg and Malsbury (1969) report, several pathways were revealed following a lesion at a self-stimulation site. It is difficult, at the outset, to attempt to isolate a particular pathway since the lesion at the self-stimulation site will show several pathways that course by the electrode tip. In this case, one pathway was to the motor nucleus of V, presumably because the lesion destroyed part of the mesencephalic root of V. Another pathway which we observed involved two components of the ascending brachium conjunctivum. One component, the uncrossed ascending limb of the brachium conjunctivum (UALBC), ascended in a region immediately ventrolateral to the central gray, sending terminals into the central gray, particularly into the nucleus of Darkschewitsch. The crossed ascending limb of the brachium conjunctivum (CALBC) passed through and apparently demonstrated preterminal degeneration in the contralateral red nucleus. No degeneration was seen in the ipsilateral red nucleus. The most salient feature of these results was that several self-stimulation placements observed in the mapping study appeared to follow CALBC. Since we did not have placements in the mapping study which were exclusively in the UALBC, we could not be sure of the importance of this pathway. We also could not be sure whether activation of the motor nucleus of V was important in mediating self-stimulation.

This experiment, then, was a valuable first step in understanding the anatomy of self-stimulation since it demonstrated involvement of a brainstem system which had not been anticipated and hence indicated the need for a more extensive examination of the problem of the anatomy of self-stimulation than had heretofore been performed. It also allowed us to see the importance of using techniques other than examination of the deepest penetration of the electrode tip. Finally, from an empirical point of view, we were exposed to a set of findings which suggested the unsuspected importance of the extrapyramidal system in the mediation of self-stimulation. These experiments forced us to reconsider self-stimulation obtained from the lateral hypothalamic focus (Olds and Olds, 1964) in relation to brainstem extrapyramidal self-stimulation.

B. HYPOTHALAMIC SELF-STIMULATION

The evidence which we had obtained from the brainstem mapping experiment suggested the involvement of extrapyramidal structures. It seemed possible, however, that other pathways might be coursing through the brainstem regions which supported self-stimulation. One possibility which we considered was that brainstem self-stimulation was a derivative of pathways descending through the brainstem originating from lateral hypothalamus. According to this view, self-stimulation effects which Malsbury and I obtained from the brachium conjunctivum, substantia nigra, and ventral tegmental decussation involved the descending fibers of passage, or perhaps, terminals from lateral hypothalamic self-stimulation sites. Huang (1970) in our laboratory, proceeded to test this assumption in a series of experiments using both anatomical and electrophysiological methods. The latter findings will be reported in a subsequent section.

At this time we decided that the size of the electrode that we had been using was too large and so employed a smaller one. Two important consequences of using a finer electrode wire need to be mentioned. First, as noted earlier, the amount of current required to sustain self-stimulation was not as great, since the current density from the smaller electrodes was greater. Hence, instead of using $25 \mu A$ as we had in the brainstem mapping study, we used only $10 \mu A$. A second consequence related to our Nauta studies of orthograde degeneration. It may be seen (Routtenberg and Malsbury, 1969, Fig. 3) that the lesion created by the electrode tract itself was quite extensive. By using a smaller wire, the overlying tract lesion would be smaller, hence the amount of degeneration created by the electrode tract itself would be considerably reduced. Put another way, a greater ratio between the signal, that is, the lesion, and the noise, the electrode tract, could be achieved with the smaller electrode.

The area of uninsulated metal surface forming an interface with the tissue is smaller by a factor of 10 with the electrode that we now use, as compared to that which has been, and for the most part still is, typically employed. If one assumes a minimum effective elliptical area, with the long axis twice the diameter of the wire and the short axis equal to the wire diameter, then with the 78.7-μ wires that we use in bipolar configuration, the exposed area is $9.7 \times 10^3 \ \mu^2$. The typically used wire, $254 \ \mu$ in diameter, yields an effective surface of approximately $101.3 \times 10^3 \ \mu^2$. Since this electrode surface is more than 10 times as large in area, it may be appreciated that the size of the electrode is reduced considerably. In addition, the reduction of current level by a factor of 2.5 should be reemphasized as yet another gain consequent to reducing the exposed tip of the electrode.

1. Mapping

Since a different type of electrode was used, it seemed important to determine whether self-stimulation placements observed with the larger wire would also be obtained with the small electrode (Huang and Routtenberg, 1971). This was particularly critical for those structures in the extrapyramidal area where self-stimulation was seen, since it was possible that the larger

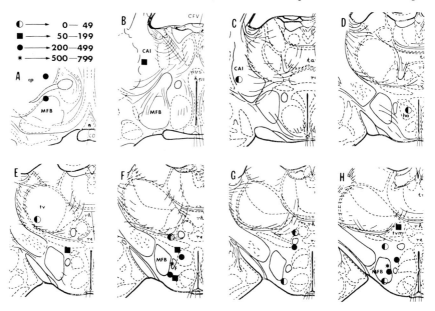

Fig. 1. Drawings showing sites of stimulation and associated self-stimulation (SS) rates. The legend at A, indicating SS scores and symbols, applies to all sections of Figs. 1–4. The symbols are associated with the following classifications of SS: half-filled circles, neutral; filled squares, low; filled circles, moderate; filled stars, high. Selected abbreviations: CAI, internal capsule; cp, nucleus caudatus putamen; F, fornix; ha, anterior hypothalamus; MFB, medial forebrain bundle; tv, ventral thalamus. (Sections A–H are from König and Klippel, 1963; Figs. 17b, 26b, 30b–34b.) Reprinted by permission of Pergamon Publishing Company, Elmsford, New York.

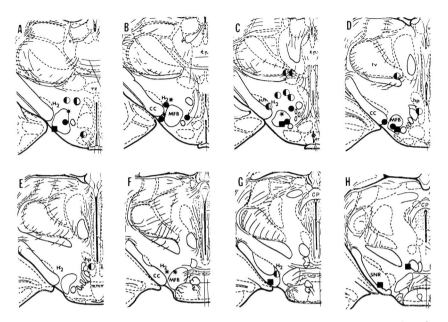

Fig. 2. Drawings showing sites of stimulation and associated SS rates. Symbols as in Fig. 1. Selected abbreviations: CC, crus cerebri; H_2, H_2 field of Forel; MFB, medial forebrain bundle; SNR, substantia nigra, zona reticulata; sut, subthalamus; tv, ventral thalamus. (Sections A–H are from König and Klippel, 1963, Figs. 37b–44b.) Reprinted by permission of Pergamon Publishing Company, Elmsford, New York.

electrodes and the more intense current levels had led to a current spread which blurred the accuracy of our localization of the electrode tip.

Figures 1–4 demonstrate, however, that self-stimulation was, in fact, obtained both from regions that have typically been implicated in self-stimulation, mainly the medial forebrain bundle (MFB), and those that have not, namely the extrapyramidal system. Figures 1 and 2 show that high rates of self-stimulation were obtained from MFB, and surrounding areas. Self-stimulation was obtained in the H_2 region, particularly well seen in Figs. 2(B) and (F). This confirmed our finding with large-diameter wire (Routtenberg and Huang, 1968). Self-stimulation was also obtained from the most medial part of the internal capsule and the most lateral edge of MFB [Figs. 2(D) and (B)]. As shown in Figs. 1(A) and (B), self-stimulation was obtained from the internal capsule in the region of the caudate/putamen complex.

Figure 3 shows that self-stimulation was indeed obtained with smaller electrodes from substantia nigra. In fact, high rates of self-stimulation were obtained from a region on the most medial aspect of substantia nigra, pars compacta (SNC) [Fig. 3(C)]. Moderate rates of self-stimulation were obtained routinely from SNC [Fig. 3(D)]. Figures 4(B) and (C) demonstrate that

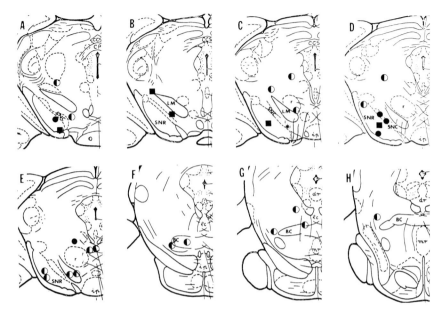

Fig. 3. Drawings showing sites of stimulation and associated SS rates. Symbols as in Fig. 1. Selected abbreviations: BC, brachium conjunctivum; MFB, medial forebrain bundle; r, red nucleus; SNC, substantia nigra, zona compacta; SNR, substantia nigra, zona reticulata. (Sections A–H are from König and Klippel, 1963; Figs. 45b–49b, 51b–52b, 54b.) Reprinted by permission of Pergamon Publishing Company, Elmsford, New York.

self-stimulation can be obtained near or in the brachium conjunctivum, although other placements near or in the brachium conjunctivum [Figs. 3(F, G) and 4(C)] demonstrated, indeed, that self-stimulation was not inevitably obtained from this fiber bundle. An interesting locus of self-stimulation, adjacent to the ventrolateral edge of the interstitial nucleus of Cajal, and immediately dorsal to the red nucleus, is observed in Fig. 3(E). Figure 3(H) shows that self-stimulation was not obtained from direct stimulation of nucleus interpositus and nucleus dentatus.

In summary, the results demonstrated clearly that self-stimulation with fine wire electrodes can be obtained from extrapyramidal structures as in the Routtenberg and Malsbury (1969) experiment, where the electrodes were larger and the current levels more intense.

It is likely, then, that these placements are not an artifact of electrode size of current intensity. Although the field of current cannot be specified until some method is devised for directly measuring current spread, it is certainly reasonable to assume that the spread is much reduced with the smaller electrode and lower current level.

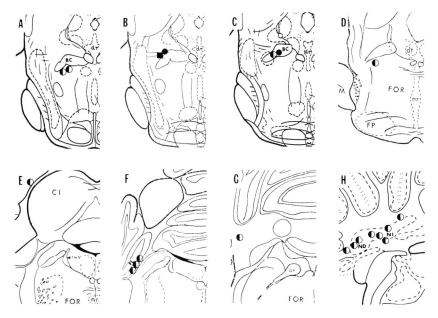

Fig. 4. Drawing showing sites of stimulation and associatated SS rates. Symbols as in Fig. 1. Selected abbreviations: BC, brachium conjunctivum; FL, flocculus; ND, dentate nucleus; NI, interpositus nucleus. (Sections A–C are from König and Klippel, 1963; Figs. 55b–57b. Sections D–G are from Routtenberg and Malsbury, 1969; Fig. 2B–D, F. Section H is from Pelligrino and Cushman, 1967; Fig. 80.) Reprinted by permission of Pergamon Publishing Company, Elmsford, New York.

2. Degeneration Following Lesions at Self-Stimulation Sites

Following the mapping experiment, Huang made lesions at self-stimulation sites in lateral hypothalamus and observed whether brainstem extrapyramidal self-stimulation sites might overlap with the pathways revealed by degeneration observed following lesions at lateral hypothalamic self-stimulation sites. If such occurred, one might consider the possibility of a relation between the self-stimulation observed in the lateral hypothalamus and that derived from brainstem extrapyramidal sites.

Before observing degeneration from self-stimulation sites, the confounding effects of degeneration created by the slender electrode tract were taken into account by placing electrodes immediately dorsal to the lateral hypothalamus and observing such degeneration. Electrodes were also placed at an angle, so that a different pattern of degeneration would be created by the electrode tract while maintaining the same lesion site. These two procedures were used, then, to enhance the distinction between the degeneration from the tract and that from the lesion itself, providing thereby the least ambiguous interpretation of the degeneration from the lesion site.

In order to obtain an overview of the observed pattern of degeneration from lateral hypothalamus, it is useful to chart first the pathways from a large lesion (Fig. 5) which destroyed the entire MFB at midhypothalamic levels [Fig. 5(D)].

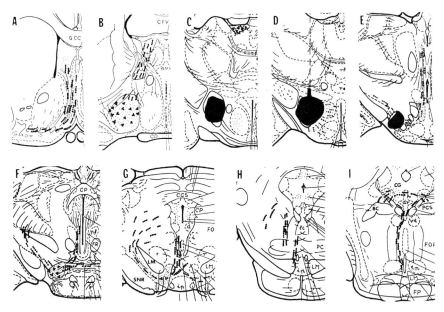

Fig. 5. Drawings of degenerated fibers which originated from lesions of MFB and surrounding areas. Coarser dots indicate degenerating fibers of passage; finer dots indicate areas of degenerating terminal axon ramifications. Selected abbreviations: BC, brachium conjunctivum; CG, central gray; LM, medial lemniscus; r, red nucleus; SNR, substantia nigra, zona reticulata. (The drawings are from König and Klippel, 1963; Figs. 14b, 25b, 30b, 33b, 40b, 43b, 47b, 51b, 56b.)

Ascending projections through the entire course of MFB may be seen; terminal degeneration is seen to be intermixed with fiber degeneration [Fig. 5(B)]. The primary target of these fibers is the medial septal area, although some terminals go to the lateral septal area [Fig. 5(A)] as well. Some of the fibers take a dorsal course and ascend in the stria medullaris to terminate in the habenula nucleus [Fig. 5(B, C)].

In the caudal direction, fibers move laterally to the H_2 field of Forel [Fig. 5(E, F)]; some move medially into the supramammillary decussation [Fig. 5(F)], others pass more caudally and terminate in the ventral tegmental area of Tsai [Fig. 5(G)]. A group of fibers move laterally at this anterior mesencephalic level, with terminations in the substantia nigra pars compacta, as well as distributing fibers to the reticular formation [Fig. 5(G)]. A more medial group of fibers is seen to ascend to the central gray [Fig. 5(G)]. In summary, three pathways [Fig. 5(H)] from the lateral hypothalamus to the brainstem and central gray may be seen: a medial, an intermediate, and a lateral pathway, all of which seem to terminate, at least in part, in various regions of the central gray.

One should note that in the case just considered that the lesion itself extends beyond the boundaries of MFB as defined by König and Klippel (1963). Hence, this lesion, although it is remarkably restricted to MFB, does overlap to some extent with adjacent structures. Thus, the pathways revealed with the larger lesion were studied with regard to their origin within MFB by using smaller lesions in other subjects.

A few examples of such attempts are shown in the charts of Figs. 6 and 7. We will consider three placements: medial, dorsal, and lateral. The medial placement [Fig. 6(C)] immediately adjacent to the fornix is in a region sometimes referred to as the "perifornical" area. The lesion made at this self-stimulation site produced ascending degeneration in the medial part of MFB. Descending degeneration in MFB is observed to occupy the most medial position of MFB

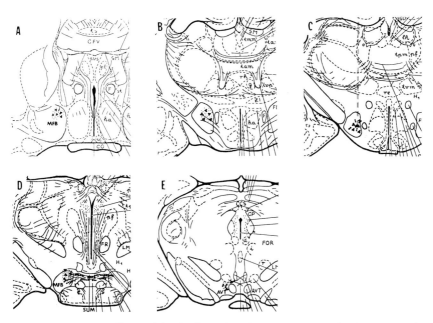

Fig. 6. Degenerated fibers originating from the lesioned medial part of MFB. Symbols for degenerated fibers and for degenerated terminal ramifications are as in Fig. 5. Selected abbreviations: AVT, ventral tegmental area of Tsai; MFB, medial forebrain bundle; SUM, supramammillary decussation. (The drawings are from König and Klippel, 1963; Figs. 24b, 31b, 37b, 42b, 46b.) Reprinted by permission of Pergamon Publishing Company, Elmsford, New York.

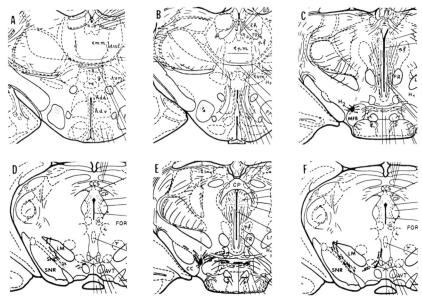

Fig. 7. Degenerated fibers originating from the lesioned dorsolateral part of MFB (A–D) and in the lesioned H_2 (E–F). Symbols for degenerating fibers and for degenerated terminal ramifications are as in Fig. 5. Selected abbreviations: CC, crus cerebri; H_2, H_2 field of Forel; LM, medial lemniscus; MFB, medial forebrain bundle; SNC, substantia nigra, zona compacta; SNR, substantia nigra, zona reticulata. (The drawings are from König and Klippel, 1963; Figs. 35b, 38b, 42b, 43b, 46b.) Reprinted by permission of Pergamon Publishing Company, Elmsford, New York.

with some fibers crossing in the supramammillary decussation. At the most posterior level where degeneration could be discerned, some fibers are observed to terminate in the ventral tegmental area of Tsai.

The dorsal placement [Fig. 7(C)] on the dorsolateral edge of MFB demonstrated degeneration which, like the medial placement, also terminated in the ventral tegmental areas of Tsai. Fibers were seen to terminate in substantia nigra pars compacta [SNC; Fig. 7(D)] in the medial position and to pass laterally. The lateral placement in the H_2 field of Forel [Fig. 7(E)] shows no degeneration into the ventral tegmental area of Tsai, but does show terminal degeneration into, and fiber degeneration passing through, SNC [Fig. 7(F)]. Two of the three major descending pathways, namely the lateral and the medial pathways, are also seen [Fig. 7(F)]. The intermediate pathway, however, is not observed.

These results indicate that degeneration from the lateral hypothalamus can pass through, or terminate in, certain placements in the brainstem which were shown by Routtenberg and Huang (1968), Routtenberg and Malsbury (1969), and Huang and Routtenberg (1971) to yield self-stimulation. This is particularly relevant to self-stimulation obtained from ventral tegmental decussation and substantia nigra. The case with regard to the brachium conjunctivum is less clear, since our mapping data did not have sufficient self-stimulation placements in this fiber bundle. In addition, small lesions in the lateral hypothalamus did not seem to lead to degeneration in the more posterior parts of the midbrain and anterior pons, where the brachium conjunctivum is most discernible. With the large lesion of Fig. 5 it can be seen that degeneration does pass through the brachium conjunctivum [Fig. 5(H, I)]. Hence, it is still possible, but not demonstrated, that self-stimulation from the brachium conjunctivum could be derivative of this lateral hypothalamic pathway. With the exception of the brachium, then, evidence would indicate the potential relation of the lateral hypothalamic self-stimulation mechanisms to brainstem extrapyramidal sites.

3. Retrograde Degeneration Following Lesions at Extrapyramidal Sites

Self-stimulation was obtained from the brachium conjunctivum by Routtenberg and Malsbury (1969) and, indeed, in the experiment by Huang and Routtenberg (1971). Self-stimulation, however, was not obtained by direct stimulation of nucleus interpositus or dentatus. That being the case, the cells of origin of brachium self-stimulation remain unknown. One can always assume that the self-stimulation obtained from the brachium conjunctivum was not derivative of the cerebellar subcortical nuclei but, in fact, came from fibers of passage perforating through the brachium conjunctivum. If this were the case, then perhaps the Fink-Heimer method was not altogether adequate to demonstrate the presence of such fibers. In order to determine, then, whether brachium conjunctivum self-stimulation was related to lateral hypothalamic mechanisms, it seemed worthwhile to attempt another approach to this problem.

The logic of this next experiment was as follows: if self-stimulation in brainstem, or from extrapyramidal sites were a derivative of the descending fibers from lateral hypothalamic cells of origin, then lesions at self-stimulation sites in the extrapyramidal system should produce retrograde chromatolytic changes in lateral hypothalamic cell bodies. To study this, then, we observed self-stimulation in extrapyramidal sites in the substantia nigra and the brachium conjunctivum (Fig. 8). One can see that self-stimulation was obtained using fine wires from direct stimulation of the brachium conjunctivum, but not when the electrode was slightly dorsal or ventral to the brachium.

A small lesion in the substantia nigra, pars compacta [Fig. 8(B)], but not one in the pars reticulata [Fig. 8(C, D)], produced retrograde chromatolysis in the lateral hypothalamus. Small lesions in the brachium conjunctivum, however, did not produce retrograde changes in the lateral hypothalamus, but rather produced retrograde changes in the nucleus interpositus and dentatus. This was not

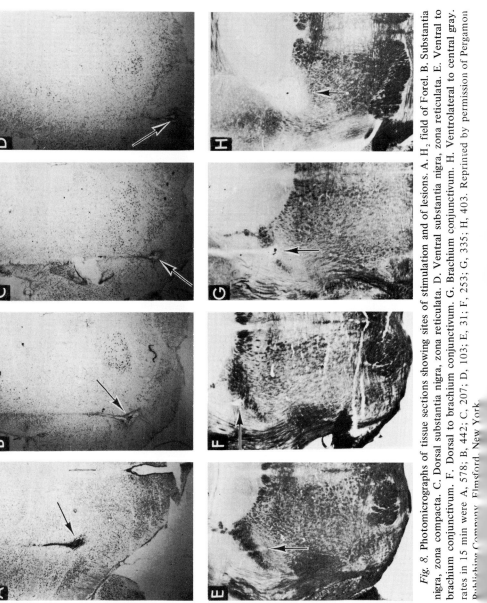

Fig. 8. Photomicrographs of tissue sections showing sites of stimulation and of lesions. A. H₂ field of Forel. B. Substantia nigra, zona compacta. C. Dorsal substantia nigra, zona reticulata. D. Ventral substantia nigra, zona reticulata. E. Ventral to brachium conjunctivum. F. Dorsal to brachium conjunctivum. G. Brachium conjunctivum. H. Ventrolateral to central gray. rates in 15 min were A, 578; B, 442; C, 207; D, 103; E, 31; F, 253; G, 335; H, 403. Reprinted by permission of Pergamon Publishing Company, Elmsford, New York.

surprising from an anatomical point of view. From our earlier experiments, however, we were faced with a dilemma, based on apparently contradictory data: (1) Stimulation of the brachium conjunctivum did support self-stimulation. (2) Lesions at such sites caused prograde degeneration in certain components of the brachium. (3) Retrograde changes were observed in the nucleus interpositus and dentatus following lesions of brachium conjunctivum self-stimulation sites. (4) But direct stimulation of dentatus or interpositus did not support self-stimulation. Since no chromatolytic changes were observed in the lateral hypothalamus, which was one region where such changes were suspected to be observed, the possibility that some other, undetected region of retrograde chromatolytic changes occurred should be considered.

We wish to retain the assumption, however, that the brachium conjunctivum is, in fact, a major fiber system involved with self-stimulation, and that the difficulty considered above concerns direct stimulation of its cell bodies of origin (point 4). The paradox then is that stimulation of the axons of nucleus interpositus and dentatus supports self-stimulation, but direct stimulation of the cell bodies does not. The answer to this problem may be found in the presumed nature of the difference between stimulation of cell bodies and axons. If the threshold for activation is lower for axons than for the cell bodies, then one might consider the terminal axons coming from the cerebellum which have been defined as inhibitory by Eccles, Ito, and Szentagothai (1967). An electrode placed in the cell bodies of interpositus might therefore preferentially activate the inhibitory axons of termination from Purkinje cells on interpositus cell bodies. Stated another way, although the stimulation of cell bodies may lead to activation for 10–20 msec (Toyama, Tsukawara, Kosaka, and Matsunami, 1970), the inhibitory action of Purkinje terminals may dominate for a longer period, perhaps 480–490 msec. This latter consequence would be of considerable importance in the behavioral response of the animal to the stimulation. Thus, EPSPs may be observed in red nucleus following activation of interpositus or dentatus, but this may be followed by a depression of that system. Such evidence was not shown in the Toyama *et al.* (1970) study. If this depression occurred, then the lack of self-stimulation from interpositus or dentatus may be simply that the net effect of stimulation there is inhibition of cellular activity by stimulation of the inhibitory axon terminals. Although this explanation requires confirmation, the considerations above do recommend detailed analysis of the consequences of the stimulation in the context of the morphology in which the exposed electrode tip is embedded.

C. TELENCEPHALIC SELF-STIMULATION

Our experiments on the projections from self-stimulation sites both from brainstem and lateral hypothalamus indicated that it was not feasible to take a limited view of the sites of self-stimulation; that is, each self-stimulation site had to be considered in terms of projections from both ascending and descending systems. It seemed important, in order to complete this initial survey, to obtain information concerning self-stimulation from forebrain regions, particularly the septal area, cingulate, and pregenual cortex. The experiment, then, followed exactly the same procedure as that described for the experiment by Huang and Routtenberg (1971). We first mapped the sites of self-stimulation in the anterior forebrain, and then studied degeneration from such self-stimulation sites (Routtenberg, 1971a).

1. Mapping Study

As can be seen in Fig. 9(A, B), self-stimulation was obtained from anterior cortical regions and from the intermediate olfactory tract. In Fig. 9(C), self-stimulation was derived from the cingulum and adjoining regions in the anterior hippocampus and in frontal and pregenual cortex. In Fig. 9(G, H), where the genu of the corpus callosum in observed, self-stimulation was seen in the caudate nucleus, as well as in the anterior commissure. Self-stimulation was also derived from the lateral septal region. Some placements did not yield self-stimulation in the central and dorsal regions of the caudate nucleus [Fig. 9(C, H)]. It would appear certain that the major self-stimulation from the caudate nucleus is along the medial edge. Self-stimulation is observed in the

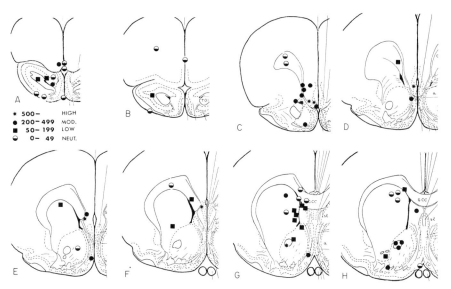

Fig. 9. Electrode point and self-stimulation rate indicated by symbols in A. (Sections A–H are from König and Klippel, 1963; Figs. 4b, 6b, 8b, 10b–14b.)

region of the anterior commissure and the most anterior parts of MFB. Self-stimulation is also observed from electrodes in the stria terminalis.

In summary, the pattern of points yielding self-stimulation suggested (Routtenberg, 1971a) that at least two clusters or groupings of self-stimulation loci could be distinguished. The first group of points were considered olfactory. These included the olfactory tract and nuclei, septal area, anterior commissure, medial forebrain bundle, stria medullaris, and stria terminalis. The other group was termed extraolfactory (Routtenberg, 1971a). The structures included in this classification were the frontal cortex, cingulum, and caudate nucleus.

2. Degeneration from Self-Stimulation Sites

The distinction between olfactory and extraolfactory sites of self-stimulation was based, in part, on consideration of the pathways from frontal cortex self-stimulation sites. Figure 10 shows the pattern of degeneration following lesions made at self-stimulation sites in the frontal cortex. This area is variously defined (see Leonard, 1969 for discussion), but it can be considered frontal cortex, at least on the basis of its receiving afferents from the dorsomedial nucleus of the thalamus.

Four placements in this region which supported self-stimulation were studied for degeneration. The pattern of the projection was similar in all cases; thus in the subsequent panels of Fig. 10 the chart from one representative subject is

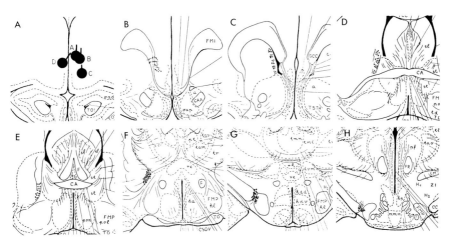

Fig. 10. Section A is a schematic summary of lesions of four subjects used in a silver impregnation experiment. Self-stimulation is 15 min for each subject. A, 527; B, 465; C, 475; D, 390. Sections B–H contain schematic reconstruction of degeneration patterns resulting from lesion at D. (Sections A–H are taken from König and Klippel, 1963; Figs. 6b, 8b, 11b, 18b, 21b, 28b, 36b, 40b.)

presented. Degeneration charted in panels B–H of Fig. 10 passed in a caudal and then lateral direction through the cingulum and into the medial aspect of the caudate nucleus [Fig. 10(C)]. It remained in that region, and then moved ventrally through the caudate nucleus in the fibers of the internal capsule, assuming a position immediately dorsal to the anterior commissure and medial to the globus pallidus [(Fig. 10(E)]. These fibers interdigitated with MFB, occupying the most medial edge of the internal capsule [Fig. 10(F, G)]. Degeneration was followed to the mesodiencephalic junction in the region of H_2. Axonal and terminal degeneration into the midbrain could not be documented with certainty.

These results point to a most important set of conclusions and considerations concerning the telencephalic anatomy of self-stimulation. First, in the forebrain, it seems worthwhile to differentiate between olfactory and extraolfactory self-stimulation systems. This distinction is based solely on anatomical grounds. Thus, self-stimulation obtained from the olfactory bulb, septal area, diagonal band of Broca is related to an olfactory system. The extraolfactory system, which has been delineated by the degeneration experiment, has its cells of origin in the frontal cortex of the rat, and projects through the caudate nucleus down into the most medial part of the internal capsule probably terminating, in part, in the area of the H_2 field of Forel.

A second point of importance is that many of the self-stimulation sites observed in the mapping experiment do indeed overlap with the degeneration pathways described following lesions at hypothalamic self-stimulation sites. This point is particularly important both with regard to self-stimulation sites in this forebrain study, and those reported in the prior experiment by Huang and Routtenberg (1971). With regard to the present results, self-stimulation sites in cingulum and caudate nucleus can be related to the trajectory of the pathway observed following lesions at frontal cortex self-stimulation sites. It will be recalled in the hypothalamic mapping study that there were several self-stimulation sites [see in particular, Fig 2(B)] in the lateral part of MFB which would activate the fibers originating from the frontal cortex. Considering the self-stimulation literature in general, then, self-stimulation that has been attributed to MFB fibers, may, in fact, be related to activation of these fibers from frontal cortex.

Whether self-stimulation derived from the ventrolateral hypothalamic region is truly activating MFB or the corticofugal fibers originating from pregenual cortex is an issue only when one has a precise definition of MFB (see Millhouse, 1969). Certainly one could define this frontodiencephalic pathway as part of MFB. This does not seem to be advisable, however, on several grounds. Descending MFB has typically been associated with cells of origin in the septal area, in the olfactory-related amygdaloid region, and perhaps directly from the hippocampus. It has not been viewed as having origins in the frontal cortex. One might be concerned about whether this frontal cortex is related to the cingulate cortex, but its lack of projection to hippocampus and its reception of dorsomedial thalamus (DMT) afferents does not recommend this view. It is difficult to place this fiber system along with MFB as typically defined, since these frontdiencephalic fibers are heavily myelinated relative to MFB. The caliber of the fiber is also different. These fibers appear in clusters, rather than diffusely spread throughout it. Observation of sections stained according to Weil (1928) shows that these clusters can be observed in normal material. These clusters do not appear to be part of the main body of the internal capsule, but in terms of their location, occupy a position intermediate between the internal capsule and MFB. In sum, although in close spatial proximity to MFB, it appears that this frontodiencephalic pathway should be distinguished from it.

A third point that should be emphasized is the fact that self-stimulation can be obtained from the frontal cortex. According to Leonard (1969) this region receives input from the anterior portion of the dorsomedial nucleus of the thalamus (DMT). It may be possible that the electrodes which yielded the highest rates of self-stimulation were activating simultaneously the efferents from DMT and from the frontdiencephalic fibers. Preliminary data suggest, indeed, that self-stimulation can be obtained from DMT efferents[1]. Since the projection to DMT from the hypothalamus is well known (Guillery, 1957), one may have the beginning of a circuit: hypothalamus-thalamus-cortex-H_2 field of Forel-brainstem. The present results recommend such a view, but further anatomical and physiological study will be required to prove it.

D. Overview of Experiments to Date: Self-Stimulation Anatomy

Considering the results from the brainstem, hypothalamic, and telencephalic self-stimulation experiments so far reviewed, two major conclusions, one methodological the other empirical, must be emphasized.

1. Methodological Summary

Perhaps the most important consequence of the present strategy is that it provides the basis for establishing the pathways related to self-stimulation. This means, as stated earlier, that the seemingly infinite catalog of points which have

---

[1] We have begun investigation of the self-stimulation in DMT in rat and have obtained low rates from this region (Huang and Routtenberg, unpublished). Until Fink-Heimer degeneration, retrograde study, and microelectrode work is performed, it will not be possible to specify the DMT involvement with certainty. Another study tracing degeneration from self-stimulation sites in rhesus monkey (Routtenberg, Gardner, and Huang, 1971) also indicates the involvement of DMT in self-stimulation.

been reported in the literature can be replaced eventually by a set of pathways, finite in number, which may then be understood in terms of their physiology and functional organization. The identification of structural organization will lead, then, to the understanding of function.

Another methodological point is the apparent paradoxical conclusion that one cannot infer the site of action of an electrode solely by the knowledge of the deepest penetration of the electrode tip. That is, one cannot be certain of the true site of action of the electrode by its site of activation. Our experience with self-stimulation at various levels of the neuraxis suggests that it is important to take a broad view in defining the site of activation of a self-stimulation electrode. The use of several anatomical techniques involving observation of the site of deepest penetration of the electrode, and degeneration from self-stimulation sites, both orthograde and retrograde, will be useful in understanding the organization of self-stimulation. We still have to consider the physiological attributes of this anatomical organization, but the former should be understood in terms of the structural basis of self-stimulation.

2. Empirical Findings

The major conclusion to be made at this time is that a relation exists among self-stimulation sites in forebrain, in lateral hypothalamus, and in extrapyramidal structures. This relation, however, has yet to be defined precisely. One suggested organization based on the data obtained so far will be presented following the discussion of the physiological data.

Before turning to the physiological data, however, it is important to point out a few important directions for future research. First, the uncertainty with regard to the role of the cerebellum remains, despite several attempts to implicate or refute its role in self-stimulation. More detailed study of the three subcortical cerebellar nuclei seems necessary as well as a more careful study of the fiber systems as they leave these nuclear groups. Second, the issue of stimulation of cell bodies as opposed to axons remains unclear. This problem must be resolved if we are to understand the organization, both structural and functional, of the fiber systems which mediate self-stimulation. Perhaps consideration of this issue will provide another route to understanding the functional relations among nuclear groups; for the present, however, this remains a problem which will best be solved with electrophysiological methods. Third, the role of the dorsomedial nucleus of the thalamus in self-stimulation, which has been suggested above, remains to be established. To our knowledge this structure has not been previously implicated in self-stimulation.

VI. Electrophysiology of Self-Stimulation

The data considered up to this point have been anatomical in nature in an effort to suggest the self-stimulation substrate location in the central nervous system. These connections do not, however, suggest a great deal concerning the function of the systems involved since the function of the fiber systems which mediate self-stimulation cannot be understood solely by acquiring detailed knowledge of those fiber pathways which mediate self-stimulation. Were all these pathways and their termination sites known, it would still not be sufficient. It was necessary to obtain physiological data that would define the functional attributes of this structural system.

We embarked, therefore, upon a series of experiments to relate the physiological activity in the brain to the activation that occurs during brain self-stimulation. We have taken two approaches to this problem. One approach involved the study of hippocampal activity derived with macroelectrodes. A second approach involved forebrain and brainstem activity observed with tungsten microelectrodes. Microelectrode studies were initiated in an attempt to define individual monosynaptic relationships revealed by silver impregnation methods in terms of their facilitatory or suppressing influence. Thus, anatomical projections would reveal the existence of a relationship, and microelectrode study would define the nature of the relationship.

Hippocampal activity was used to consider the polysynaptic relationships among the self-stimulation fiber systems defined by anatomical and micro-electrode methods. It was presumed that observation of hippocampal activity might represent a "summarizing statement" of the activity occurring in these fiber systems. When we consider data from the hippocampus in detail we will discuss this view further. The study of hippocampal activity was initiated also in the hope that some relation could then be detected between the activity observed in the hippocampus during brain stimulation and that observed during normal patterns of behavior. It was thought that comparison of the activity observed in the two situations might provide an important clue concerning the function of the fibers mediating self-stimulation.

In summary, then, the integration of the anatomical, microelectrode, and macroelectrode data was to proceed by defining (1) the anatomical projections, (2) the nature of the projection as revealed by microelectrode studies, (3) the overall operation of the system as revealed by hippocampal activity, and (4) the relation of this hippocampal activity to normal behavior. It would then be possible to arrive at an understanding of the function of the fibers which mediate the self-stimulation phenomenon based on (1) experimental anatomical and microelectrode definitions of monosynaptic relationships, and (2) poly-synaptic combinations leading to certain patterns of hippocampal macro-electrode activity.

The relationship of such hippocampal patterns to those observed during behavioral activities would allow an understanding of the role that self-stimulation pathways play in behavior, and the neurobiological bases for the behavioral activities in terms of anatomically and physiologically defined systems. It should be noted that an explanation for self-stimulation itself would not necessarily be achieved. One would, rather, understand the function of the fiber pathways which mediate self-stimulation. With this overview, then, the physiological data that we have collected in recent years will now be reviewed.

A. MICROELECTRODE RECORDING

The purpose of recording neuronal activity was to define the cellular relationships among the various nuclear groups that are important in self-stimulation. The results obtained to date have been interesting but disappointing, since we have not been able with the microelectrode technique to characterize unequivocally the functional relationships among nuclear groups revealed with anatomical methods. The evidence that will be presented does suggest that this approach can yield important results. There should, however, be no illusions with regard to the research here. The time and effort already extended has been considerable and in our view, not commensurate with the amount of information that has been gained. Nonetheless, we are encouraged by certain of our findings and hope by reviewing current facts as well as future prospects to encourage appropriate exploration of the electrophysiological organization of self-stimulation.

Our first research effort along these lines investigated the role of reticular formation in self-stimulation. As discussed earlier, Glickman (1960) and Olds and Peretz (1960) indicated that reticular formation supported self-stimulation. Others (Sharpless, 1958) argued that the reticular formation represented a convergent site for self-stimulation. It was in this context, then, that we initiated our research.

1. Brain Stimulation and Neuronal Activity

Since self-stimulation obtained from the hypothalamus and that observed in the septal area were dissimilar in several respects (Routtenberg, 1968a), it was thought that the similar observed behavior in the two cases, the bar-pressing itself, might be mediated by convergences at some distant site, perhaps the reticular formation (RF). With this view, then, Huang and I looked at the effects of stimulation in posterior hypothalamus and in the septal region on unitary activity in the brainstem.

The methods used have been detailed in the experimental report (Routtenberg and Huang, 1968). Briefly, animals were chronically implanted with two electrodes, one in the septal area, one in the posterior hypothalamus. Following recovery from the implantation and subsequent self-stimulation testing, animals were anesthetized with ether and placed in a semiacute experiment. Ether anesthesia was replaced with *d*-tubocurarine paralysis and procaine local anesthesia. The effects of stimulation at both sites on unitary activity of several brainstem sites was studied with tungsten microelectrodes. If more than one session was required of an individual animal, it was recovered from paralysis and used again. In other experiments (Routtenberg and Vern, 1968) we have similarly tested for self-stimulation and then performed an acute experiment following behavioral testing. We have not, however, evaluated the effects of prior behavioral training on the responsiveness of neurons to stimulation.

The types of responses evoked by stimulation in the septal area and the hypothalamus are noted in the next two figures (Figs. 11 and 12). It may be seen that five different types of responses were observed. Because we recorded from only 150 neurons throughout the brainstem, we did not attempt to establish relationships between the type of response observed and the site of recording. In our analysis of the influence of septal and hypothalamic stimulation on unitary activity we did not then distinguish between the various

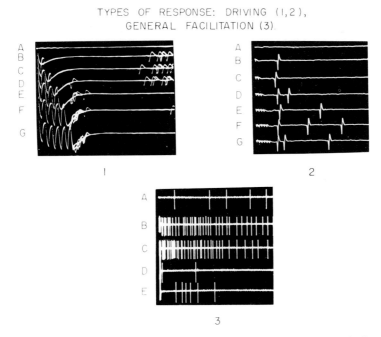

Fig. 11. Part 1 was recorded from reticularis parvocellularis, part 2 from the interpeduncular nucleus, part 3 from reticularis gigantocellularis. For parts 1 and 2, A was without stimulation; B–G with posterior diencephalic (PD) stimulation where the number of stimulus pulses increased from 1 to 6. In part 1, each record was 10 superimposed traces. Note that the response latency was decreased in a single discrete step as the stimulus strength was increased. For part 3, A was without stimulation, B–C with PD stimulation, D–E with septal-limbic stimulation. Calibrations for part 1, 2 msec and 2 mV; for part 2, 5 msec and 2 mv; for part 3, 100 msec and 1 mV. Reprinted by permission of Pergamon Publishing Company, Elmsford, New York.

TYPES OF RESPONSE: INHIBITION (4,5), DRIVING
AND INHIBITION (6,7), ANTICIPATION (8).

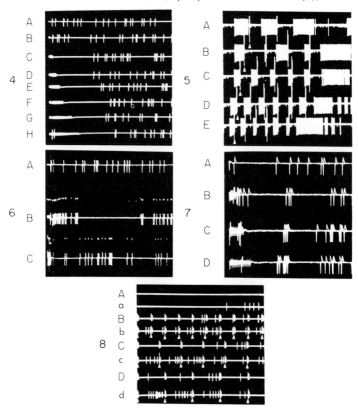

Fig. 12. For part 4, which was taken from the inferior colliculus, A was spontaneous activity, B–H were taken following PD stimulation, the train duration of which was increased successively. In part 5, obtained from reticularis parvocellularis, all records involved repetitive PD stimulation. Interstimulus interval for A was 1000; B, 800; C, 630; D, 500; and E, 400 msec. Only the second stimulus artifact of each sweep is indicated by an arrow. Note the long-lasting bursts at the end of sweeps B–E as the stimulation was withheld. In part 6, obtained from interpeduncular nucleus, each record was 10 traces superimposed. A was for spontaneous activity; B, for the effect of PD stimulation; C, for the effect of septal-limbic stimulation. In part 7, recorded from reticularis pontis caudalis, all records were taken following PD stimulation, the number of stimulus pulses increasing from A to D. In part 8, recorded from mesencephalic reticular formation, A and a were spontaneous activity, B-d, with PD stimulation. In each pair of B and b, C and c, D and d, the first record shows the effect of the initial stimulation, the second the effect of the later stimulation. Interrecord interval for each pair was 10 times interstimulus interval (5, 8, and 10 sec). Interstimulus interval was 500, 800, and 1000 msec for Bb, Cc, and Dd respectively, the stimulus artifact indicated by an arrow on the second record of each pair. Calibration for part 4, 20 msec and 5 mV; for part 5, 500 msec and 2 mV; for part 6, 20 msec and 2 mV; for part 7, 10 msec and 2 mV; for part 8, 500 msec and 5 mV. Reprinted by permission of Pergamon Publishing Company, Elmsford, New York.

types of responses observed. Such distinctions will be required if we are to understand fully the relationship between stimulation at self-stimulation sites and the nature of the influence at selective nuclear groups. For the present analysis, however, we were able to draw certain conclusions relevant to the initial purposes of the experiment.

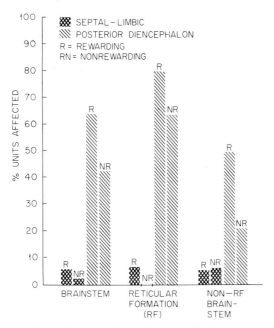

Fig. 13. Influence of septal-limbic and posterior diencephalic stimulation upon brainstem unitary activity. Comparison of the percentage units affected (ordinate) as a function of the locus of recording electrode (abscissa). Within each recording locus, comparisons are presented both between site of stimulation (septal-limbic *vs.* posterior diencephalon) and behavioral effect of stimulation (rewarding *vs.* nonrewarding). Reprinted by permission of Pergamon Publishing Company, Elmsford, New York.

As can be seen in Fig. 13, hypothalamic stimulation had a considerably greater influence on brainstem unitary activity than did stimulation of the septal area. Stimulation at both reward (R) and nonreward (NR) sites in the hypothalamus equally affected a high percentage of the units that were recorded.[2] A greater influence of R than NR was discerned if and only if brainstem or brainstem without RF was considered. This was not the case with self-stimulation in the septal area where there was no difference between nonreticular formation brainstem units in terms of their influence by R and NR

[2] Use of the term reward in this context is for convenience and should be read as a shorthand form for "electrode sites, which when tested in a behavioral situation, supported self-stimulation."

brain stimulation. There was, however, a considerable difference between R and NR brain stimulation with regard to RF only. Thus, one can conclude that septal area and posterior hypothalamus are different, not only with regard to a wide variety of autonomic and behavioral measures (Routtenberg, 1968a) but with regard to their influence on brainstem neuronal activity. One can also conclude that the reticular formation does not discriminate between R and NR since loci in septal area and hypothalamus which both supported self-stimulation produced different responses in RF, while R and NR loci in the hypothalamus both caused similar responses. Hence, it seems unlikely that RF represents an important structure in coding for the self-stimulation effect. This is supported by the results of Lorens (1966) which showed that lesions of the reticular formation did not attenuate MFB self-stimulation.

In the Routtenberg and Huang (1968) study self-stimulation in the posterior hypothalamus was obtained from two different regions, the medial forebrain bundle (MFB) and the adjacent H_2 field of Forel (H_2). When we compared the units influenced by stimulation in these two regions it was found that stimulation in H_2 and MFB influenced RF units equally; MFB 25 of 31 units and H_2, 12 of 15 units. However, when we analyzed the response of non-RF brainstem, MFB stimulation influenced only 7 of 29 units whereas H_2 influenced 23 of 30. Thus, H_2 stimulation appears to have a more pervasive influence on nonreticular structures. Whatever the significance of that finding, it is clear that the microelectrode recording method used here can indeed differentiate between spatially adjacent, but functionally dissimilar, self-stimulation sites.

A recent study by Keene and Casey (1970) has confirmed our initial finding that stimulation in the posterior hypothalamus at self-stimulation sites can evoke facilitatory activity in the nucleus gigantocellularis (Fig. 13, part 3). Keene and Casey (1970) have shown, in addition, that gigantocellularis neurons respond to aversive stimuli such as pinching and foot shock. Further, they report that chronic stimulation in this region produced escape behavior. Although we have had placements in this region (Routtenberg and Malsbury, 1969, Fig. 2; Fig. 2 in this paper), escape behavior was not observed. Different levels of stimulation or stimulus parameters may account for the different results obtained. It would be of considerable interest to understand why stimulation at a so-called reward site activates a site which seems to respond as well to aversive stimuli such as pinching or peripheral shock to the feet. These results are consistent with the Olds and Olds (1962) report that stimulation in the lateral hypothalamus facilitated escape to aversive dorsal midbrain stimulation and with Stein's (1965) report of facilitation of avoidance to peripheral shock by hypothalamic stimulation. These findings suggest a possible neuronal substrate for this facilitation by brain stimulation of behavioral response to aversive stimulation. It leaves unexplained, however, why stimulation at the posterior hypothalamic site should support self-stimulation, since presumably this activates a region which mediates aversion.

In a more recent microelectrode investigation in our laboratory using the fine wire stimulating electrodes and barbiturate anesthesia, it has been demonstrated (Huang and Routtenberg, 1971) that stimulation at self-stimulation sites in the hypothalamus produces suppression of activity in the substantia nigra, pars compacta. This region was not studied during the first experiment by Routtenberg and Huang (1968) and such results suggest an important link between the so-called limbic system self-stimulation sites and the extrapyramidal system. It is worth recalling that Huang and Routtenberg (1971) demonstrated that lesions of self-stimulation sites in lateral hypothalamus led to orthograde degeneration in the substantia nigra pars compacta (SNC) and that lesions at self-stimulation sites in SNC produced retrograde cell chromatolytic changes in the lateral hypothalamus. All of these data recommend the view that an important relation exists between substantia nigra, pars compacta, and the lateral hypothalamus.

Another microelectrode experiment indicated that there was an ascending influence of stimulation at hypothalamic sites on neurons of the cingulate region and septal area (Routtenberg and Vern, 1968). Stimulation at R-sites in the hypothalamus provoked, as in the study with Huang, a wide variety of responses (Fig. 14) from 158 neurons recorded in septal area, cingulate cortex, and adjacent regions. A summary of the responses obtained is presented in Table I. One response which is characteristic for the medial septal area is shown in Fig. 14, panels G and H. This demonstrates the burst pattern originally described by Petsche *et al.* (1962). This activity is characteristic of the medial septal region when hippocampal theta is observed. We attempted to study R and NR

TABLE I

NUMBER OF UNITS RESPONDING AND RESPONSE PATTERN FOLLOWING STIMULATION AT REWARDING AND NONREWARDING SITES

Type of response pattern	Rewarding		Nonrewarding	
	Number	%	Number	%
A. Drive	15	17	14	21
B. Drive-suppression	17	19	14	21
C. Suppression-drive-suppression	8	9	0	0
D. Simple inhibition	12	13	16	23
E. Drive-suppression-drive	3	3	2	3
F. Complete inhibition	4	5	3	4
G. Septal bursts	12	13	7	10
No effect	19	21	12	18

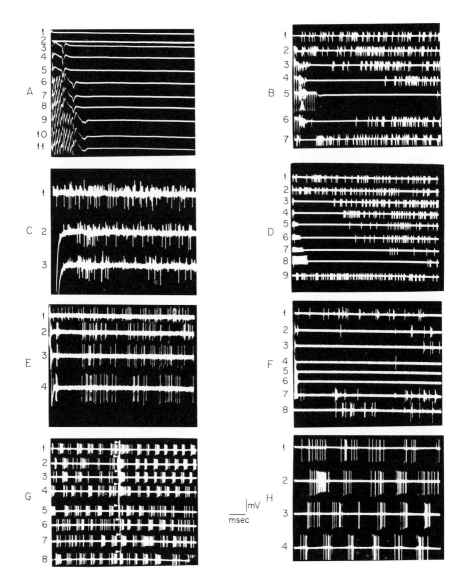

Fig. 14. A. Drive: Traces 1, 2–spontaneous level; 3–5–1 pulse; 6–8–5 pulses; 9–11–8 pulses. Calibration: 2 mV and and 5 msec 1 sweep. Unit from cingulate cortex. In this and succeeding traces, positivity is down. B. Drive-suppression: Trace 1–spontaneous; (note unitary response during stimulation in traces 4 and 5) 2–6–1, 2, 4, 10, and 4 pulses; Trace 7–spontaneous. Calibration: 2 mV and 20 msec 20 sweeps. Unit from cingulate cortex. C. Suppression-drive-suppression: Trace 1–spontaneous; Trace2–5 pulses; Trace 3–10 pulses. Calibration: 0.2 mV and 20 msec 20 sweeps. Unit from cingulate cortex. D. Simple

stimulation sites in terms of their effectiveness in facilitating bursting in the septal area. No difference was observed. We did observe that stimulation of R-sites produced a particular pattern, suppression-drive-suppression, which was not elicited by NR stimulation. The significance of this finding may reside in the fact that, at sites which supported self-stimulation, the consequence of activation of a particular set of pathways, ascending and descending, produced this particular pattern; NR placements simply did not have access to this set of pathways.

2. Implications and Discussion

One can gather from the microelectrode experiments reviewed above that stimulation produces a complicated set of responses at distant brain sites. One must be cautious, therefore, in the interpretation of the effects of brain stimulation since there are quite clearly, direct monosynaptic effects, polysynaptic effects, and rebound or disinhibition effects as a result of stimulation. These results indicate that the kind of neuronal activity that is being generated during self-stimulation is complex. One should be cautious, therefore, in interpreting the relation between the behavioral patterns caused by the stimulation and the type of electrophysiological patterns that are generated during the stimulation. A recent series of experiments studying the behavioral refractory period by Coon and colleagues (e.g., Smith and Coons, 1970) may be susceptible to several alternative interpretations because of this problem.

The results obtained with microelectrode recording also indicate that there is considerable detailed information that is yet to be gained. One would, for example, have preferred more information with regard to the comparison of the effects of MFB and field of Forel stimulation on brainstem unitary activity. It is clear that our anatomical techniques are not demonstrating what the physiological techniques have shown. Thus, stimulation of either field of Forel or MFB can activate reticular formation neurons with short latency mono-synaptic responses. The Fink-Heimer technique, however, has not been capable of demonstrating unequivocally the presence of terminals on reticular neurons (Huang and Routtenberg, 1971).

---

suppression: Trace 1—spontaneous; Traces 2–8–1, 5, 10, 30, 50, 70, 100 pulses; 9—spontaneous. Calibration: 5 mV and 100 msec 25 sweeps. Unit from cingulate cortex. E. Drive-suppression-drive: Trace 1—spontaneous; Traces 2–4–1, 5, 10 pulses. Calibration: 0.2 mV and 50 msec 20 sweeps. Unit from diagonal band of Broca. F. Complete suppression: Trace 1—spontaneous; Traces 2–6–1, 2, 4, 12, 20 pulses; 7–8—spontaneous. Calibration: 1 mV and 200 msec 25 sweeps. Unit from lateral septal nucleus. G. Septal bursts: Traces 1–8—stimulation applied to animal at approximately midway point across trace (indicated by arrows); 1–4–50 pulses; 5–8–10 pulses. Calibration: 2 mV and 500 msec 1 sweep. Unit from medial septal nucleus. H. Septal bursts: Traces 1–2—spontaneous; 3–4—stroking back. Calibration: 0.5 mV and 200 msec 1 sweep. Unit from medial septal nucleus.

At the time when we performed the initial microelectrode experiment (Routtenberg and Huang, 1968) we did not differentiate between the medial and lateral parts of MFB. It is possible that part of MFB stimulation was activating the fibers of origin from the frontal cortex. Nonetheless, it was demonstrated that MFB had considerably less effect, whereas the field of Forel had a much greater effect on nonreticular neurons. This influence may be related to the lateral and intermediate pathways which arise from the field of Forel (Huang and Routtenberg, 1971).

Of considerable interest is the effect of stimulation in the lateral hypothalamus on neurons of substantia nigra, pars compacta. According to our results, it may be suggested that activation in the frontal cortex will suppress the activity of the substantia nigra. This proposal is based on two findings: (1) stimulation of lateral hypothalamus suppresses SNC neuronal activity, (2) lesions at self-stimulation sites in frontal cortex lead to degeneration through lateral hypothalamus. Because of other anatomical data suggesting a frontal-nigral projection (e.g., Harting and Martin, 1970), it may be suggested that frontal cortical fibers, in part, may have played a role in suppressing SNC neuronal activity. This type of suppression may be similar to the control mechanisms that have been described in the cerebellum (Eccles *et al.*, 1967), in which the primary output from the cerebellum, the Purkinje cell, inhibits neurons of the subcortical cerebellar nuclei. It would be particularly interesting then, if this corticopetal tract is an important descending forebrain pathway concerned with motor output control.

One final issue concerning the relation of self-stimulation sites producing aversive behavioral responses is worth mentioning. This relationship has not been clarified by microelectrode recordings to date, although Keene and Casey (1970) have suggested that one output from the lateral hypothalamus is to the medial brainstem in the medulla, in the nucleus reticularis gigantocellularis. These results, they suggest, support the idea that self-stimulation can enhance response to aversive brain stimulation. It is interesting, but disappointing, that we have not been able to trace a degeneration into nucleus reticularis gigantocellularis, although one should have expected such degeneration on the basis of their research.

B. HIPPOCAMPAL ACTIVITY

We have investigated the relationship of hippocampal activity to self-stimulation primarily because evidence that preceded our work suggested that the hippocampus is remarkably sensitive to behavioral activities of the vertebrate, particularly the cat (Grastyan, 1959; Adey and Tokizane, 1967). The importance of the relation of hippocampal electrophysiology to behavior had not been emphasized, however, until the work of Green and Arduini (1954) demonstrated that stimulation of the reticular formation produces a characteristic EEG pattern termed hippocampal theta of synchronized, regularized waves in the hippocampus. Jung and Kornmüller (1938) had early recognized the presence of these waves but it was not until the investigation by Green and Arduini (1954) that their functional importance was emphasized.

Green and Arduini showed that stimulation of the brainstem reticular formation produced hippocampal theta, a synchronized activity, while producing neocortical desynchronization, a pattern considered to reflect arousal (Moruzzi and Magoun, 1949). It was thought that the relation between hippocampus and cerebral cortex was reciprocal: when one showed the activation pattern of desynchronization, the other one showed the synchronized pattern of suppressed activity. This reciprocal relation was supported by Adey (1961) who demonstrated that stimulation in the hippocampus itself can suppress the activity of reticular transmission of evoked potentials generated in the lower brainstem and recorded in the midbrain reticular formation. The fact that stimulation of the reticular formation which produced neocortical arousal also produced theta activity led Green and Arduini (1954) to suggest that theta activity represented a hippocampal arousal pattern. This was the first major theory concerning the significance of hippocampal theta. This view, like many that followed it, was questioned on several grounds. For example, Jouvet (1967) and others demonstrated hippocampal activity in the theta mode during sleep with rapid eye movements. Thus, a simple explanation of theta activity as an arousal pattern seemed to be inadequate. Several experiments, particularly from Adey's laboratory, have attempted to define theta activity in terms of its role in learning. Elazar and Adey (1967) have suggested, in fact, that these waves are themselves related to some form of information processing.

Our own view of recording from hippocampus was that it represented an invaluable approach to the understanding of hippocampal function with regard to behavior. It was felt, however, that the behavior being observed was too complex, not allowing for a clear statement of the hippocampal activity-behavior relationship. It was felt, also, that an investigation of the relation of the hippocampus to basic motivational conditions and simple behavioral patterns of the animal would yield unambiguous information. Such information could be related, perhaps subsequently, to these complex patterns.

That such an investigation was indeed necessary was indicated by the uncertain information concerning hippocampal activity and food deprivation. Since interest had been generated with regard to the hippocampus and arousal, and between the relation of arousal and drive (Hebb, 1955), it was of interest to observe hippocampal activity during a drive state such as food deprivation. If drive and arousal were related, theta activity should occur in hippocampus during food deprivation. Hockman (1964), however, did not find this result. It seemed worthwhile, because of this discrepancy, to observe the activity of the hippocampus under food deprivation conditions and to relate EEG activity changes to the variety of behavioral patterns which the rodent typically displays.

1. Observed Behavior

In a freely moving, unanesthetized animal, exploring and sniffing about a novel environment, a continuous record of synchronized, regularized activity in the hippocampus with a 7–8 Hz frequency is observed (Routtenberg, 1968b). If the animal is allowed to stay in that environment, exploratory activity decreases and hippocampal activity in the theta mode also diminishes. Following food deprivation, the animal shows a high level of exploratory activity, perhaps searching for food, and this is accompanied by theta activity during the entire observation period. This persistence of theta activity is in contrast to the record of an animal that is observed during *ad libitum* conditions. If the food-deprived animal is presented with food, there is a marked alteration in the record when the animal begins to eat (Fig. 15, traces 1–4). During eating there is a "theta

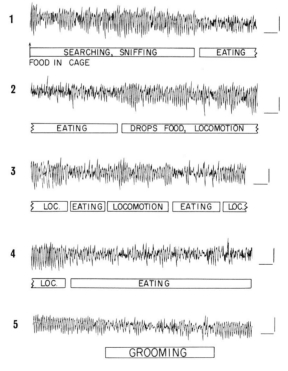

Fig. 15. Traces 1–4: Shifts in hippocampal activity between theta and theta "blocking" parallel shifts in behavior between exploration and eating. Calibration: 1 sec and 20 μV. Trace 5: Shift to theta "blocking" during grooming behavior. Calibration: 1 sec and 40 μV. Reprinted by permission of Pergamon Publishing Company, Elmsford, New York.

blocking" which occurs during mastication. Brief, sporadic episodes of theta are observed (Fig. 15, trace 4) during eating, and these appear to be related to those times when the animal interrupts actual chewing and raises its head, prior to again biting on the rat chow biscuit. Hippocampal desynchronization of theta blocking is also observed when a water-deprived animal is presented with water and licks a water tube. During the licking behavior the theta activity is blocked and one sees a considerable amount of desynchronization. A similar blocking of activity in the theta mode is also observed during grooming behavior (Fig. 15, trace 5).

These results point to two major conclusions. First, theta activity does, indeed, occur during food deprivation, particularly when the recording electrode is in the CA2/3 region of the hippocampus. Differences in our experiment and that reported by Hockman (1964) may perhaps be related to differences in the location of recording sites. A second conclusion that our results point to is that two major patterns of activity, one synchronized, the other desynchronized, appear in hippocampus. The two patterns of activity seem to be, at least on the basis of visual inspection of the polygraph records in relation to specific observable behavioral patterns, reciprocally related to one another.

This view of reciprocal relation between hippocampal theta and hippocampal desynchronization was first suggested by Grastyan et al. (1966). They proposed that hippocampal theta represents a reward process and hippocampal desynchronization an aversive process and that reward and aversion are represented by these two states of hippocampal activity. This view is hard to reconcile, however, with our results of the relation of the observed behavior and hippocampal activity discussed above. We have demonstrated, for example, that desynchronization, which is presumably an aversive state for the animal, according to Grastyan, occurs during feeding and drinking as well as grooming behavior. It is difficult to imagine that eating, drinking, and grooming represent punishment or an aversive state. It would seem, then, that the position of Grastyan et al. (1966) may be incorrect, or at least not capable of being generalized to other conditions.

2. Punishing Brain Stimulation

Since the proposal of Grastyan et al. (1966) was based on aversive hypothalamic brain stimulation data, we endeavored to assess the generality of their view using punishing brain stimulation in the dorsal midbrain on the lateral border of the central gray (Routtenberg and Kramis, 1968). In Fig. 16 it can be seen that stimulation of the dorsal midbrain produced a marked hippocampal synchronization as high as 10–13 Hz. The generality of Grastyan's findings may, therefore, be questioned. It should be noted that while Grastyan reported desynchronization with aversive stimulation in hypothalamus, it was only obtained with extremely high voltage levels.

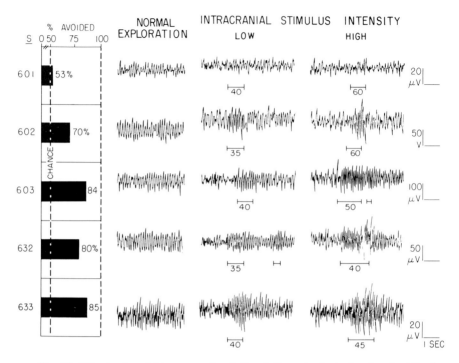

Fig. 16. Behavioral and hippocampal activity of five animals during dorsal midbrain stimulation. Behavioral response is summarized by the bar graphs, which represent the mean percent of stimuli avoided during the last four sessions. Hippocampal response observed in three conditions: A. Normal exploration, 7–9 Hz. B. Low-intensity aversive stimulation employed during shuttle box trials, 8–10 Hz. C. High-intensity aversive stimulation employed in the freely moving animal after completion of shuttle box trials, 10–13 Hz. The stimulus duration is indicated by the length of the markers under the records in comparison with the length of the 1-sec lines at far right. The numbers under these markers indicate the intensity of the stimuli, in microamperes. Reprinted by permission of the American Association for the Advancement of Science, Washington, D.C.

When paralysis was used with the same animals, hippocampal theta of a lower frequency, 6–8 Hz, was observed. This demonstrates that theta activity can be driven to higher frequency levels in freely moving animals using brain stimulation, and that paralysis by virtue of reducing blood pressure, proprioceptive feedback (Hodes, 1962), or other internal centrifugal stimuli may lead to the reduction of the theta response frequency to brain stimulation. It was clear, then, that not only was hippocampal desynchronization not necessarily related to the aversive state, but rather hippocampal synchronization (theta) appeared to be related to such a state, at least as generated by stimulation in the dorsal midbrain.

3. Gerbil Foot-Stomping

Another line of research provided a different perspective on the functions associated with each type of hippocampal activity. This work involved the species-typical response of "foot-stomping" in the gerbil (Routtenberg and Kramis, 1967). Kramis and I had demonstrated in this animal that rewarding brain stimulation was followed, as a rebound effect, by a rhythmic tapping of its hind feet. We demonstrated subsequently that this rhythmic tapping or foot-stomping is present during reproductive behavior. Kuhn and Zucker (1968) have replicated these findings and have demonstrated in addition that this behavior is sexually dimorphic, being most prominent in males. Of interest to us, particularly with regard to the reciprocal relation between hippocampal theta activity and hippocampal desynchronization suggested in our initial study, was that foot-stomping occurred as a rebound effect. In order to relate these findings to the reciprocal relation suggested by our hippocampal data, we recorded from the gerbil hippocampus during this species-typical behavior (Kramis and Routtenberg, 1969). We observed that during foot-stomping behavior in the gerbil, hippocampal desynchronization was present. Grooming behavior was also associated with hippocampal desynchronization, as we had shown in the rat. Finally, self-stimulation in the gerbil generated theta activity in the hippocampus. These results indicate, then, that during self-stimulation one observes hippocampal theta activity and during foot-stomping, which occurs as a rebound following such stimulation, one observes hippocampal desynchronization. These results support the suggested reciprocity between these two types of hippocampal activity.

Although we have not pursued the rebound characteristics of this foot-stomping behavior in any detail, it is worthwhile mentioning some observations which we have not reported in the literature. A 2-sec train of brain stimulation is followed by foot-stomping activity with a latency dependent on the stimulation intensity. The latency is 10–20 sec using a moderate intensity of stimulation, and as much as 1–2 min when a high level of stimulation is used. This remarkable result requires explanation and perhaps is related to the anatomical circuitry which was described in the first section of this paper. It is not related to epileptiform activity, at least as indicated by hippocampal EEG records. Other possible mechanisms related to neurohumoral events may also be considered. This rebound foot-stomping should not be viewed as an experimental artifact since a similar rebound foot-stomping is seen in the male gerbil following physiological stimulation by the female during sexual behavior. If these two results are considered to be closely related, then further study of this unique response to brain self-stimulation seems warranted.

We wish to conclude that a reciprocal relation exists between brain stimulation effects at self-stimulation sites and this foot-stomping behavior. A similar type of relationship has been described by Black and Vanderwolf (1969) for aversive brain stimulation in the rabbit. This animal presents a single thump of the hind feet following such a stimulus. Although Black and Vanderwolf did not record hippocampal activity, it would be predicted that during aversive brain stimulation hippocampal theta would be present and during the foot-thump hippocampal desynchronization would be observed. Based on such considerations one would expect to observe foot-stomping following aversive brain stimulation in the gerbil. That such may occur is suggested by our finding (Routtenberg and Kramis, 1967) that aversive peripheral shock engendered gerbil foot-stomping behavior.

In summary, then, it would appear that synchronized hippocampal patterns correspond to certain behavioral activities while hippocampal desynchronization corresponds with other behavioral acts. Those observed during hippocampal desynchronization appear to be, in general, organized motor activities, specifically, eating, drinking, grooming, and a species-typical response, foot-stomping. Pickenhain and Klingberg (1967) and Vanderwolf (1969) have reported results which support the view that during organized or automatic motor activities, hippocampal desynchronization appears to be prominent.

The type of behavior related to hippocampal theta seems less clear. In the rat the synchronized activity is often related to movement, though this is by no means always the case (Pickenhain and Klingberg, 1967). The work of Adey (1967) and our own work suggesting the sensitivity of the hippocampus to the presence of novel environmental stimuli (Routtenberg, 1968b) recommends the view that the hippocampus is important in the processing of stimuli or input processing. Pickenhain and Klingberg (1967) suggest that hippocampal theta occurs during the comparison of present sensory stimuli with past information and Adey (1967) suggests that the hippocampus is involved in information processing and storage. We prefer to take the more general position that the function occurring during hippocampal theta is best described as input processing.

It is worthwhile emphasizing the fact that hippocampal theta is observed during three dissimilar events: Rewarding brain stimulation, aversive brain stimulation, and exploratory activity. These three different conditions may be related by the view that such stimuli are fundamental to an organism in understanding and manipulating his environment. Under any of these three conditions it is important that the animal process accompanying stimuli in the environment so that it can know the conditions under which it should (1) move forward or repeat the activity in the case of appetitive stimuli; (2) withdraw or refrain from repeating the activity in the case of aversive stimuli; and (3) gain further information concerning the stimulus environment to decide between (1) or (2) in the case of novel stimuli.

The reciprocal relation between hippocampal theta activity and hippocampal desynchronization is diagrammed in Fig. 17, which proposes that each type of activity reflects the function of a single system. The activity of system I is involved with motor organization or output processing and is reflected by hippocampal desynchronization. System II, which is an input processing system, is active when hippocampal theta activity occurs. The figure further suggests the reciprocal relation between these two systems. Further theoretical arguments concerning the anatomical and physiological bases for these two systems have been discussed elsewhere (Routtenberg, 1966, 1968a, 1971b). The involvement of the extrapyramidal system will be considered in the next section.

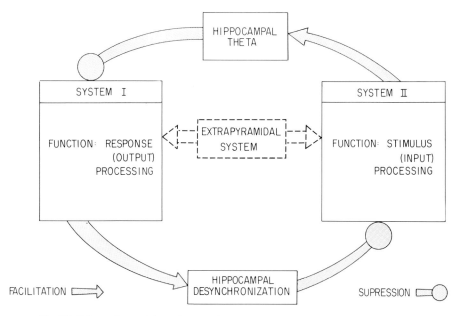

Fig. 17. Schematic model to show reciprocal relation between system I and system II and the indication of each by hippocampal activity.

It is worthwhile to consider an example of the type of evidence which the present view may help to explain. Paxinos and Bindra (1970) have shown that hippocampal theta activity typically produced during brain self-stimulation will be blocked if the animal is required to render itself immobile in order to receive the brain stimulation from the same electrode. This suggests that the immobility or freezing response which is related to hippocampal desynchronization (Routtenberg, Zechmeister, and Benton, 1970) seems to shift the balance from system II to system I. That is, the primary system in control becomes the motor organization system. Put another way, brain stimulation without enforced immobility tends to provide the primary emphasis on the activity of system II. When the animal now is required to withhold responding and to exert a specific organized pattern of motor activity such as holding still, this shifts the balance of activity to system I, hence the activity in the hippocampus is seen as hippocampal desynchronization or at least as a reduction in hippocampal theta.

It is not apparent, at least on the basis of our own data, that the behavior correlated with each type of hippocampal activity requires that EEG activity for its occurrence. It would appear to be the case that such hippocampal activity generally reflects, or is a consequence of, the behavior observed, rather than being the causal agent. Thus, for example, theta activity does not appear to be a necessary or sufficient condition for self-stimulation, nor does it appear to be a necessary or sufficient condition for punishment (Kramis, 1972). It should be emphasized, then, that hippocampal activity is an indicator of two processes, which we have referred to as system I and system II. Put another way, hippocampal activity is a consequence of these behaviors and does not appear to be related in any specific fashion to their causation. Reconsidering the early hippocampal theta arousal theory of Green and Arduini (1954), one sees that both types of hippocampal activity, rather than theta only, occur when the animal is in an alert or aroused condition. In one case the animal is engaged in a specific, organized, or species-typical motor pattern; in the other case, it is engaged primarily in the process of gaining information about the environment.

4. Brainstem Self-stimulation

The results of the mapping experiment demonstrated the involvement of the extrapyramidal system in self-stimulation. The hippocampal data suggested (1) that self-stimulation and punishment loci typically produce theta activity and (2) that hippocampal activity had two components, conceptually viewed as representing input and output processing. What, then, might be expected to occur in hippocampus during activation of brainstem extrapyramidal sites which mediate self-stimulation? If one takes the strict classical view of the extrapyramidal system related to motor function, then one should observe hippocampal desynchronization during stimulation. If, on the other hand, one views the extrapyramidal system as related to sensory processing, as has been emphasized more recently (Routtenberg, 1971b), one would expect stimulation to generate hippocampal theta activity.

With these considerations in mind we observed hippocampal responsivity, in paralyzed unanesthetized animals, to stimulation applied at 0.5 mm steps through the brainstem. When a response, typically theta activity, to the brain stimulation was observed, the electrode was cemented in place; the animal was recovered using Tensilon (edrophonium hydrochloride), and given an injection of Wycillin. One week after this procedure, each subject was tested both for self-stimulation and for aversive effects using a situation identical to that reported by Routtenberg and Kramis (1968).

The major results of this experiment (Routtenberg, 1970) are shown in the next three figures. In Fig. 18 one can see that hippocampal theta activity is generated by aversive stimulation in the central gray (trace a) and by stimulation in and around the red nucleus. A rebound effect is also seen. Desynchronization-synchronization occurred following stimulation in the rubrospinal tract (trace g). One sees an enhancement of theta activity, following stimulation, although there appears to be synchronization during the stimulation as well. The most prominent synchronization, however, appears to be after the stimulation, rather than during it.

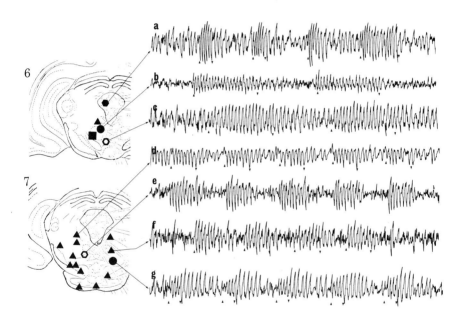

Fig. 18. In this and the following figures symbols indicate both site of stimulation and behavioral response to stimulation. Outlined hexagon: 500–999 self-stimulation responses in 15 min; filled circle; 200–499 responses; filled square: 50–199 responses; filled triangle: 0–49 responses; filled hexagon: aversive (less than 100 stimuli received in tilt cage). Arrows leading from stimulation loci indicate typical hippocampal response pattern. Onset of stimulation indicated by upward arrowhead, offset by downward arrowhead. Mesencephalic placements. Calibration: 1 sec and 50 μV (a, g), 100 μV (b, f, e), 200 μV (c), 500 μV (d). Onset and offset of stimuli in e the same as in d. (All sections but the last (11) were taken from König and Klippel, 1963.) (Section 6 is Fig. 49b and Section 7 is Fig. 50b of König and Klippel, 1963.) Reprinted by permission of the American Psychological Association, Washington, D.C.

Figure 19 shows that aversive brain stimulation in traces b[3] and c produces synchronization, which in the case of the central gray persists after the stimulus. Stimulation of the superior cerebellar peduncle which supports self-stimulation produces theta activity both in a and d. In Fig. 20 theta activity is observed following stimulation of both the dorsal and the deep tegmental nuclei. These areas did not support self-stimulation. Stimulation in the reticular formation also produces theta activity, which typically habituated after several presentations.

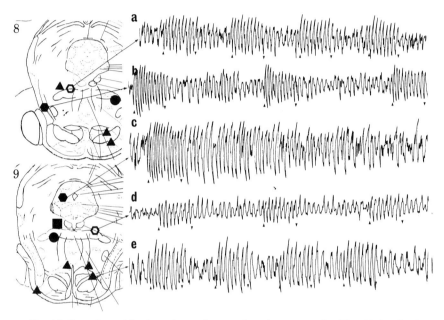

Fig. 19. Posterior midbrain and anterior pontine placements. See Fig. 18 for further explanation. Calibration: 1 sec and 50 μV (c, e), 100 μV (a, d), and 200 μV (b). Section 8 is Fig. 53b and Section 9 is Fig. 54b of König and Klippel, 1963.) Reprinted by permission of the American Psychological Association, Washington, D.C.

Two such cases where frequency and amplitude of the response were reduced may be seen in Fig. 20 (traces d and e); no self-stimulation was obtained from these sites. Such data confirm and extend our earlier reports (Routtenberg and Kane, 1965; Routtenberg and Malsbury, 1969) that activation of reticular formation does not appear to support self-stimulation.

This experiment was a first step in attempting to define a relationship between brainstem self-stimulation and hippocampal activity. Several extensions

[3] The aversive effects of stimulation of the lateral lemniscus have not, to my knowledge been reported before. Since the intensity of stimulation is quite low, this indicates the sensitivity of this fiber system to abnormal forms of stimulation. Perhaps these data may be useful in determining the physiological substrates for noise.

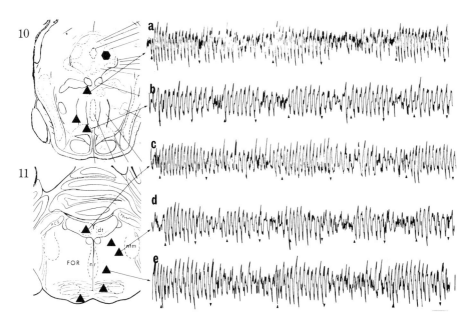

Fig. 20. Pontine placements. Section 11 is approximately 1.0 mm posterior to Section 10. See Fig. 18 for further explanation. Calibration: 1 sec and 40 μV (d), 100 μV (a, c, e), and 200 μV (b). (Section 10 is Fig. 55b of König and Klippel, 1963.) Reprinted by permission of the American Psychological Association, Washington, D.C.

of this experiment are indicated. First, since only one current level was used to facilitate comparisons between electrode placements in brainstem and electrophysiological responses in hippocampus (see section IV, B, 1–3), future study should use several different current levels. Second, since subsequent work (Kramis, 1972) demonstrated that sites which do not support self-stimulation tend to show a diminution of the theta response as the stimulus is repeated, future study should repeat the stimulus sufficiently to determine whether habituation occurs. This will minimize confusion between sites which support self-stimulation and those that do not.

The use of higher intensities of stimulation is important in the context of the results reported by Torii (1961). He showed that stimulation at low voltages in the ventromedial part of the brainstem produced a moderate amount of theta activity. As the intensity of the stimulation was increased, from 1 to 4 V, the synchronization was completely replaced by desynchronized activity. This suggests that we did not observe desynchronization because we were using low level stimulation. For anatomical localization, however, it was necessary to use such levels. Since it is difficult to resolve this issue concerning the intensity of current level without compromising anatomical localization, a systematic exploration of a few brainstem sites using multiple current levels seems indicated.

When stimulation was applied to dorsomedial parts of the brainstem, Torii (1961) found that stimulation which evoked an unambiguous theta at low levels of stimulation continued to produce this synchronized pattern when as much as 4 V was applied to the stimulating electrode. The placements found to provoke such effects were likely in aversive brain loci.

Another area where we opted for an unambiguous finding concerned recording of hippocampal activity under paralysis. We did not record during self-stimulation itself since we had shown (Kramis and Routtenberg, 1969) that the behavior related to self-stimulation, not only the stimulation, can alter the response in the hippocampus to the brain stimulation. This would have given us another factor to deal with in interpreting data. Having obtained the present results, it would now appear worthwhile to observe hippocampal activity during stimulation at extrapyramidal sites in the chronic preparation.

In view of our earlier anatomical findings (Routtenberg and Malsbury, 1969), it will be of interest to determine the hippocampal response to stimulation in the substantia nigra. It would be expected that the response characteristics of hippocampus to stimulation in substantia nigra, as compared to hypothalamic placements, will be different. The nature of these differences will allow further understanding of the place which the substantia nigra occupies in the organization of the pathways of self-stimulation.

3. Overview of Hippocampal Activity

In considering the range of results obtained with brain stimulation and hippocampal activity, it seems most important to emphasize certain key features of the data. First, hippocampal activity is, indeed, remarkably sensitive to moment-to-moment behavior (e.g., Fig. 15). This conclusion was reinforced by a recent experiment (Routtenberg et al., 1970) in which no change in hippocampal activity related to memory consolidation could be discerned. Although activity in hippocampus was altered, we concluded that the changes in hippocampal activity were related to the behavior of the animal rather than to the learning experience itself.

Second, the observed hippocampal activity may be conveniently considered as having two discernible components, synchronization and desynchronization. Despite the fact that regional differences in hippocampus have not been studied systematically, each of these components reliably occurred during particular behavioral patterns. We have suggested that the two types of activity represent the functioning of two systems, system I and system II, each one of which involves certain nuclear groups at each level of the neuraxis.

Third, the contribution of several structures to the functioning of system I and to system II suggests that the type of activity observed in hippocampus will be a function of the relative contribution of those structures within a system as well as the relative contribution of each of the two systems. Thus, recording from hippocampus may provide a summary of these interactions, whether during electrical stimulation at self-stimulation sites or during observed behavior.

Fourth, the evidence suggests that a reciprocal relation does exist between the two systems. This relationship, shown in Fig. 17, indicates two systems, reciprocally related one to the other, with the reciprocity indicated by the alterations between synchronized and desynchronized hippocampal activity. The extrapyramidal system, according to this scheme, appears to have the properties of both system I and system II; it can produce both hippocampal theta and hippocampal desynchronization activity. Within the context of the two-system hypothesis proposed here, it is clear that the extrapyramidal system in our experiment shows more of the system II-hippocampal theta-producing properties. In terms of classical literature it is quite clear that the extrapyramidal system has system I or motor organization properties. Thus, the extrapyramidal system is viewed as having properties of both system I and system II (Routtenberg, 1971a).

VII. Final Overview

A. METHODOLOGY

1. A Functional Approach

In this section I would like to suggest that the experimental approach that has been used here does not necessarily have to be limited to the study of self-stimulation, but rather, may be applied to other brain-behavior functions. It may be used by those researchers interested in defining neurological systems other than in terms of the anatomical system itself.

The pure anatomist, like the descriptive zoologist, is oblivious to all philosophical curiosity. When he has proclaimed that a crossing of the optic tracts is an anatomical rule in the vertebrates, he rests fully satisfied. This is incomprehensible mental inertia, for if anatomy and histology are to aspire to the rank of true sciences, it is essential that, like chemistry and astronomy, they concern themselves with the development of phenomena and become ever more dynamic and more causal (Ramon y Cajal, 1937, pp. 470–471).

We may arrive at an anatomical organization of input-output substrates, then, based on the description of anatomical pathways in the context of the behavioral activities or function that they mediate.

The same approach can be used to advantage with regard to electro-physiology. Thus, microelectrode data collected in terms of anatomical mapping alone lack a functional attribute as would the strict anatomical approach. If one could establish relationships based on microelectrode data as has been demonstrated between the lateral hypothalamus and substantia nigra (Huang, 1970) and between the lateral hypothalamus and the nucleus reticularis gigantocellularis (Keene and Casey, 1970), then it would be possible to provide the basis for a functionally based understanding of electrophysiological data.

Up to this point, it should be noted, electrophysiological study has been most useful in those areas which have been less complex in terms of conceptual thinking; on the input side as exemplified by the Hubel and Wiesel research program (e.g., 1970), and on the output side, as exemplified by the studies of Evarts and colleagues (Evarts and Thach, 1969). It has been less fruitful to attempt to establish such relationships within the central nervous system, although one can point to the approach of Eccles *et al.* (1967) in attempting to define these relationships in the cerebellum in both anatomical and physiological terms. Their work could provide, in addition, a most important basis for electrophysiological recording in the chronic, freely moving animal.

2. *Convergence between Methods*

Another virtue of the approach suggested here is the convergent use of several methods. One example relates to our research concerning the substantia nigra, pars compacta (SNC). We have shown that lesions at self-stimulation sites in the lateral hypothalamus produce terminal degeneration in SNC. Additionally, lesions at self-stimulation sites in SNC produce retrograde degeneration into the lateral hypothalamus. Finally, stimulation of the lateral hypothalamus produces a suppression of SNC neuronal activity recorded with tungsten microelectrodes (Huang and Routtenberg, 1971). Whatever the interpretation of these results, it is clear that there is an intimate relation between SNC and the lateral hypothalamus revealed by the use of several different methods.

Convergence of information has been helpful in describing the anatomical loci which support the highest rates of self-stimulation (Routtenberg and Malsbury, 1969). One such locus is in the ventral tegmentum, immediately above the ventral tegmental area of Tsai. In comparison with sites throughout the rat brain, we have found the highest rates of self-stimulation in this region. This may be attributed to the fact that several fiber systems passing through this region are related to self-stimulation. In fact, the three major outputs from the lateral hypothalamus (Fig. 5) do pass through this region. The location of these fiber pathways also suggests that some of the placements attributed to the ventral tegmental decussation and the red nucleus (Routtenberg and Malsbury, 1970), and to the interstitial nucleus of Cajal (Huang and Routtenberg, 1971), may most likely be related to these lateral hypothalamic output fibers. Since their termination in the central gray region corresponds closely to the central gray self-stimulation reported by Margules (1969), this provides convergent evidence that this fiber pathway mediates self-stimulation along its entire trajectory.

B. Theoretical Considerations: Stimulus-Response Organization of Self-Stimulation Pathways

It has been emphasized that it is difficult to point out the major anatomical features of self-stimulation in a particular region of the brain without discussion of the self-stimulation pathways revealed in other regions. Thus, in summarizing our results gained to date, we must view the organization of self-stimulation in terms of all three major areas—brainstem, hypothalamus, and forebrain—that have been discussed. To do so, however, will require hypothetical constructs where anatomical projections or physiological data are not yet available. It seems worthwhile, nonetheless, to provide a first approximation based on data currently available.

It will be convenient in summarizing these data, then, to consider the anatomical organization of self-stimulation in terms of an input-output organization. It should be realized that such an approach will ultimately be required if an understanding of the fiber systems which mediate self-stimulation is to be achieved. The use of input-output terminology is also of assistance in discussing data gained from other disciplines or fields of study. The present section will demonstrate one organization based primarily on the self-stimulation anatomical data and electrophysiological results.

For this purpose, then, a four-stage model (Fig. 21) will be considered. The hypothalamus in this model is considered important during the initial stage. It receives sensory input initially processed through olfactory, gustatory, visual, auditory, and somesthetic sense organs and classical sensory pathways. The focus of sensory inputs to the hypothalamus is certainly not a classical picture of sensory anatomy and physiology. Nonetheless, it is the case that these modalities have inputs to the hypothalamus as indicated by data elsewhere (Routtenberg, 1971b). In general, input processing can be of inputs which are external, in the sense that irrespective of whether they are proximal or distal, they are imposed onto the surface of the body.

A second input system, an internal one, should be considered as having inputs from the striated and smooth musculature. In this discussion attention will be focused on the proprioceptive system, particularly as it relates to the position of the body in space. According to the scheme in Fig. 21, this system is represented as having pathways to the cerebellum which then convey impulses to the thalamus. In summary of the input stage, then, two systems, external and

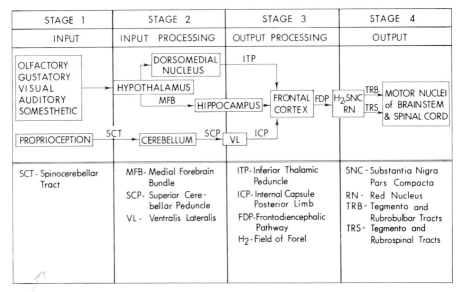

STAGE 1	STAGE 2	STAGE 3	STAGE 4
INPUT	INPUT PROCESSING	OUTPUT PROCESSING	OUTPUT

| SCT - Spinocerebellar Tract | MFB- Medial Forebrain Bundle
SCP- Superior Cerebellar Peduncle
VL - Ventralis Lateralis | ITP- Inferior Thalamic Peduncle
ICP- Internal Capsule Posterior Limb
FDP-Frontodiencephalic Pathway
H_2- Field of Forel | SNC - Substantia Nigra Pars Compacta
RN - Red Nucleus
TRB- Tegmento and Rubrobulbar Tracts
TRS- Tegmento and Rubrospinal Tracts |

Fig. 21. Four-stage input-output model which relates the anatomical organization of self-stimulation both to the patterns of hippocampal activity generated during brain stimulation and to the hippocampal activity observed in freely behaving animals.

internal, convey sensory stimuli to two nodal relay points, the hypothalamus and the cerebellum.

During the second, or input processing stage, activity is conducted from the hypothalamus and cerebellum, leading eventually to frontal cortex (Fig. 21). Two pathways from the hypothalamus are considered. One route leaves the hypothalamus and terminates in the dorsomedial nucleus of the thalamus (Guillery, 1959). It then goes to the frontal cortex (Leonard, 1969). The other leaves the hypothalamus and terminates in the septal area and hippocampus (Guillery, 1957). The pathway then leads to the frontal cortex.

A second pathway that is active during the input processing stage is the cerebellar output, the superior cerebellar peduncle, which goes to and through the red nucleus, terminating in the ventralis lateralis of the thalamus. Projections then go to the cortex via the internal capsule.

The third stage, or output processing (Fig. 21) involves conduction of activity from the frontal cortex to the H_2 field of Forel (H_2), substantia nigra, pars compacta (SNC), and to the red nucleus (RN). Based on the charting of degeneration from medial placements in MFB (Huang and Routtenberg, 1971) and degeneration from the forebrain (Routtenberg, 1971a; Leonard, 1969; Harting and Martin, 1970) there are at least two pathways that can be considered to pass caudally through the lateral hypothalamus: (1) a lateral hypothalamic pathway passing just dorsal to and through the substantia nigra, pars compacta (SNC) which distributes terminals to central gray and perhaps reticular formation; and (2) a corticofugal pathway originating in frontal cortex and terminating, in part, in H_2, the substantia nigra, and RN. It is this latter pathway which is thought to be active during stage 3 output processing.[4]

In the final output stage, H_2, SNC, and RN modulate the activity of the reticular formation, so that output systems from the tegmentum and the red nucleus, which form tegmentobulbar and tegmentospinal tracts, rubrobulbar and rubrospinal tracts, then influence cranial nerve and spinal cord motor nuclei.

It has been the purpose of this section to provide a conceptual framework for the anatomical organization of self-stimulation in terms of ongoing behavior. This means that typical behavioral activities should be considered ultimately in terms of neural activity in certain anatomical structures. The focus, then, is on mechanisms of behavior, in general, not on self-stimulation and its methods. That is, the anatomy of self-stimulation may now be focused on the behavioral function of the fiber systems rather than the behavior of self-stimulation itself. This view will enable the study and use of self-stimulation anatomy and physiology in pointing to critical systems underlying behavior without the necessity of placing special importance on the particular behavior used to reveal such pathways.

In this context, then, it may be recalled that activation of a wide variety of input pathways produce hippocampal theta activity. It is not clear whether hippocampal theta activity should appear with respect to brain stimulation that supports self-stimulation. This is particularly difficult when any stimulation that will produce a response should inevitably produce the proprioceptive feedback, which we have suggested is the major condition for activation of one of the fiber pathways that support self-stimulation. Thus, either type of hippocampal pattern may occur during self-stimulation (Routtenberg, 1970).

Of major importance, then, is the view that the understanding of the relationships among the anatomical pathways that have been discussed up to this time may be clarified by careful understanding of the patterns of activity in the hippocampus, both with regard to hippocampal theta and with regard to hippocampal desynchronization. Thus hippocampal theta activity would be presumed to occur following the input (stage 1) mode, during the input processing (stage 2) mode, as the elaboration occurs toward frontal cortex. It is during the initiation of the output processing mode (stage 3), from frontal

---

[4] This fiber pathway occupies the lateral aspect of MFB. If the sensory input system is viewed as occupying the medial aspects of MFB (Guillery, 1957), then it may be the case that two different systems related to self-stimulation are activated by a single electrode placed in MFB. The reason that high rates of self-stimulation are obtained from MFB, then, may be related to the fact that stimulation in MFB simultaneously activates two systems that can support self-stimulation.

cortex to the H_2, SNC, and RN and from these structures to motor nuclei of brainstem and spinal cord (stage 4), that desynchronization in the hippocampus is observed. According to this scheme, during stage 2 activity, system II is engaged. As the mode shifts from input processing to output processing, from stage 2 to stage 3, the shift occurs from system II to system I.

VIII. Summary

The early history of intracranial self-stimulation was reviewed in an effort to clarify certain difficulties with terminology, techniques, and untested assumptions. It was concluded that the identification of the behavior as "rewarding" was not a fruitful approach and that alternative formulations must await detailed information concerning the anatomical and physiological organization of the pathways which mediate self-stimulation.

The author's work in this area was reviewed. First, the anatomical pathways revealed by making lesions at self-stimulation sites and then using Nauta and Fink-Heimer methods demonstrated the involvement of several heretofore unsuspected regions which supported self-stimulation. It appears that such methods will be capable of replacing the infinite catalog of self-stimulation points with a finite set of pathways. Second, the response of neurons recorded with tungsten microelectrodes to electrical activation of self-stimulation sites was considered. The data obtained, although not as detailed as the anatomical work, have provided a functional definition of certain anatomical projections. Progress along this line of research will enable specification of the described anatomical pathways in terms of activation and suppression at synaptic junctions. Finally, hippocampal responses derived with macroelectrodes to brain stimulation were observed in an effort to relate experimental anatomical data and microelectrode specification of monosynaptic relations to the mode and pattern of response in hippocampus.

These three lines of research were summarized in schematic form. The basic assumption was that the self-stimulation pathways could be organized into an input-output configuration. A four-stage model was proposed in which the anatomical foci of activity were indicated by hippocampal activity.

Acknowledgment

The research presented in this chapter, and the preparation of the manuscript was supported by Public Health Service Research Grant MH 17255. The author is grateful to Peter Frey and Ronald Kramis for reading an initial draft of this chapter.

References and Author Index*

Abbie, A. A. The brain-stem and cerebellum of *Echidna aculeata*. *Philosophical Transactions of the Royal Society (London)*, 1934, **B224**, 1–74. [76]

Addens, J. L., and Kurotsu, T. Die Pyramidenbahn von Echidna. *Proceedings Koninklijke Nederlandse Akademie van Wetenschappen*, 1936, **39**, 1142–1151. [73, 76]

Adey, W. R. Studies of hippocampal electrical activity during approach learning. In J. F. Delafresnaye (Ed.), *Brain mechanisms and learning*. Oxford: Blackwell, 1961. [301]

Adey, W. R. Hippocampal states and functional relations with cortico-subcortical systems in attention and learning. In W. R. Adey and T. Tokizane (Eds.), *Progress in brain research: structure and function of the limbic system*. Vol. 27. Amsterdam: Elsevier, 1967. [306]

Adey, W. R., Segundo, J. P., and Livingston, R. B. Corticofugal influences on intrinsic brainstem conduction in cat and monkey. *Journal of Neurophysiology*, 1957, **20**, 1–16. [132, 133]

Adey, W. R., and Tokizane, T. (Eds.) *Progress in brain research: structure and function of the limbic system*. Vol. 27. Amsterdam: Elsevier, 1967. [300]

Afifi, A., and Kaelber, W. W. Eferent connections of the substantia nigra in the cat. *Experimental Neurology*, 1965, **11**, 474–482. [154, 167, 168]

Akert, K. Diencephalon. In D. E. Sheer (Ed.), *Electrical stimulation of the brain*. Austin, Texas: University of Texas Press, 1961. Pp. 288–320. [261]

Albino, R. C., and Lucas, J. W. Mutual facilitation of self-rewarding regions within the limbic system. *Journal of Comparative and Physiological Psychology*, 1962, **55**, 182–185. [272]

Alexander, F. *Psychosomatic medicine: Its principles and applications*. New York: Norton, 1950. [56]

Alexander, L. The fundamental types of histopathologic changes encountered in cases of athetosis and paralysis agitans. *Research Publications of the Association for Research in Nervous and Mental Diseases*, 1942, **21**, 334–493. [138]

Allen, G. I., Korn, H., and Oshima, T. Monosynaptic pyramidal activation of pontine nuclei cells projecting to the cerebellum. *Brain Research*, 1969, **15**, 272–275. [83, 88]

Allen, G. I., Korn, H., Oshima, T., and Toyama, K. Time course of pyramidal activation of pontine nuclei cells in the cat. *Brain Research*, 1970, **19**, 291–294. [88]

Altman, J. Some fiber projections to the superior colliculus in the cat. *Journal of Comparative Neurology*, 1962, **119**, 77–96. [166]

Anand, B. K. and Pillai, R. V. Activity of single neurons in the hypothalamic feeding centres: Effect of gastric distention. *Journal of Physiology*, 1967, **192**, 63–77. [221]

Anand, B. K. and Brobeck, J. R. Hypothalamic control of food intake in rats and cats. *Yale Journal of Biology and Medicine*, 1951, **24**, 123–140. [210]

* Numbers in brackets indicate pages where references are cited.

Andén, N. E., Carlsson, A., Dahlstrom, A., Fuxe, K., Hillarp, N. A., and Larsson, K. Demonstration and mapping out of nigro-neostriatal dopamine neurons. *Life Sciences,* 1964, **3**, 523–530. [137, 155]

Andén, N. E., Dahlstrom, A., Fuxe, K., and Larsson, K. Functional role of the nigro-neostriatal dopamine neurons. *Acta Pharmacologica,* 1966, **24**, 263–274. [168]

Andy, O. J., and Brown, J. S. Diencephalic coagulation in the treatment of hemiballismus. *Surgical Forum,* 1960, **10**, 795–799. [165]

Ansell, S. D., Waisbrot, A. J., and Smith, K. U. Real-time hybrid computer analysis of self-regulation feedback control of cardiac activity. *Proceedings of the First Institute of Science and Technology in Criminology.* New York: Thomson, 1967. Pp. 403–418. [58, 59]

Aprison, M. H., Shank, R. P., and Davidoff, R. A. A comparison of the concentration of glycine, a transmitter suspect, in different areas of the brain and spinal cord in seven different vertebrates. *Comparative Biochemistry and Physiology,* 1969, **28**, 1345–1355. [215]

Asmussen, E. Exercise and the regulation of ventilation. Supplement to *Circulation Research,* 1967, **XX, XXI,** 132–145. [21, 35, 54]

Asmussen, E., Christensen, E. H., and Nielsen, M. Die O_2-Aufnahme der ruhenden und der arbeitenden Skelettmuskeln. *Skandinavian Archives of Physiology,* 1939, **82**, 212–220. [27, 31]

Atkinson, D. E. Biological feedback control at the molecular level. *Science,* 1965, **150**, 851–862. [30]

Atkinson, D. E. Regulation of enzyme activity. *Annual Review of Biochemistry,* 1966, **35**, 85–124. [30]

Auer, J. Terminal degeneration in the diencephalon after ablation of frontal cortex in the cat. *Journal of Anatomy,* 1956, **90**, 30–41. [169]

Baenninger, R. Visual reinforcement, habituation, and prior social experience of Siamese Fighting Fish. *Journal of Comparative and Physiological Psychology,* 1970, **71**, 1–5. [17]

Bagley, C., Jr. Cortical motor mechanism of the sheep brain. *Archives of Neurology and Psychiatry,* 1922, **7**, 417–453. [73, 74, 77, 83, 84, 95]

Bagley, C., and Richter, C. P. Electrically excitable region of the forebrain of the alligator. *Archives of Neurology and Psychiatry,* 1924, **11**, 257–263. [95]

Bard, P. A diencephalic mechanism for the expression of rage with special reference to the sympathetic nervous system. *American Journal of Physiology,* 1928, **84**, 490–515. [100]

Bard, P., and Macht, M. B. The behavior of chronic decerebrate cats. In G. E. W. Wolstenholme and C. M. O'Conner (Eds.), *Ciba Foundation Symposium on the Neurological Basis of Behavior.* London: Churchill, 1958. [109, 110, 111, 129, 261]

Bard, P., and Mountcastle, V. B. Some forebrain mechanisms involved in expression of rage with special reference to suppression of angry behavior. *Research Publications of the Association of Nervous and Mental Diseases,* 1948, **27**, 362–404. [105]

Bard, P., and Rioch, D. McK. A study of four cats deprived of neocortex and additional portions of the forebrain. *Bulletin of the Johns Hopkins Hospital,* 1937, **60**, 73–147. [102, 105, 106, 107, 109, 111]

Barnard, J. W., and Woolsey, C. N. A study of localization in the corticospinal tracts of monkey and rat. *Journal of Comparative Neurology,* 1956, **105**, 25–50. [74, 75, 76]

Bates, J. A. V. The individuality of the motor cortex. *Brain,* 1960, **83**, 654–667. [95]

Barrett, J. N., and Crill, W. E. Specific membrane resistivity of dye-injected cat motoneurons. *Brain Research,* 1971, **28**, 556–561.

Battig, K., Rosvold, H. E., and Mishkin, M. Comparison of the effects of frontal and caudate lesions on delayed response and alternation in monkeys. *Journal of Comparative and Physiological Psychology,* 1960, **53**, 400–404. [130]

Battig, K., Rosvold, H. E., and Mishkin, M. Comparison of the effects of frontal and caudate lesions on discrimination learning in monkeys. *Journal of Comparative and Physiological Psychology,* 1962, **55,** 458–463.[130]

Bautista, N. S., and Matzke, H. A. A degeneration study of the course and extent of the pyramidal tract of the opossum. *Journal of Comparative Neurology,* 1965, **124,** 367–376. [74, 76, 96]

Bazett, H. C., and Penfield, W. G. A study of the Sherrington decerebrate animal in the chronic as well as the acute condition. *Brain,* 1922, **45,** 185–265. [105, 109, 111]

Beach, F. A. The neural basis of innate behavior: I. Effects of cortical lesions upon the maternal behavior pattern in the rat. *Journal of Comparative Psychology,* 1937, **24,** 393–440. [260]

Beach, F. A. Effect of cortical lesions upon the copulatory behavior of male rats. *Journal of Comparative Psychology,* 1940, **29,** 193–246. [260]

Beatty, W. W., and Schwartzbaum, J. S. Enhanced reactivity to quinine and saccharine solutions following septal lesions in the rat. *Psychonomic Science,* 1967, **8,** 483–484.[15]

Beatty, W. W., and Schwartzbaum, J. S. Commonality and specificity of behavioral dysfunctions following septal and hippocampal lesions in rats. *Journal of Comparative and Physiological Psychology,* 1968, **66,** 60–68. [15]

Benson, G., Shapiro, D., Tursky, B., and Schwartz, G. E. Decreased systolic blood pressure through operant conditioning in patients with essential hypertension. *Science,* 1971, **173,** 740–742.[5]

Berger, B. D., Wise, C. D., and Stein, L. Norepinephrine: Reversal of anorexia in rats with lateral hypothalamic damage. *Science,* 1971, **172,** 282–284. [221]

Bergman, L. E. Neue Untersuchungen zur Kenntnis der Pyramidenbahn. 2. Die Oblongata-pyramide des Elephanten. *Anatomischer Anzeiger,* 1915, **48,** 235–240. [73]

Biedenbach, M. A., and Towe, A. L. Fiber spectrum and functional properties of pyramidal tract neurons in the American opossum. *Journal of Comparative Neurology,* 1970, **140,** 421–430.[74, 76, 79, 96]

Bischoff, E. Beitrag zur Anatomie des Igelgehirnes. *Anatomischer Anzeiger,* 1900, **18,** 348–358.[76, 77]

Bizzi, E. Discharge of frontal eye field neurons during saccadic and following eye movements in unanesthetized monkeys. *Experimental Brain Research,* 1968, **6,** 69–80. [70].

Black, A. H. The direct control of neural processes by reward and punishment. *American Scientist,* 1971, **59,** 236–245. [230]

Black, A. H., Young, G. A., and Batenchuk, C. Avoidance training of hippocampal theta waves in Flaxedilized dogs and its relation to skeletal movement. *Journal of Comparative and Physiological Psychology,* 1970, **70,** 15–24. [230]

Black, S. L., and Vanderwolf, C. H. Thumping behavior in the rabbit. *Physiology and Behavior,* 1969, **4,** 445–450.[306]

Bland, B. H. Diencephalic and hippocampal mechanisms of motor activity in the rat. Unpublished Ph.D. thesis, University of Western Ontario, 1971.

Bland, B. H., and Vanderwolf, C. H. Electrical stimulation of the hippocampal formation: Behavioral and bioelectrical effects. *Brain Research,* 1972, **43,** 67–88. (a) [230, 237, 238, 239, 240]

Bland, B. H., and Vanderwolf, C. H. Diencephalic and hippocampal mechanisms of motor activity in the rat: Effects of posterior hypothalamic stimulation on behavior and hippocampal slow wave activity. *Brain Research,* 1972, **43,** 89–106. (b) [230, 251, 254, 255]

Bland, B. H., Wishart, T. B., Altman, J. L., Whishaw, I. Q., and Vanderwolf, C. H. Electroencephalographic correlates of behavior elicited by electrical stimulation of the septum: Seizure induced feeding. Unpublished manuscript, 1971. [239]

Blum, R. A. Effects of subtotal lesions of frontal granular cortex on delayed reaction in monkeys. *Archives of Neurology and Psychiatry,* 1952, **67**, 375–386. [191]

Bogacz, J., St. Laurent, J., and Olds, J. Dissociation of self-stimulation and epileptiform activity. *Electroencephalography and Clinical Neurophysiology.* 1965, **19**, 75–87. [266]

Bolles, R. C. Species-specific defense reactions and avoidance learning. *Psychological Review,* 1970, **77**, 32–48. [2,8]

von Bonin, G., and Bailey, P. *The Neocortex of Macaca mulatta.* Urbana, Illinois: University of Illinois Press, 1947. [170]

Bowsher, D. Projections of the gracile and cuneate nuclei in *Macaca mulatta:* An experimental degeneration study. *Journal of Comparative Neurology,* 1958, **110**, 135–155. [171]

Bowsher. D. The termination of secondary somatosensory neurons within the thalamus of *Macaca mulatta:* An experimental degeneration study. *Journal of Comparative Neurology,* 1961, **177**, 213–227. [171]

Brady, J. V., and Nauta, W. J. H. Subcortical mechanisms in emotional behavior: Affective changes following septal forebrain lesions in the albino rat. *Journal of Comparative and Physiological Psychology,* 1953, **46**, 339–346.

Brady, J. V., and Nauta, W. J. H. Subcortical mechanisms in emotional behavior: The duration of affective changes following septal and habenular lesions in the albino rat. *Journal of Comparative and Physiological Psychology,* 1955, **48**, 412–420.

Brady, J. V., Schreiner, L., Geller, I., and Kling, A. Subcortical mechanisms in emotional behavior: The effect of rhinencephalic injury upon the acquisition and retention of a conditioned avoidance response in cats. *Journal of Comparative and Physiological Psychology,* 1954, **49**, 179–186. [132]

Breland, K., and Breland, M. The misbehavior of organisms. *American Psychologist,* 1961, **16**, 681–684. [6]

Bremner, F. J. Hippocampal electrical activity during classical conditioning. *Journal of Comparative and Physiological Psychology,* 1968, **66**, 35–39. [248]

Bromiley, R. B. Conditioned responses in a dog after removal of neocortex. *Journal of Comparative and Physiological Psychology,* 1948, **41**, 102–110. [105, 107, 110, 111, 117, 129, 130]

Brown, C. W., and Ghiselli, E. E. Subcortical mechanisms in learning. II. The Maze. *Journal of Comparative Psychology,* 1938, **26**, 27–44. [131]

Brown, J. L. Neuro-ethological approaches to the study of emotional behavior: Stereotype and variability. *Annals of the New York Academy of Science,* 1969, **159**, Art. 3, 1084–1095. [6]

Brutkowski, S. Functions of prefrontal cortex in animals. *Physiological Reviews,* 1965, **45**, 721–746. [14]

Brutkowski, S., and Dąbrowska, J. Disinhibition after prefrontal lesions as a function of duration of intertrial intervals. *Science,* 1963, **139**, 505–506. [182, 185, 186]

Brutkowski, S., and Dąbrowska, J. Prefrontal cortex control of differentiation behavior in dogs. *Acta Biologiae Experimentalis,* 1966, **26**, 425–439. [182, 185, 186]

Brutkowski, S., Konorski, J., Ławicka, W., Stępień, I., and Stępień, L. The effect of the removal of frontal poles of the cerebral cortex on motor conditioned reflexes in dogs. *Acta Biologiae Experimentalis,* 1956, **17**, 167–188. [181, 182]

Brutkowski, S., and Mempel, E. Disinhibition of inhibitory conditioned responses following selective brain lesions in dogs. *Science,* 1961, **134**, 2040–2041. [183]

Brutkowski, S., Mishkin, M., and Rosvold, H. E. Positive and inhibitory motor conditioned reflexes in monkeys after ablation of orbital or dorsolateral surface of the frontal cortex. In E. Gutman and P. Hnik (Eds.), *Central and Peripheral Mechanisms of Motor Functions.* Prague: Publishing House of the Czechoslovak Academy of Sciences, 1963. Pp. 133–141. [183]

Buchwald, J. S., Beatty, D., and Eldred, E. Conditioned responses of gamma and alpha motoneurones in cat trained to conditioned avoidance. *Experimental Neurology,* 1961, **4,** 91–105. [118]

Buchwald, J. S., and Eldred, E. Conditioned responses in the gamma efferent system. *Journal of Nervous and Mental Disease,* 1961, **132,** 146–152. [118, 123]

Buchwald, J. S., and Grover, F. S. Amplitudes of background fast activity characteristic of specific brain sites. *Journal of Neurophysiology,* 1970, **33,** 148–159. [118]

Buchwald, J. S., Halas, E. S., and Schramm, S. A comparison of multiple-unit and EEG activity recorded from the same brain site in chronic cats during behavioral conditioning. *Nature,* 1965, **205,** 1012–1014. [118]

Buchwald, J. S., Halas, E. S., and Schramm, S. Changes in cortical and subcortical unit activity during behavioral conditioning. *Physiology and Behavior,* 1966, **1,** 11–22. [120, 121, 122]

Buchwald, J. S., and Humphrey, G. L. An analysis of habituation in the specific sensory systems. In E. Stellar and J. Sprague (Eds.), *Progress in Physiological Psychology.* Vol. 5. New York: Academic Press, 1971. [118, 126, 133]

Buchwald, J. S., and Schramm, S. A study of conditioning in chronically spinalized kittens. *Physiologist,* 1965, **8,** 115. [114]

Buchwald, J. S., Standish, M., Eldred, E., and Halas, E. S. Contribution of muscle spindle circuits to learning as suggested by training under Flaxedil. *Electroencephalography and Clinical Neurophysiology,* 1964, **16,** 582–594. [118]

Buchwald, J. S., Weber, D. S., Holstein, S. B., and Schwafel, J. A. Quantified unit background activity in the waking cat during paralysis, anesthesia and cochlear destruction. *Brain Research,* 1969, **15,** 465–482. [118]

Buchwald, N. A., Wyers, E. J., Lauprecht, C. W., and Heuser, G. The "caudate-spindle". IV: A behavioral index of caudate-induced inhibition. *Electroencephalography and Clinical Neurophysiology,* 1961, **13,** 531–537. [124, 130]

Bucy, P. C., Ladpli, R., and Ehrlich, A. Destruction of the pyramidal tract in the monkey. The effects of bilateral section of the cerebral peduncles. *Journal of Neurosurgery,* 1966, **25,** 1–20. [71, 89, 97]

Buerger, A. A., and Dawson, A. M. Spinal kittens: Long-term increases in electromyograms due to a conditioned routine. *Physiology and Behavior,* 1968, **3,** 99–103. [114]

Buerger, A. A., and Fennessy, A. Learning of leg position in chronic spinal rats. *Nature,* 1970, **225,** 751–752. [114]

Bumke, O. C. E. Ueber Variationen im Verlauf der Pyramidenbahn. *Archiv für Psychiatrie,* 1907, **42,** 1–18. [74, 75]

Buresová, O., Bureš, J., Bohdanecký, Z., and Weiss, T. Effect of atropine on learning, extinction, retention, and retrieval in rats. *Psychopharmacologia,* 1964, **5,** 255–263. [233]

Butter, C. M. Perseveration in extinction and in discrimination reversal tasks following selective frontal ablations in *Macaca mulatta. Physiology and Behavior,* 1969, **4,** 163–171. [196]

Butter, C. M., Mishkin, M., and Rosvold, H. E. Conditioning and extinction of a food-rewarded response after selective ablations of frontal cortex in Rhesus monkeys. *Experimental Neurology,* 1963, **7,** 65–75. [195]

Butters, N., and Rosvold, H. E. Effect of septal lesions on resistance to extinction and delayed alternation in monkeys. *Journal of Comparative and Physiological Psychology,* 1968, **66,** 389–395. [131]

Buxton, D. F., and Goodman, D. C. Motor functions and the corticospinal tracts in the dog and raccoon. *Journal of Comparative Neurology,* 1967, **129,** 341–360. [75]

Campbell, C. B. G., Yashon, D., and Jane, J. A. The origin, course, and termination of corticospinal fibers in the slow loris, *Mycticebus coucang* (Boddaert). *Journal of Comparative Neurology,* 1966, **127,** 101–112. [74, 75, 83]

Cannon, W. B. *Bodily changes in pain, hunger, fear and rage.* (2nd Ed.) New York: Appleton-Century-Crofts, 1929. [207]

Cannon, W. B. Organization for physiological homeostasis. *Physiological Reviews,* 1929, **9**, 399–468. [24]

Cannon, W. B. Hunger and thirst. In C. Murchison (Ed.), *Handbook of general experimental psychology.* Worcester, Massachusetts: Clark University Press, 1934. [24]

Cannon, W. B., and Britton, S. W. The influence of emotion on medulliadrenal secretion. *American Journal of Physiology,* 1927, **79**, 433–465. [105]

Caplan, M. Effects of withheld reinforcement on timing behavior of rats with limbic lesions. *Journal of Comparative and Physiological Psychology,* 1970, **71**, 119–135. [15]

Carey, J. H. Certain anatomical and functional interrelations between the tegmentum of the midbrain and the basal ganglia. *Journal of Comparative Neurology,* 1957, **108**, 57–90. [131]

Carli, G. Dissociation of electrocortical activity and somatic reflexes during rabbit hypnosis. *Archives Italiennes de Biologie,* 1962, **100**, 48–85. [250]

Carlton, P. L. Cholinergic mechanisms in the control of behavior by the brain. *Psychological Review,* 1963, **70**, 19–39. [204, 208, 228]

Carlton, P. L. Brain-acetylcholine and inhibition. In J. T. Tapp (Ed.), *Reinforcement and behavior.* New York: Academic Press, 1969. [204, 205, 224]

Carman, J. B., Cowan, W. M., and Powell, T. P. S. The organization of cortico-striate connexions in the rabbit. *Brain,* 1963, **86**, 525–562. [139, 159, 172]

Carman, J. B., Cowan, W. M., Powell, T. P. S., and Webster, K. E. A bilateral cortico-striate projection. *Journal of Neurology, Neurosurgery, and Psychiatry,* 1965, **28**, 71–77. [159, 172]

Carmel, P. W. Efferent projections of the ventral anterior nucleus of the thalamus in the monkey. *American Journal of Anatomy,* 1970, **128**, 159–184. [166]

Carpenter, M. B. Brain stem and infratentorial neuraxis in experimental dyskinesia. In *Extrapyramidal system and neuroleptics.* Univ. de Montreal. Montreal: Therien Frères, 1960; *Revue Canadienne de Biologie,* 1961, **20**, 107–136. [172]

Carpenter, M. B. Ventral tier thalamic nuclei. In D. Williams (Ed.), *Modern trends in neurology.* Vol. 4. London: Butterworths, 1967. [165]

Carpenter, M. B., Fraser, R. A. R., and Shriver, J. E. The organization of pallidosubthalamic fibers in the monkey. *Brain Research,* 1968, **11**, 522–559. [139, 169]

Carpenter, M. B., and Hanna, G. R. Fiber projections from the spinal trigeminal nucleus in the cat. *Journal of Comparative Neurology,* 1961, **117**, 117–132. [171]

Carpenter, M. B., and McMasters, R. E. Lesions of the substantia nigra in the rhesus monkey. Efferent fiber degeneration and behavioral observations. *American Journal of Anatomy,* 1964, **114**, 293–320. [152, 161, 167, 168]

Carpenter, M. B., and Strominger, N. L. Efferent fiber projections of the subthalamic nucleus in the rhesus monkey. A comparison of the efferent projections of the subthalamic nucleus, substantia nigra and globus pallidus. *American Journal of Anatomy,* 1967, **121**, 41–72. [138, 149, 150, 152, 161, 165, 167, 168, 169, 173]

Carpenter, M. B., Whittier, J. R., and Mettler, F. A. Analysis of choreoid hyperkinesia in the rhesus monkey. Surgical and pharmacological analysis of hyperkinesia resulting from lesions in the subthalamic nucleus of Luys. *Journal of Comparative Neurology,* 1950, **92**, 293–332. [164, 165]

Casey, K. L., and Towe, A. L. Cerebellar influence on pyramidal-tract neurones. *Journal of Physiology (London),* 1961, **158**, 399–410. [88]

Cazard, P., and Buser, P. Modification des réponses sensorielles corticales par stimulation de l'hippocampe dorsal chez le lapin. *Electroencephalography and Clinical Neurophysiology,* 1963, **15**, 413–425. [133]

Chang, H. T. High level decussation of the pyramids in the pangolin, *Manis pentadactyla* Dalmanii. *Journal of Comparative Neurology,* 1944, **81,** 333–338. [73]

Chow, K. L. Lack of behavioral effects following destruction of some thalamic association nuclei in monkey. *American Medical Association Archives of Neurology and Psychiatry,* 1954, **71,** 762–771. [131]

Christopher, M., and Butter, C. M. Consummatory behaviors and locomotor exploration evoked from self-stimulation sites in rats. *Journal of Comparative and Physiological Psychology,* 1968, **66,** 335–339. [206, 208]

Clare, M. H., Landau, W. M., and Bishop, G. H. Electrophysiological evidence of a collateral pathway from the pyramidal tract to the thalamus in the cat. *Experimental Neurology,* 1964, **9,** 262–267. [72, 83]

Clark, W. E. L. The termination of ascending tracts in the thalamus of the macaque monkey. *Journal of Anatomy,* 1936, **72,** 1–40. [165, 171]

Clemente, C. D., Sterman, M. B., and Wyrwicka, W. Post-reinforcement EEG synchronization during alimentary behavior. *Electroencephalography and Clinical Neurophysiology,* 1964, **16,** 355–365. [236]

Clough, J. F. M., Kernell, D., and Phillips, C. G. A distribution of monosynaptic excitation from the pyramidal tract and from primary spindle afferents to motoneurons of the baboon's hand and forearm. *Journal of Physiology (London),* 1968, **198,** 145–166. [90, 92]

Cole, M., Nauta, W. J. H., and Mehler, W. R. The ascending efferent projections of the substantia nigra. *Transactions of the American Neurological Association,* 1964, **89,** 74–78. [154, 167, 168]

Cooper, E. R. A. The development of the substantia nigra. *Brain,* 1946, **69,** 22–23. [171]

Cooper, I. S. Relief of juvenile involuntary movement disorders by chemopallidectomy. *Journal of the American Medical Association,* 1957, **164,** 2197–1301. [165]

Cowan, W. M., and Powell, T. P. S. Striopallidal projection in the monkey. *Journal of Neurology, Neurosurgery, Psychiatry,* 1966, **29,** 426–439. [139, 172]

Culler, E., and Mettler, F. A. Conditioned behavior in a decorticate dog. *Journal of Comparative Psychology,* 1934, **18,** 291–303. [104, 112]

Curtis, D. R., Duggan, A. W., and Johnston, G. A. R. Glycine, strychnine, picrotoxin and spinal inhibition. *Brain Research,* 1969, **14,** 759–762. [216]

Curtis, D. R., Hösle, L., Johnston, G. A. R., and Johnston, I. H. The hyperpolarization of spinal motoneurons by glycine and related amino acids. *Experimental Brain Research,* 1968, **5,** 235–258. [214, 215]

Dąbrowska, J. Reversal learning in frontal rats. *Acta Biologiae Experimentalis,* 1964, **24,** 19–26. [198]

Dąbrowska, J. Dissociation of impairment after lateral and medial prefrontal lesions in dogs. *Science,* 1971, **171,** 1037–1038. [185, 186, 189]

Dafney, N., and Feldman, S. Effects of stimulating reticular formation, hippocampus and septum on single cells in the posterior hypothalamus. *Electroencephalography and Clinical Neurophysiology,* 1969, **26,** 578–587. [16]

Dahl, D., Ingram, W. R., and Knott, J. R. Diencephalic lesions and avoidance learning in cats. *Archives of Neurology,* 1962, **7,** 314–319. [131]

Dahlström, A., and Fuxe, K. Evidence for the existence of monoamine-containing neurons in the central nervous system. I. Demonstration of monoamines in the cell bodies of brain stem neurons. *Acta Physiologica Scandinavica (Supplement 232),* 1964, **62,** 1–5. [137, 155, 168]

Dalton, A., and Black, A. H. Hippocampal electrical activity during the operant conditioning of movement and refraining from movement. *Communications in Behavioral Biology,* 1968, **2,** 267–273. [230]

Dart, R. A. The dual structure of the neopallium: Its history and significance. *Journal of Anatomy (London)*, 1934, **69**, 3–19. [95]

Dejours, P. Regulation of breathing during muscular exercise in man: A neuro-humoral theory. In N. J. C. Cunningham and B. B. Lloyd (Eds.), *Regulation of Human Respiration*. Oxford: Blackwell Scientific Publications, 1964, Pp. 535–547. [54]

Delgado, J. M. R., Roberts, W. W., and Miller, N. E. Learning motivated by electrical stimulation of the brain. *American Journal of Physiology*, 1954, **179**, 587–593. [211]

DeMyer, W. Number of axons and myelin sheaths in the adult human medullary pyramids. Study with silver impregnation and iron hematoxylin staining methods. *Neurology (Minneapolis)*, 1959, **9**, 42–47. [79]

DeMyer, W., and Russell, J. The number of axons in the right and left medullary pyramidal of macaca rhesus and the ratio of axons to myelin sheaths. *Acta Morphologica Neerlando-Scandinavica*, 1958, **2**, 134–139. [79]

Denny-Brown, D. *The cerebral control of movement.* Liverpool, England: Liverpool University Press, 1966.

Deutsch, J. A. Higher nervous function: The physiological basis of memory. *Annual Review of Physiology*, 1962, **24**, 259–286. [129]

DeVito, J. L. Projections from the cerebral cortex to intralaminar nuclei in monkey. *Journal of Comparative Neurology*, 1969, **136**, 193–202. [170]

Dewey, J. The reflex arc concept in psychology. *Psychological Review*, 1896, **3**, 357–370.

Dexler, H., and Margulies, A. Über die Pyramidenbahn des Schafes und der Ziege. *Morphologisches Jahrbuch*, 1906, **35**, 413–449. [77]

Diamond, I. T., Goldberg, J. M., and Neff, W. D. Tonal discrimination after ablation of auditory cortex. *Journal of Neurophysiology*, 1962, **25**, 223–285. [103]

Diamond, I. T., Jones, E. G., and Powell, T. P. S. The projections of the auditory cortex upon the diencephalon and brain stem in the cat. *Brain Research*, 1969, **15**, 305–340. [171]

Diamond, I. T., and Neff, W. D. Ablation of temporal cortex and discrimination of auditory patterns. *Journal of Neurophysiology*, 1957, **20**, 300–315. [103]

Divac, I. Functions of the caudate nucleus. *Acta Biologiae Experimentalis*, 1968, **28**, 107–120.   (a)

Divac, I. Effects of prefrontal and caudate lesions on delayed responses in cats. *Acta Biologiae Experimentalis*, 1968, **28**, 149–167.   (b)

Dobrzecka, C., and Konorski, J. Qualitative versus directional cues in differential conditioning. I. Left leg-right leg differentiation to cues of a mixed character. *Acta Biologiae Experimentalis*, 1967, **27**, 163–168. [187]

Dobrzecka, C., and Konorski, J. Qualitative versus directional cues in differential conditioning. II. Left leg-right leg differentiation to nondirectional cues. *Acta Biologiae Experimentalis*, 1968, **28**, 61–69. [187]

Doty, R. W. Conditional reflexes formed and evoked by brain stimulation. In D. E. Sheer (Ed.), *Electrical stimulation of the brain.* Austin, Texas: University of Texas Press, 1961. [103]

Doty, R. W., Rutledge, L. T., and Larsen, R. M. Conditioned reflexes established to electrical stimulation of cat cerebral cortex. *Journal of Neurophysiology*, 1956, **19**, 401–415. [103]

Douglas, A., and Barr, M. L. The course of the pyramidal tract in rodents. *Revue Canadienne de Biologie.* 1950, **8**, 118–122. [76]

Douglas, R. J. The hippocampus and behavior. *Psychological Bulletin*, 1967, **67**, 416–442. [16, 132, 133]

Dräseke. J. Zur mikroskopischen Kenntnis der Pyramidenkreuzung der Chiropteren. *Anatomischer Anzeiger*, 1903, **23**, 449–456. [73, 76]

Dräseke, J. Zur Kenntnis des Rückenmarks und der Pyramidenbahnen von Talpa europaea. *Monatsschrift für Psychiatrie Neurologie,* 1904, **15,** 401–409. [76]

Dresel, K., and Rothman, H. Völliger Ausfall der Substantia nigra nach Exstirpation von Grosshirn und Striatum. *Zeitschrift für die Gesamte Neurologie und Psychiatrie,* 1925, **94,** 781–789. [154]

Dresse, A. Importance du système mesencephalo-telencéphalique noradrénergique comme substratum anatomique du comportement d'autostimulation. *Life Sciences,* 1966, **5,** 1003–1014. [208, 225, 226]

Dubois, E. Sur le rapport du poids de l'encéphale avec la grandeur du corps chez les mammiféres. *Bulletin Société d'Anthropologie (Paris),* 1897, **8,** 337–376. [81]

Dudar, J. D., and Szerb, J. C. The effect of topically applied atropine on resting and evoked cortical acetylcholine release. *Journal of Physiology (London),* 1969, **203,** 741–762. [236]

Dusser de Barenne, J. G. Récherches expérimentales sur les fonctions du système nerveux central, faites en particuliur sur deux chats dont le neopallium avait été enlévé. *Archives Néerlandaises de Physiologie.* 1920, **4,** 30–123. [102]

Dykman, R. A., and Shurrager, P. S. Successive and maintained conditioning in spinal carnivores. *Journal of Comparative and Physiological Psychology,* 1956, **49,** 27–35. [113, 114, 115]

Eccles, J. C., Ito, M., and Szentagothai, J. *The cerebellum as a neuronal machine.* New York: Springer-Verlag, 1967. [285, 300, 314]

Eidelberg, E., White, J. C., and Brazier, Mary A. B. The hippocampal arousal pattern in rabbits. *Experimental Neurology,* 1959, **1,** 483–490. [247]

Elazar, Z., and Adey, W. R. Spectral analysis of low frequency components in the electrical activity of the hippocampus during learning. *Electroencephalography and Clinical Neurophysiology,* 1967, **23,** 225–240. [301]

Elftman, H. Work done by muscle in running. *American Journal of Physiology,* 1940, **129,** 672. [21, 37]

Ellen, P., and Wilson, A. S. Perseveration in the rat following hippocampal lesions. *Experimental Neurology,* 1963, **8,** 310–317. [14]

Ellen, P., Wilson, A. S., and Powell, E. W. Septal inhibition and timing behavior in the rat. *Experimental Neurology,* 1964, **10,** 120–132. [14]

Ellison, G. D., Sorenson, C. A., and Jacobs, B. L. Two feeding syndromes following surgical isolation of the hypothalamus in rats. *Journal of Comparative and Physiological Psychology,* 1970, **70,** 173–188. [206]

Emmers, R., Chun, R. W. M., and Wang, G. H. Behavior and reflexes of chronic thalamic cats. *Archives Italiennes de Biologie,* 1965, **103,** 178–193. [106]

Evarts, E. V. Temporal patterns of discharge of pyramidal tract neurons during sleep and waking in the monkey. *Journal of Neurophysiology,* 1964, **27,** 152–171. [93]

Evarts, E. V. Relation of discharge frequency to conduction velocity in pyramidal tract neurons. *Journal of Neurophysiology,* 1965, **28,** 216–228. [93, 94]

Evarts, E. V. Relation of pyramidal tract activity to force exerted during voluntary movement. *Journal of Neurophysiology,* 1968, **31,** 14–27. [70, 93, 94]

Evarts, E. V. Activity of pyramidal tract neurons during postural fixation. *Journal of Neurophysiology,* 1969, **32,** 375–385. [70, 93, 94]

Evarts, E. V., and Thach, W. T. Motor mechanisms of the CNS: cerebrocerebellar interrelations. *Annual Review of Physiology,* 1969, **31,** 451–498. [314]

Evarts, E. V., Bizzi, E., Burke, R. E., DeLong, M., and Thach, W. T., Jr. Central control of movement. *Neurosciences Research Program Bulletin,* 1971, **9,** 170 pp. [13]

Faull, R. L. M., and Carman, J. B. Ascending projections of the substantia nigra in the rat. *Journal of Comparative Neurology,* 1968, **132,** 73–92. [154, 155, 167, 168]

Felix, D., and Wiesendanger, M. Pyramidal and non-pyramidal motor cortical effects on distal forelimb muscles of monkeys. *Experimental Brain Research,* 1971, **12,** 81–91. [92]

Fenn, W. D. Relation between the work performed and the energy liberated in muscular contraction. *Journal of Physiology,* 1924, **58,** 373–395. [21]

Fenn, W. D. Frictional and kinetic factors in the work of spring running. *American Journal of Physiology,* 1930, **92,** 583–611. [36, 37]

Fernandez de Molina, A., and Hunsberger, R. W. Central representation of affective reactions in forebrain and brain stem: Electrical stimulation of amygdala, stria terminals, and adjacent structures. *Journal of Physiology (London),* 1959, **145,** 251–256. [211]

Ferraro, A. Contributa sperimentale allo studio della substantia nigra normale e dei suoi rapporti con la corteccia cerebrale e con il corpo striato. *Archives of General Neurology and Psychiatry,* 1925, **6,** 26–117. [154]

Fetz, E. E. Pyramidal tract effects on interneurons in the cat lumbar dorsal horn. *Journal of Neurophysiology,* 1968, **31,** 69–80. [84]

Fetz, E. E. Operant conditioning of cortical unit activity. *Science,* 1969, **163,** 955–958. [70, 93, 94]

Fetz, E. E., and Finocchio, D. V. Operant conditioning of specific patterns of neural and muscular activity. *Science,* 1971, **174,** 431–435. [70, 93]

Fink, R. P., and Heimer, L. Two methods for selective silver impregnation of degenerating axons and their synaptic endings in the central nervous system. *Brain Research,* 1967, **4,** 369–374. [273]

Fisher, A. M., Harting, J. K., Martin, G. F., and Stuber, M. I. The origin, course, and termination of corticospinal fibers in the armadillo. *Journal of Neurological Sciences,* 1969, **8,** 347–361. [77, 83]

Foerster, O. Motorisch Felder und Bahnen. In O. Bumke and O. Foerster (Eds.), *Handbuch*

Fonberg, E. The role of the hypothalamus and amygdala in food intake, alimentary motivation and emotional reactions. *Acta Biologiae Experimentalis,* 1969, **29,** 335–358. [179, 183]

Forbes, A., and Mahan, C. Attempts to train the spinal cord. *Journal of Comparative and Physiological Psychology,* 1963, **56,** 36–40. [114]

Forbes, A., and Sherrington, C. S. Acoustic reflexes in the decerebrate cat. *American Journal of Physiology,* 1914, **35,** 367–376. [108, 110, 111]

Fox, S. S., Liebeskind, J. C., O'Brien, J. H., and Dingle, R. D. H. Mechanisms for limbic modification of cerebellar and cortical afferent information. In W. R. Adey and T. Tokizane (Eds.), *Progress in brain research. Structure and function of the limbic system.* Vol. 27. Amsterdam: Elsevier, 1967. [133, 239]

Freeman, W. J. The electrical activity of a primary sensory cortex: Analysis of EEG waves. *International Review of Neurobiology,* 1963, **5,** 53–119. [231]

Freud, S. *General introduction to psychoanalysis.* New York: Boni and Liveright, 1920. [21]

Frigyesi, T. L., and Purpura, D. P. Electrophysiological analysis of reciprocal caudato-nigral relations. *Brain Research,* 1967, **6,** 440–456. [168]

Fritsch, G., and Hitzig, E. Über die elektrische Erregbarkeit des Grosshirns (On the electrical excitability of the cerebrum). *Archiv für wissenschaftliche Medizin,* pp. 300-332. In K. H. Pribram (Ed.), *Brain and behaviour 2: Perception and action.* Baltimore, Maryland: Penguin Books, 1969. [9]

Fruton, J. S., and Simmonds, S. *General biochemistry.* New York: Wiley, 1960. [28]

Fulton, J. F., and Sheehan, D. Uncrossed lateral pyramidal tract in higher primates. *Journal of Anatomy (London),* 1935, **69,** 181–187. [75]

Fuse, G. Vergleichend-anatomische Beiträge zur Kenntnis über die sog. obere, zweite oder proximale Pyramidenkreuzung bei Endentaten, sowie bie einigen fliegenden Säugern. *Arbeiten aus anatomischen Instituten Sendai,* 1926, **12**, 47–92.   (a) [73, 76]

Fuse, G. Zur Frage nach dem Ursprung und Verlauf der sog. Zonalfasern der spinalen Quintuswurzel bei Echidna (Kölliker). *Arbeiten aus anatomischen Instituten Sendai,* 1926, **12**, 92–97.   (b) [76]

Fuse, G. Uber eine bisher unbekannte Kreuzungs- und Verlaufsart der Pyramidenbahn bei den Säugetieren: Der ventrale Seitenstrangtypus der sog. Distalen Pyramidenkreuzung beim Zweisehenfaultier (*Choloepus didactylus*). *Arbeiten aus anatomischen Instituten Sendai,* 1926, **12**, 98–164.   (c) [77]

Fuse, G. Eine neue Kreuzungsart der Pyramidenbahn bei den Säugern: Mittlerer Seitenstrangtypus der sog. proximalen Pyramidenkreuzung beim grossen Ameisenbären (Myrmecophaga tridactyla). *Arbeiten aus anatomischen Instituten Sendai,* 1926, **12**, 165–168.   (d) [73, 77]

Fuxe, K. Distribution of monoamine terminals in the central nervous system. *Acta Physiologica Scandinavica (Supplement 247),* 1965, **64**, 41–85. [207, 224, 225]

Fuxe, K., and Andén, N. E. Studies on central monoamine neurons with special reference to the nigro-neostriatal dopamine neuron system. In E. Costa *et al.* (Eds.), *Biochemistry and pharmacology of the basal ganglia.* Hewlett, New York: Raven Press, 1966. [139, 168]

Fuxe, K., Hökfelt, T., and Nilsson, O. Observations on the cellular localization of dopamine in the caudate nucleus of the rat. *Zeitschrift für Zellforschung und Mikroskopische Anatomie,* 1964, **63**, 701–706. [155]

Fuxe, K., Hökfelt, T., and Ungerstedt, U. Morphological and functional aspects of central monoamine neurons. *International Review of Neurobiology,* 1970, **13**, 93–126. [207]

Gaito, J. Macromolecules and brain function. In J. Gaito (Ed.), *Macromolecules and behavior.* New York: Appleton-Century Crofts, 1966. [129]

Gall, F. J., and Spurzheim, C. *Anatomie et Physiologie du Système Nerveux en Général et du Cerveau en Particulier.* Paris, 1810. [71]

Gambarian, L. S., Garibian, A. A., Sarkisian, J. S., and Garadian, V. O. Conditioned motor reflexes in cats with damage to the globus pallidus. *Experimental Brain Research,* 1971, **12**, 92–104. [131]

Garey, L. M., Jones, E. G., and Powell, T. P. S. Interrelationships of the striate and extrastriate cortex with the primary relay sites of the visual pathways. *Journal of Neurology, Neurosurgery and Psychiatry,* 1968, **31**, 135–157. [166]

Gastaut, H. Some aspects of the neurophysiological basis of conditioned reflexes and behavior. In G. E. W. Wolstenholme and C. M. O'Connor (Eds.), *Ciba Foundation Symposium on the Neurological Basis of Behaviour.* Boston, Massachusetts: Little, Brown, 1958.   (a) [110]

Gastaut, H. The role of the reticular formation in establishing conditioned reactions. In H. H. Jasper, L. D. Proctor, R. S. Knighton, W. C. Noshay, and R. T. Costello (Eds.), *The Reticular Formation of the Brain.* Boston, Massachusetts; Little, Brown, 1958.   (b) [110, 129]

Geller, I., and Seifter, J. The effects of meprobamate, barbiturates, d-amphetamine and promazine on experimentally induced conflict in the rat. *Psychopharmacologia,* 1960, **1**, 482–492. [206, 209, 210]

Gerben, M. J. Running elicited by hypothalamic stimulation. *Psychonomic Science,* 1968, **12**, 19–20. [253]

Gerben, M. J. Elicited locomotor behavior during hypothalamic self-stimulation. *Communications in Behavioral Biology,* 1969, **3**, 223–231. [253]

Gerbner, M., and Pásster, E. The role of the frontal lobe in conditioned reflex activity. *Acta Physiologica Academiae Scientiarum Hungaricae,* 1965, **26,** 89–95.[179]

Gerbrandt, L. K. Generalizations from the distinction of passive and active avoidance. *Psychological Reports,* 1964, **15,** 11–22.[14]

Gerbrandt, L. K. Neural systems of response release and control. *Psychological Bulletin,* 1965, **64,** 113–123.[14]

Gibson, W. E., Reid, L. D., Sakai, M., and Porter, P. B. Intracranial reinforcement compared with sugar-water reinfocement. *Science,* 1965, **148,** 1357–1359.[266]

Girden, E., Mettler, F. A., Finch, G., and Culler, E. Conditioned responses in a decorticate dog to acoustic, thermal and tactile stimulation. *Journal of Comparative Psychology,* 1936, **21,** 367–385.[104, 106, 110, 129]

Gladfelter, W. E., and Brobeck, J. R. Decreased spontaneous locomotor activity in the rat induced by hypothalamic lesions. *American Journal of Physiology,* 1962, **203,** 811–817. [9]

Glees, P., Gole, J., Liddel, E. G. T., and Phillips, C. G. Beobachtungen über die motorische Rinde des Affen (Rhesus, Papio strepitus and Papio papio). *Archives Psychiatry und Atschr. für Neurology,* 1950, **185,** 675–689. [75]

Glickman, S. E. Reinforcing properties of arousal. *Journal of Comparative and Physiological Psychology,* 1960, **53,** 68–71. [271, 292]

Glickman, S. E. Perseverative neural processes and consolidation of the memory trace. *Psychological Bulletin,* 1961, **58,** 218–233. [129]

Glickman, S. E., and Schiff, B. B. A biological theory of reinforcement. *Psychological Review,* 1967, **74,** 81–109. [6, 10, 12, 17, 264]

Gloor, P., Vera, C. L., and Sperti, L. Electrophysiological studies of hippocampal neurons. I. Configuration and laminar analysis of the "resting" potential gradient, of the main-transient response to perforant path, fimbrial and mossy fibre volleys and of "spontaneous" activity. *Electroencephalography and Clinical Neurophysiology,* 1963, **15,** 353–378. [238]

Gobbel, W. G., Jr., and Liles, G. W. Efferent fibers of parietal lobe of cat (*Felis domesticus*). *Journal of Neurophysiology,* 1945, **8,** 257–266.[74]

Goddard, G. V. Functions of the amygdala. *Psychological Bulletin,* 1964, **62,** 89–109. [14]

Goldby, F. An experimental investigation of the motor cortex and pyramidal tract of *Echidna aculeata. Journal of Anatomy (London),* 1939, **73,** 509–524. (a). [73, 76]

Goldby, F. An experimental investigation of the motor cortex and its connections in the phalanger, *Trichosurus vulpecula. Journal of Anatomy (London),* 1939, **74,** 12–33. (b) [76]

Goldby, F., and Kacker, G. N. A survey of the pyramidal system in the coypu rat, *Myocastor coypus. Journal of Anatomy (London),* 1963, **97,** 517–531.[76]

Goldman, P., and Rosvold, H. E. Localization of function within the dorsolateral prefrontal cortex of the rhesus monkey. *Experimental Neurology,* 1970, **27,** 291–304. [189, 190, 191]

Goldstein, K. Zur vergleichenden Anatomie der Pyramidenbahn. *Anatomischer Anzeiger,* 1904, **24,** 451–454. [76]

Goltz, F. M. Der Hund ohne Grosshirn. *Pflügers Archiv für die Gesamte Physiologie,* 1892, **51,** 570–614. [104, 112]

Granit, R. (Ed.) *Muscular afferents and motor control.* Nobel Symposium I. Stockholm: Almqvist and Wiksell, 1966.[264]

Granit, R. *The basis of motor control.* New York: Academic Press, 1970. [7, 10, 35]

Granit, R., and Kaada, B. R. Influence of stimulation of central nervous structures on muscle spindles in cat. *Acta Physiologica Scandinavica,* 1952, **27,** 130–160.[261]

Grastyán, E. The hippocampus and higher nervous activity. In M. A. B. Brazier (Ed.), *The central nervous system and behavior.* New York: Josiah Macy, Jr. Foundation, 1959. [300]

Grastyán, E., Karmos, G., Vereczkey, and Kellenyi, L. The hippocampal electrical correlates of the homeostatic regulation of motivation. *Electroencephalography and Clinical Neurophysiology,* 1966, **21**, 34–53. [250, 303]

Grastyán, E., Lissák, K., Madarász, I., and Donhoffer, H. Hippocampal electrical activity during the development of conditioned reflexes. *Electroencephalography and Clinical Neurophysiology,* 1959, **11**, 409–430. [132, 236]

Grastyán, E., Szabó, I., Molnar, P., and Kolta, P. Rebound reinforcement, and self-stimulation. *Communications in Behavioral Biology,* 1968, **A2**, 235–266. [2]

Gray, P. A., Jr. The cortical lamination pattern of the opossum, *Didelphys virginiana. Journal of Comparative Neurology,* 1924, **37**, 221–263. [74, 96]

Green, J. D. The Hippocampus. In J. Field, H. W. Magoun, and V. E. Hall (Eds.), *Handbook of Physiology, Neurophysiology,* Vol. 2. Washington, D.C.: American Physiological Society, 1960. [132]

Green, J. D., and Arduini, A. H. Hippocampal electrical activity in arousal. *Journal of Neurophysiology,* 1954, **17**, 533–557. [236, 300, 301, 308]

Green, J. D., and Machne, X. Unit activity of rabbit hippocampus. *American Journal of Physiology,* 1955, **181**, 219–221. [132]

Green, J. D., Maxwell, D. S., Schindler, W. J., and Stumpf, C. Rabbit EEG "theta" rhythm: Its anatomical source and relation to activity in single neurons. *Journal of Neurophysiology,* 1960, **23**, 403–420. [230]

Griffiths, E., Chapman, N., and Campbell, D. An apparatus for detecting and monitoring movement. *American Journal of Psychology,* 1967, **80**, 438–441. [230]

Gross, Ch. A comparison of the effects of partial and total lateral frontal lesions on test performance by monkeys. *Journal of Comparative and Physiological Psychology,* 1963, **56**, 41–47. [186]

Gross, Ch., and Weiskrantz, L. Evidence for dissociation between impairment on auditory discrimination and delayed response in frontal monkeys. *Experimental Neurology,* 1962, **5**, 453–476. [186]

Gross, Ch., and Weiskrantz, L. Some changes in behavior produced by lateral frontal lesions in the macaque. In J. M. Warren and K. Akert (Eds.), *The frontal granular cortex and behavior.* New York: McGraw-Hill, 1964. Pp. 74-101. [191]

Grossman, S. P. Direct adrenergic and cholinergic stimulation of hypothalamic mechanisms. *American Journal of Physiology,* 1962, **202**, 872–882. [221]

Grossman, S. P. *A textbook of physiological psychology.* New York: Wiley, 1967. [129, 130, 131]

Grossman, S. P. Avoidance behavior and aggression in rats with transections of the lateral connections of the medial or lateral hypothalamus. *Physiology and Behavior,* 1970, **5**, 1103–1108. [11]

Groves, P. M., and Thompson, R. F. Habituation: A dual process theory. *Psychological Review,* 1970, **77**, 419–450. [115]

Guillery, R. W. Degeneration in the hypothalamic connexions of the albino rat. *Journal of Anatomy (London),* 1957, **91**, 91–115. [289, 316, 317]

Guillery, R. W. Afferent fibers to the dorsomedial thalamic nucleus in the cat. *Journal of Anatomy (London),* 1959, **93**, 403–419. [316]

Haartsen, A. B. The fibre content of the cord in small and large mammals. *Acta morphologica Neerlando-Scandinavica,* 1961, **3**, 331–340. [77]

Haartsen, A. B., and Verhaart, W. J. C. Cortical projections to brain stem and spinal cord in the goat by way of the pyramidal tract and the bundle of Bagley. *Journal of Comparative Neurology,* 1967, **129,** 189–202. [73, 74, 77, 84, 85]

Hamilton, C. L. Problems of refeeding after starvation in the rat. *Annals of the New York Academy of Sciences,* 1969, **157,** 1004–1017. [205]

Hamilton, L. W., McCleary, R. A., and Grossman, S. P. Behavioral effects of cholinergic septal blockade in the cat. *Journal of Comparative and Physiological Psychology,* 1968, **66,** 563–668. [222]

Hammond, L. J. Increased responding to CS⁻ in differential CER. *Psychonomic Science,* 1966, **5,** 337–338. [4]

Hardin, W. B., Jr. Spontaneous activity in the pyramidal tract of chronic cats and monkeys. *Archives of Neurology,* 1965, **13,** 501–512. [93, 94]

Harper, R. *Behavioral and electrophysiological studies of sleep and animal hypnosis.* Unpublished doctoral dissertation, McMaster University, Hamilton, Ontario, 1968. [250]

Harris, F., Jabbur, S. J., Morse, R. W., and Towe, A. L. Influence of the cerebral cortex on the cuneate nucleus of the monkey. *Nature (London),* 1965, **208,** 1215–1216. [88, 92]

Harting, J. K., and Martin, G. F. Neocortical projections to the mesencephalon of the armadillo, *Dasypus novemcinctus. Brain Research,* 1970, **17,** 447–462. [300, 316]

Hassler, R. Motorische und sensible Effekte umschriebener Reizungen und Ausschaltungen im menschlichen Zwischenhirn. *Deutsche Zeitschrift für Nervenheilkunde,* 1961, **183,** 148–171. [138]

Hatchek, R. Über eine eigentümliche Pyramidenvariation in Säugetierreihe. *Arbeiten Neurologie Institut, Universität Wien,* 1903, **10,** 48–57. [76]

Hebb, D. O. Drives and the C.N.S. *Psychological Review,* 1955, **62,** 243–254. [265, 271, 301]

Hern, J. E. C., Landgren, S., Phillips, C. G., and Porter, R. Selective excitation of corticofugal neurones by surface-anodal stimulation of the baboon's motor cortex. *Journal of Physiology (London),* 1962, **161,** 73–90. [91]

Herz, A. Drugs and the conditioned avoidance response. *International Review of Neurobiology,* 1960, **2,** 229–277. [254]

Hess, W. R. *The Functional Organization of the Diencephalon.* New York: Grune and Stratton, 1957. [206, 207, 211, 261]

Hill, A. V. The maximum work and mechanical efficiency of human muscles and their most economical speed. *Journal of Physiology,* 1922, **56,** 19–41. [36]

Hill, A. V. Production and absorption of work by muscle. *Science,* 1960, **131,** 897–903. [36]

Hinde, R. A. *Animal behaviour: A synthesis of ethology and comparative psychology.* 2nd ed. New York: McGraw-Hill, 1970. [5, 6]

Hirano, T., Best, P., and Olds, J. Units during habituation, discrimination learning, and extinction. *Electroencephalography and Clinical Neurophysiology,* 1970, **28,** 127–135. [132]

Hockman, C. H. EEG and behavioral effects of food deprivation in the albino rat. *Electroencephalography and Clinical Neurophysiology,* 1964, **17,** 420–427. [301, 303]

Hodes, R. Electrocortical synchronization resulting from reduced proprioceptive drive caused by neuromuscular blocking agents. *Electroencephalography and Clinical Neurophysiology,* 1962, **14,** 220–232. [304]

Hoebel, B. G. Feeding and self-stimulation. *Annals of the New York Academy of Sciences,* 1969, **157,** 758–778. [205, 221]

Hoebel, B. G. Feeding: Neural control of intake. *Annual Review of Physiology,* 1971, **33,** 533–568. [219]

Hoff, E. C. The distribution of the spinal terminals (Boutons) of the pyramidal tract, determined by experimental degeneration. *Proceedings of the Royal Society,* 1932, **B111,** 226–237.[83]

Hoff, E. C., and Hoff, H. E. Spinal termination of the projection fibers from the motor cortex of primates. *Brain,* 1934, **57,** 454–473.[83]

Holdstock, T. L. Autonomic reactivity following septal and amygdaloid lesions in white rats. *Physiology and Behavior,* 1969, **4,** 603–607. [13]

Holmes, G. The nervous system of the dog without a forebrain. *Journal of Physiology,* 1901–1902, **27,** 1–25. [104, 110, 112, 154]

Holstein, S. B., Buchwald, J. S., and Schwafel, J. A. Progressive changes in auditory response patterns to repeated tone during normal wakefulness and paralysis. *Brain Research,* 1969, **16,** 133–148.[118]

Homma, S. Firing of the cat motoneurone and summation of the excitatory postsynaptic potential. In R. Granit (Ed.), *Nobel Symposium I: Muscular Afferents and Motor Control.* New York: Wiley, 1966. Pp. 235–244. [90]

Hornykiewicz, O. Metabolism of brain dopamine in human Parkinsonism: Neurochemical and clinical aspects. In E. Costa *et al.* (Eds.), *Biochemistry and Pharmacology of the Basal Ganglia.* Hewlett, New York: Raven Press, 1966. [137, 155, 168]

Hösli, L., Tebécis, A. K., and Filias, N. Effects of glycine, beta-alanine and GABA, and their interaction with strychnine, on brain stem neurons. *Brain Research,* 1969, **16,** 293–295. [215]

Huang, Y. H. Self-stimulation pathways from the lateral hypothalamus. Unpublished doctoral dissertation, Northwestern University, 1970. [275, 314]

Huang, Y. H., and Routtenberg, A. Lateral hypothalamic self-stimulation pathways in *Rattus norvegicus. Physiology and Behavior,* 1971, **7,** 419–432. [276, 283, 286, 288, 297, 299, 300, 314, 316]

Hubel, D. H., and Wiesel, T. N. The period of susceptibility to the physiological effects of unilateral eye closure in kittens. *Journal of Physiology,* 1970, **206,** 419–436.[314]

Hughes, K. R. Dorsal and ventral hippocampus lesions and maze learning: Influence of pre-operative environment. *Canadian Journal of Psychology,* 1965, **19,** 325–332. [260]

Hull, C. L. *Principles of behavior: An introduction to behavior theory.* New York: Appleton-Century-Crofts, 1943. [24, 27]

Humphrey, G. L., Kitzes, M. I., and Buchwald, J. S. Progressive changes of the acoustic reflex in decerebrate cats. *Federation Proceedings,* 1970, **29,** 324.[118]

Huxley, H. E. The mechanism of muscular contraction. *Science,* 1969, **64,** 1356-1366. [31]

Ingram, W. R. Modification of learning by lesions and stimulation in the diencephalon and related structures. In H. H. Jasper, L. D. Proctor, R. S. Knighton, W. S. Noshay, and R. T. Costello (Eds.), *The reticular formation of the brain.* Boston, Massachusetts: Little, Brown, 1958. [131]

Ingram, W. R., Barris, R. W., Fisher, C. and Ranson, S. W. Catalepsy. An experimental study. *Archives of Neurology and Psychiatry (Chicago),* 1936, **35,** 1175–1197.[261]

Innes, I. R., and Nickerson, M. Drugs inhibiting the action of acetylcholine on structures innervated by postganglionic parasympathetic nerves (antimuscarinic or atropinic drugs). In L. S. Goodman and A. Gilman (Eds.), *The pharmacological basis of therapeutics.* New York: Macmillan, 1965. Pp. 521–545. [259]

Irwin, S. Correlation in rats between the locomotor and avoidance-suppressant potencies of eight phenothiazine tranquilizers. *Archives Internationales de Pharmacodynamie et de Thérapie,* 1961, **132,** 279–286. [258]

Ito, M. Hippocampal electrical correlates of self-stimulation in the rat. *Electroencephalography and Clinical Neurophysiology*, 1966, **21**, 261–268. [250]

Jabbur, S. J., and Towe, A. L. Analysis of the antidromic cortical response following stimulation at the medullary pyramids. *Journal of Physiology (London)*, 1961, **155**, 148–160. [74]

Jackson, J. H. Relations of different divisions of the central nervous system to one another and to parts of the body. *The Lancet*, 1898, **1**, 79–87. [100, 101]

Jacobsen, C. F. Influence of motor and premotor area lesions upon the retention of acquired skilled movements in monkeys and chimpanzees. *Research Publications of the Association for Research in Nervous and Mental Diseases*, 1934, **13**, 225–247. [198]

Jacobsen, C. F. Studies of cerebral function in primates. I. The functions of the frontal association areas in monkeys. *Comparative Psychology Monographs*, 1936, **13**, no. 63, 3–60. [191]

Jacobson, A., and Kales, A. Somnambulism: All-night EEG and related studies. *Research Publications of the Association for Nervous and Mental Disease*, 1967, **45**, 424-455. [259]

Jane, J. A., Campbell, C. B. G., and Yashon, D. The origin of the corticospinal tract of the tree shrew (*Tupaia glis*) with observations on its brain stem and spinal terminations. *Brain, Behavior and Evolution*, 1969, **2**, 160–182. [74, 75, 83]

Jane, J. A., Yashon, D., DeMyer, W., and Bucy, P. C. The contribution of the precentral gyrus to the pyramidal tract of man. *Journal of Neurosurgery*, 1967, **26**, 244–248. [74]

Jansen, J., and Brodal, A. (Eds.) *Aspects of Cerebellar Anatomy*. Oslo: Tanum, 1954. [165]

Jansen, J., and Brodal, A. Das Kleinhirn. In W. von Mollendorff (Ed.), *Handbuch der mikroskopischen Anatomie des Menschen*. Vol. III. Berlin: Springer, 1958. [165]

Jerison, H. J. Gross brain indices and the analysis of fossil endocasts. In C. R. Noback and W. Montagna (Eds.), *Advances in Primatology*, Vol. 1, The Primate Brain. New York: Appleton-Century-Crofts, 1970. Pp. 225–244. [81]

Johnston, J. B. The cell masses in the forebrain of the turtle, *Cistudo carolina. Journal of Comparative Neurology*, 1915, **25**, 393–468. [86]

Johnston, J. B. Evidence of a motor pallium in the forebrain of reptiles. *Journal of Comparative Neurology*, 1916, **26**, 475–479. [95]

Jones, E. G., and Powell, T. P. S. The projection of the somatic sensory cortex upon the thalamus in the cat. *Brain Research*, 1968, **10**, 369–391. [171]

Jouvet, M. Neurophysiology of the states of sleep. *Physiological Reviews*, 1967, **47**, 119–177. [205, 301]

Jung, R., and Kornmüller, A. E. Eine Methodik der Ableitung lokalisierter Potentialschwankungen aus subcorticalen Hirngebieten. *Archives Psychiatrie und Nervenkranken*, 1938, **109**, 1–30. [301]

Kaada, B. R. Somato-motor, autonomic and electrocorticographic responses to electrical stimulation of "rhinencephalic" and other structures in primates, cat and dog. *Acta Physiologica Scandinavica*, 1951, **24** (Suppl. 83), 1–285. [13]

Kaada, B. R., Rasmussen, E. W., and Kviem, O. Effects of hippocampal lesions on maze learning and retention in rats. *Experimental Neurology*, 1961, **3**, 333–355. [260]

Kaada, B. R., Rasmussen, E. W., and Kveim, O. Impaired acquisition of passive avoidance behavior by subcallosal, septal, hypothalamic and insular lesions in rats. *Journal of Comparative and Physiological Psychology*, 1962, **55**, 661–670. [2, 11, 211]

Kalischer, O. Weitere Mittheilung zur Grosshirnlocalisation bei den Vögeln. *Sitzungsberichte der Königlich Preussischen Akademie der Wissenschaften zu Berlin*, 1901, **1**, 428–439. [85]

Kalischer, O. Das Grosshirn der Papageien in anatomischer und physiologischer Beziehung. *Abhandlungen der Königlich Preussischen Akademie der Wissenschaften, Abhandlungen nicht zur Akademie gehöriger Gelehrter*, IV, 1905. [85, 95]

Kandel, E. R., and Spencer, W. A. Cellular neurophysiological approaches in the study of learning. *Physiological Reviews,* 1968, **48,** 63–134. [115]

Karplus, J. P., and Kreidl, A. Über Totalexstirpationen einer und beider Grosshirn-hemisphaeren an Affen (Macacus rhesus). *Archives für Anatomie und Physiologie Leipzig,* 1914, **38,** 155–212. [102]

Karten, H. J. The organization of the avian telencephalon and some speculations on the phylogeny of the amniote telencephalon. *Annals of the New York Academy of Science,* 1969, **167,** 164–179. [86]

Karten, H. J. Efferent projections of the wulst of the owl. *Anatomical Record,* 1971, **169,** 353. [86]

Katz, R. I., Chase, T. N., and Kopin, I. J. Effects of ions on stimulus-induced release of amino acids from mammalian brain slices. *Journal of Neurochemistry,* 1969, **16,** 961–967. [215, 216]

Kawamura, H., and Domino, E. F. Hippocampal slow ("arousal") wave activation in the rostral midbrain transected cat. *Electroencephalography and Clinical Neurophysiology,* 1968, **25,** 471–480. [247]

Kawamura, H., Nakamura, Y., and Tokizane, T. Effect of acute brain stem lesions on the electrical activities of the limbic system and neocortex. *Japanese Journal of Physiology,* 1961, **11,** 564–575. [247]

Keene, J. J., and Casey, K. L. Excitatory connection from lateral hypothalamic self-stimulation sites to escape sites in medullary reticular formation. *Experimental Neurology,* 1970, **28,** 155–166. [296, 300, 314]

Keesey, U. T., and Nichols, D. J. Relation between the ongoing electroencephalogram and fluctuations of visibility of a stabilized retinal image. *Journal of the Optical Society of America,* 1966, **56,** 543. [60]

Kellogg, W. N., Deese, J., Pronko, N. H., and Feinberg, M. An attempt to condition the chronic spinal dog. *Journal of Experimental Psychology,* 1947, **37,** 99–117. [113]

Kellogg, W. N., Pronko, N., and Deese, J. Spinal conditioning in dogs. *Science,* 1946, **103,** 49–50. [113]

Kelsey, J. E., and Grossman, S. P. Nonperseverative disruption of behavioral inhibition following septal lesions in rats. *Journal of Comparative and Physiological Psychology,* 1971, **75,** 302–311. [15]

Kemp, J. M. An electron microscopic study of the termination of afferent fibers in the caudate nucleus. *Brain Research,* 1968, **11,** 464–467. [159]

Kemp, J. M., and Powell, T. P. S. The cortico-striate projection in the monkey. *Brain,* 1970, **93,** 525–546. [139, 159, 172]

Kennard, M. A., and McCulloch, W. S. Motor responses to stimulation of cerebral cortex in absence of areas 4 and 6 (*Macaca mulatta*). *Journal of Neurophysiology,* 1943, **6,** 181–189. [69, 96]

Kennedy, T. T., and Towe, A. L. Identification of a fast lemnisco-cortical system in the cat. *Journal of Physiology (London),* 1962, **160,** 535–547. [74]

Kenyon, J. The effect of septal lesions upon motivated behavior in the rat. Unpublished Ph.D. dissertation. McGill University, 1962. [15]

Kernell, D., and Wu, C.-P. Responses of the pyramidal tract to stimulation of the baboon's motor cortex. *Journal of Physiology (London),* 1967, **191,** 653–672.   (a) [91]

Kernell, D., and Wu, C.-P. Post-synaptic effects of cortical stimulation on forelimb motoneurones in the baboon. *Journal of Physiology (London),* 1967, **191,** 673–690.   (b) [88, 91]

Kimble, D. P. The effects of bilateral hippocampal lesions in rats. *Journal of Comparative and Physiological Psychology,* 1963, **56,** 273–283. [260]

Kimble, D. P., Rogers, L. and Hendrickson, C. W. Hippocampal lesions disrupt maternal, not sexual behavior in the albino rat. *Journal of Comparative and Physiological Psychology,* 1967, **63**, 401–407. [260]

Kimble, D. P. Hippocampus and internal inhibition. *Psychological Bulletin,* 1968, **70**, 285–295. [4, 16, 132, 183]

Kimble, D. P. Possible inhibitory functions of the hippocampus. *Neuropsychologia,* 1969, **7**, 235–244. [4, 16]

Kimble, G. A., and Perlmuter, L. C. The problem of volition. *Psychological Review,* 1970, **77**, 361–384. [12]

King, F. A. Effects of septal and amygdaloid lesions on emotional behavior and conditioned avoidance responses in the rat. *Journal of Nervous and Mental Diseases,* 1958, **126**, 57–63. [14]

King, J. L. The cortico-spinal tract of the rat. *Anatomical Record,* 1910, **4**, 245–252. [76]

King, J. L. The pyramid tract and other descending paths in the spinal cord of the sheep. *Quarterly Journal of Experimental Physiology,* 1911, **4**, 133–149. [77]

Kitai, S. T., Oshima, T., Provini, L., and Tsukahara, N. Cerebro-cerebellar connections mediated by fast and slow conducting pyramidal tract fibers of the cat. *Brain Research,* 1969, **15**, 267–271. [83, 88]

Kitzes, M., and Buchwald, J. S. Progressive alterations in cochlear nucleus, inferior colliculus, and medial geniculate responses during acoustic habituation. *Experimental Neurology,* 1969, **25**, 85–105. [118]

Kleiner, F. B., Meyer, P. M., and Meyer, D. R. Effects of simultaneous septal and amygdaloid lesions upon emotionality and retention of a black-white discrimination. *Brain Research,* 1967, **5**, 459–468. [131]

Kleist, K. *Gehirnpathologie.* Leipzig: Barth, 1934. [138]

Klemm, W. R. Electroencephalographic-behavioral dissociations during animal hypnosis. *Electroencephalography and Clinical Neurophysiology,* 1966, **21**, 365–372. [250]

Klemm, W. R. Mechanisms of the immobility reflex ("animal hypnosis") II. EEG and multiple unit correlates in the brain stem. *Communications in Behavioral Biology,* 1969, **3**, 43–52. [250]

Knook, H. L. *The fibre-connections of the forebrain.* Leiden: van Gorcum, 1965. [154]

Knott, J. R., Ingram, W. R., and Correll, R. E. Effects of certain subcortical lesions on learning and performance in the cat. *Archives of Neurology,* 1960, **2**, 247–259. [131]

Koella, W. P., and Czicman, J. S. The mechanism of the EEG-synchronizing action of serotonin. *American Journal of Physiology,* 1966, **211**, 926–934. [205]

Kolliker, A. von. *Die medulla oblongata und die Vierhügelgegend von Ornithoryhynchus und Echidna.* Leipzig: Engelmann, 1901. [76]

Komisaruk, B. R. Synchrony between limbic system theta activity and rhythmical behavior in rats. *Journal of Comparative and Physiological Psychology,* 1970, **70**, 482–492. [17]

Komisaruk, B. R., and Olds, J. Neuronal correlates of behavior in freely moving rats. *Science,* 1968, **161**, 810–812. [10]

König, J. F. R., and Klippel, R. A. *The rat brain.* Baltimore, Maryland: Williams and Wilkins, 1963. [276, 277, 278, 279, 280, 281, 282, 286, 287, 309, 310, 311]

Konorski, J. *Integrative activity of the brain.* Chicago, Illinois: University of Chicago Press, 1970. [177, 179, 184, 188, 190]

Konorski, J., and Lawicka, W. Physiological mechanism of delayed reactions. I. The analysis and classification of delayed reactions. *Acta Biologiae Experimentalis,* 1959, **19**, 175–199. [187]

Konorski, J., and Lawicka, W. Analysis of errors by prefrontal animals on the delayed-response test. In J. M. Warren and K. Akert (Eds.), *The frontal granular cortex and behavior.* New York: McGraw-Hill, 1964. [191, 192]

Konorski, J., Stępień, L., Brutkowski, S., Ławicka, W., and Stępień, I. The effect of the removal of interprojective fields of the cerebral cortex on the higher nervous activity of animals. *Bulletin Société des Sciences et des lettres de Łódź*, 1952, **3**, 1–5. [181]

Konorski, J., and Szwejkowska, G. Chronic extinction and restoration of conditioned reflexes. IV. The dependence of the course of extinction and restoration of conditioned reflexes on the "history" of the conditioned stimulus. (The principle of the primacy of first training.) *Acta Biologiae Experimentalis*, 1952, **16**, 95–114. [184]

Kovach, J. K. Interaction of innate and acquired: Color preferences and early exposure learning in chicks. *Journal of Comparative and Physiological Psychology*, 1971, **75**, 386–398. [8]

Koyasu, Y. On the spinal conditioned reflex in the dog. *Osaka University Medical Journal*, 1957, **9**, 107–112. [113]

Kozenberg, W. *Untersuchungen über das Rückenmark des Igels*. Wiesbaden, 1899. [76, 86]

Kramis, R. C. Hippocampal synchrony and desynchrony: Frequency-specific elicitation by intracranial stimuli and relation to motivating brain stimuli and behavior. Unpublished doctoral dissertation, Northwestern University, 1972. [308, 311]

Kramis, R. C., and Routtenberg, A. Rewarding brain stimulation, hippocampal activity, and foot-stomping in the gerbil. *Physiology and Behavior*, 1969, **4**, 7–11. [305, 312]

Krasne, F. B. General disruption resulting from electrical stimulation of ventromedial hypothalamus. *Science*, 1962, **138**, 822–823. [211]

Kreiner, J. Reconstruction of neocortical lesions within the dog's brain: instructions. *Acta Biologiae Experimentalis*, 1966, **26**, 221–243. [179]

Krogh, A. *The anatomy and physiology of capillaries*. New Haven, Connecticut: Yale University Press, 1922. [31]

Kuhn, R. E., and Zucker, I. Reproductive behavior of the Mongolian gerbil, *Meriones unguiculatus*. *Journal of Comparative and Physiological Psychology*, 1968, **66**, 747–752. [305]

Kuypers, H. G. J. M. An anatomical analysis of cortico-bulbar connexions to the pons and lower brain stem in the cat. *Journal of Anatomy (London)*, 1958, **92**, 198–218. (a) [72, 75, 83]

Kuypers, H. G. J. M. Corticobulbar connections to the pons and lower brain stem in man. *Brain*, 1958, **81**, 364–388. (b) [72, 83]

Kuypers, H. G. J. M. Some projections from the pericentral cortex to the pons and lower brain stem in monkey and chimpanzee. *Journal of Comparative Neurology*, 1958, **110**, 221–255. (c) [72, 75, 83]

Kuypers, H. G. J. M. Central cortical projections to motor and somato-sensory cell groups. *Brain*, 1960, **83**, 161–184. [72, 83]

Kuypers, H. G. J. M., and Brinkman, J. Precentral projections to different parts of the spinal intermediate zone in the rhesus monkey. *Brain Research*, 1970, **24**, 29–48. [83]

Kuypers, H. G. J. M., Fleming, W. R., and Farinholt, J. W. Subcorticospinal projections in the rhesus monkey. *Journal of Comparative Neurology*, 1962, **118**, 107–137. [84]

Kuypers, H. G. J. M., and Lawrence, D. G. Cortical projections to the red nucleus and the brain stem in the rhesus monkey. *Brain Research*, 1967, **4**, 151–188. [154, 166, 167, 170, 171]

Kuypers, H. G. J. M., and Tuerk, J. R. The distribution of the cortical fibres within the nuclei cuneatus and gracilis in the cat. *Journal of Anatomy (London)*, 1964, **98**, 143–162. [83]

Landgren, S., Phillips, C. G., and Porter, R. Minimal synaptic actions of pyramidal impulses on some alpha motoneurones of the baboon's hand and forearm. *Journal of Physiology (London)*, 1962, **161**, 91–111. (a) [90, 91, 92, 93, 94]

Landgren, S., Phillips, C. G., and Porter, R. Cortical fields of origin of the monosynaptic pyramidal pathways to some alpha motoneurones of the baboon's hand and forearm. *Journal of Physiology (London)*, 1962, **161**, 112–125. (b) [90]

Lardy, H. A. Energetic coupling and regulation of metabolic rates. In C. Liebezq (Ed.), *Proceedings Third International Congress Biochemistry, Brussels.* New York: Academic Press, 1956.[31]

Larsson, K. Mating behavior in male rats after cerebral cortex ablation. I. Effects of lesions in the dorsolateral and median cortex. *Journal of Experimental Zoology,* 1962, **151,** 167–176.[260]

Larsson, K. Mating behavior in male rats after cerebral cortex ablation. II. Effect of lesions in the frontal lobes compared to lesions in the posterior half of the hemispheres. *Journal of Experimental Zoology,* 1964, **155,** 203–214.[260]

Lashley, K. S. Studies of cerebral function in learning. V: The retention of motor habits after destruction of the so-called motor areas in primates. *American Medical Association Archives of Neurology and Psychiatry,* 1924, **12,** 249–276. [103]

Lashley, K. S. *Brain mechanisms and intelligence.* Chicago, Illinois: University of Chicago Press, 1929; Dover edition, 1963.[103, 104, 129, 260]

Lashley, K. S. In search of the engram. *Proceedings of the Society for Experimental Biology, Symposium,* 1950, **4,** 454–482. [129]

Lassek, A. M. The pyramidal tract of the monkey. A Betz cell and pyramidal tract enumeration. *Journal of Comparative Neurology,* 1941, **74,** 193–202. [79]

Lassek, A. M. The pyramidal tract. A fiber and numerical analysis in a series of non-digital mammals (ungulates). *Journal of Comparative Neurology,* 1942, **77,** 399–404. (a) [79]

Lassek, A. M. Pyramidal tract: effect of pre- and postcentral cortical lesions on fiber components of pyramids in monkeys. *Journal of Nervous and Mental Disease,* 1942, **95,** 721–729. (b) [78]

Lassek, A. M. A study of the effect of complete frontal lobe extirpations on the fiber components of the pyramidal tract. *Journal of Comparative Neurology,* 1952, **96,** 121–125.[74, 78]

Lassek, A. M., Dowd, L. W., and Weil, A. The quantitative distribution of the pyramidal tract in the dog. *Journal of Comparative Neurology,* 1930, **51,** 153–163. [82]

Lassek, A. M., and Karlsberg, P. The pyramidal tract of an aquatic carnivore. *Journal of Comparative Neurology,* 1956, **106,** 425–431. [79]

Lassek, A. M., and Rasmussen, G. L. The human pyramidal tract. A fiber and numerical analysis. *Archives of Neurology and Psychiatry,* 1939, **42,** 872–876.[79]

Lassek, A. M., and Rasmussen, G. L. A comparative fiber and numerical analysis of the pyramidal tract. *Journal of Comparative Neurology,* 1940, **72,** 417–428. [79]

Lassek, A. M., and Wheatley, M. D. The pyramidal tract. An enumeration of the large motor cells of area 4 and the axons in the pyramids of the chimpanzee. *Journal of Comparative Neurology,* 1945, **82,** 299–302.[79]

Laursen, A. M. Conditional avoidance behavior of cats with pallidal lesions. *Danish Medical Bulletin,* 1962, **9,** 21–22. [131]

Laursen, A. M. Motion speed and reaction time after section of the pyramidal tracts in cats. *Bulletin of the Swiss Academy of Medical Science,* 1966, **22,** 336–340.[89]

Laursen, A. M., and Wiesendanger, M. Motor deficits after transection of a bulbar pyramid in the cat. *Acta Physiologica Scandinavica,* 1966, **68,** 118–126. [89]

Laursen, A. M., and Wiesendanger, M. The effect of pyramidal lesions on response latency in cats. *Brain Research,* 1967, **5,** 207–220.[103]

Ławicka, W. Physiological analysis of disturbances of the delayed responses in dogs after prefrontal ablation. *Bulletin of the Polish Academy of Sciences,* 1957, **5,** 107–110. (a)

Ławicka, W. The effect of the prefrontal lobectomy on the vocal conditioned reflexes in dogs. *Acta Biologiae Experimentalis,* 1957, **17**, 317–325.   (b) [181]

Ławicka, W. Physiological mechanism of delayed reactions. II Delayed reactions in dogs and cats to directional stimuli. *Acta Biologiae Experimentalis,* 1959, **19**, 199–221. [191]

Ławicka, W. The role of stimuli modality in successive discrimination and differentiation learning. *Bulletin of the Polish Academy of Sciences,* 1964, **12**, 35–38. [187]

Ławicka, W. Differing effectiveness of auditory, quality and location cues in two forms of differentiation learning. *Acta Biologiae Experimentalis,* 1969, **29**, 83–92.   (a) [187]

Ławicka, W. A proposed mechanism for delayed response impairment in prefrontal animals. *Acta Biologiae Experimentalis,* 1969, **29**, 401–414.   (b) [189, 191, 193, 194]

Ławicka, W., and Konorski, J. Physiological mechanism of delayed reactions. III. The effects of prefrontal ablations on delayed reactions in dogs. *Acta Biologiae Experimentalis,* 1959, **19**, 221–233. [188, 191]

Ławicka, W., and Konorski, J. The effects of prefrontal lobectomies on the delayed responses in cats. *Acta Biologiae Experimentalis,* 1961, **21**, 141–156. [193]

Ławicka, W., Mishkin, M., Kreiner, J., and Brutkowski, S. Delayed response deficit in dogs after selective ablation of the proreal gyrus. *Acta Biologiae Experimentalis,* 1966, **26**, 309–322. [183]

Ławicka, W., Mishkin, M., and Rosvold, H. E. Dissociation of impairment on auditory tasks following orbital and dorsolateral frontal lesions in monkeys. *Proceedings of the Congress of Polish Physiologist Society, Lublin, Poland,* 1966, **10**, 178. [183, 187, 188, 189, 191, 192]

Ławicka, W., Mishkin, M., and Rosvold, H. E. Effects of partial prefrontal lesions on auditory discriminatory tests in monkeys. *Acta Neurobiologiae Experimentalis,* 1972, **2**. [183, 187, 188, 189]

Lawrence, D. G., and Kuypers, H. G. J. M. The functional organization of the motor system in the monkey. I. The effects of bilateral pyramidal lesions. *Brain,* 1968, **91**, 1–14.   (a) [89, 103]

Lawrence, D. G., and Kuypers, H. G. J. M. The functional organization of the motor system in the monkey. II. The effects of lesions of the descending brain-stem pathways. *Brain,* 1968, **19**, 15–36.   (b) [89]

Lebedinskaia, S. I., and Rosenthal, J. S. Reactions of a dog after removal of the cerebral hemispheres. *Brain,* 1935, **58**, 412–419. [102, 103, 106, 107]

Leonard, C. M. The prefrontal cortex of the rat. I. Cortical projection of the medio-dorsal nucleus. II. Efferent connections. *Brain Research,* 1969, **12**, 321–343. [287, 289, 316]

Levin, P. M., and Bradford, F. K. The exact origin of the cortico-spinal tract in the monkey. *Journal of Comparative Neurology,* 1938, **68**, 411–422. [74]

Lewis, R., and Brindley, G. S. The extrapyramidal cortical motor map. *Brain,* 1965, **88**, 397–406. [90]

Lewis, P. R., and Shute, C. C. D. The cholinergic limbic system: Projections to hippocampal formation, medial cortex, nuclei of the ascending cholinergic reticular system and the subfornical organ and supra-optic crest. *Brain,* 1970, **90**, 521–540. [209, 224]

Leyton, A. S. F., and Sherrington, C. S. Observations on the excitable cortex of the chimpanzee, orang-utan and gorilla. *Quarterly Journal of Experimental Physiology,* 1917, **11**, 135–222. [69]

Linowiecki, A. J. The comparative anatomy of the pyramidal tract. *Journal of Comparative Neurology,* 1914, **24**, 509–530. [76]

Liss, P. The role of the hippocampus and septum in response inhibition. Unpublished Ph.D. dissertation. McGill University, 1965. [9]

Liu, C.-N., and Chambers, W. W. An experimental study of the corticospinal system in the monkey *(Macaca mulatta)*. The spinal pathways and preterminal distribution of degenerating fibers following discrete lesions of the pre- and postcentral gyri and bulbar pyramid. *Journal of Comparative Neurology,* 1964, **123,** 257–284. [74, 75, 83]

Livingston, R. B. Reinforcement. In G. C. Quarton, T. Melnechuk, and F. O. Schmitt (Eds.), *The neurosciences: a study program.* New York: Rockefeller University Press, 1967. [13]

Livingston, R. B., Fulton, J. F., Delgado, J. M. R., Sachs, E. Jr., Brendler, S. J., and Davis, G. D. Stimulation and regional ablation of orbital surface of frontal lobe. In J. F. Fulton, C. D. Aring, and S. B. Wortis (Eds.), *The frontal lobes, Research Publication of the Association for Research in Nervous and Mental Disease,* 1948, **27,** 405–420. [13]

Lloyd, A. J., Wikler, A., and Whitehouse, J. M. Non-conditionability of flexor reflex in the chronic spinal dog. *Journal of Comparative and Physiological Psychology,* 1969, **68,** 576–579. [114]

Lloyd, D. P. C. The influence of pyramidal excitation on the spinal cord of the cat. *American Journal of Physiology,* 1941, **133,** 363–364. (a) [89]

Lloyd, D. P. C. The spinal mechanism of the pyramidal system in cats. *Journal of Neurophysiology,* 1941, **4,** 525–546. (b) [89]

Lloyd, D. P. C. Note on convergence of pyramidal and primary afferent impulses in the spinal cord of the cat. *Proceedings of the New Hampshire Academy of Science,* 1968, **59,** 381–384. [89]

Loeb, C., Magni, F., and Rossi, G. F. Electrophysiological analysis of the action of atropine on the central nervous system. *Archives Italiennes de Biologie,* 1960, **98,** 293–307. [235]

Longo, V. G. Behavioral and electroencephalographic effects of atropine and related compounds. *Pharmacological Review,* 1966, **18,** 965–996. [259]

Lorens, S. A. Effect of lesions in the central nervous system on lateral hypothalamic self-stimulation in the rat. *Journal of Comparative and Physiological Psychology,* 1966, **62,** 256–262. [267, 296]

Loucks, R. B. Methods of isolating stimulation effect with implanted barriers. In D. E. Sheer (Ed.), *Electrical Stimulation of the Brain.* Austin, Texas: University of Texas Press, 1961. [103, 104]

Lubar, J. F., and Perachio, A. A. One way and two way learning and transfer of an active avoidance response in normal and cingulectomized cats. *Journal of Comparative and Physiological Psychology,* 1965, **60,** 46–52. [14]

Lundberg, A., and Voorhoeve, P. Effects from the pyramidal tract on spinal reflex arcs. *Acta Physiologica Scandinavica,* 1962, **56,** 201–219. [9]

Luschei, E. S., Johnson, R. A., and Glickstein, M. Response of neurons in the motor cortex during performance of simple repetitive arm movement. *Nature (London),* 1968, **217,** 190–191. [93, 94]

MacLean, P. D. Chemical and electrical stimulation of hippocampus in unrestrained animals. II. Behavioral findings. *American Medical Association Archives of Neurology and Psychiatry,* 1957, **78,** 128–142. [229]

Magendie, F. *Précis élémentaire de physiologie.* 4. Aufl., S. 147. Bruxelles: Dumont, 1834. [71]

Magoun, H. W. Caudal and cephalic influences of the brain stem reticular formation. *Physiological Reviews,* 1950, **30,** 459–474. [261]

Margules, D. L. Dissociation of operant behavior and feeding by cholinergic blockade of the ventromedial nucleus of the hypothalamus. *Federation Proceedings,* 1967, **26,** 2. [214, 221, 223]

Margules, D. L. Noradrenergic basis of inhibition between reward and punishment in amygdala. *Journal of Comparative and Physiological Psychology,* 1968, **66,** 329–334. [222]

Margules, D. L. Noradrenergic rather than sertonergic basis of reward in the dorsal tegmentum. *Journal of Comparative and Physiological Psychology*, 1969, **67**, 32–35. (a)[208, 315]

Margules, D. L. Noradrenergic synapses for the suppression of feeding behavior. *Life Sciences*, 1969, **1**, 693–704. (b) [205, 221]

Margules, D. L. Alpha-adrenergic receptors in hypothalamus for the suppression of feeding behavior by satiety. *Journal of Comparative and Physiological Psychology*, 1970, **73**, 1–12. (a)[205, 221]

Margules, D. L. Beta-adrenergic receptors in the hypothalamus for learned and unlearned taste aversions. *Journal of Comparative and Physiological Psychology*, 1970, **73**, 13–21. (b)[205, 221]

Margules, D. L. Control of punished behavior by endogenous acetylcholine in the hypothalamus. *Twenty-fifth International Congress of Physiological Sciences*, Munich, Germany, 1971. (a)[212]

Margules, D. L. Localization of the anti-punishment actions of norepinephrine and atropine in amygdala and entopeduncular nucleus. *Brain Research*, 1971, **35**, 177–184. (b) [219, 225]

Margules, D. L. Alpha and beta adrenergic receptors in amygdala: Reciprocal inhibitors and facilitators of punished operant behavior. *European Journal of Pharmacology*, 1972, in press. [222, 225]

Margules, D. L., and Margules, A. S. Cholinergic receptors in the ventromedial hypothalamus govern operant response strength. *American Journal of Physiology*, submitted. [224]

Margules, D. L., and Stein, L. Neuroleptic vs. tranquilizers: Evidence from animal studies of mode and site of action. In H. Brill *et al.* (Eds.), *Neuro-psychopharmacology*, New York: Excerpta Medica Foundations, 1967. [204, 210, 212, 214, 218, 221]

Margules, D. L., and Stein, L. Facilitation of Sidman avoidance by positive brain stimulation. *Journal of Comparative and Physiological Psychology*, 1968, **66**, 182–184. [208]

Margules, D. L., and Stein, L. Cholinergic synapses in the ventromedial hypothalamus for the suppression of operant behavior by punishment and satiety. *Journal of Comparative and Physiological Psychology*, 1969, **67**, 327–335. (a)[214, 221, 223]

Margules, D. L., and Stein, L. Cholinergic synapses of a periventricular punishment system in the medial hypothalamus. *American Journal of Physiology*, 1969, **217**, 2. (b) [211, 212, 214, 219, 221]

Margules, D. L., and Lowes, G. Anti-punishments effects of direct placement of *l*-norepinephrine hydrochloride and atropine methyl nitrate in the hippocampal gyrus and dentate gyrus. In preparation.[219]

Martin, G. F., and Fisher, A. M. A further evaluation of the origin, the course and the termination of the opossum corticospinal tract. *Journal of Neurological Science*, 1968, **7**, 177–187. [74, 76, 96]

Martin, J. P., and McCaul, I. R. Acute hemiballismus treated by ventrolateral thalamolysis. *Brain*, 1959, **82**, 104–108. [165]

Maser, J. D. A deficit in response initiation and suppression on an operant discrimination task by septally damaged rats. Unpublished Ph.D. dissertation. Temple University, 1970. [9, 14]

Maspes, P. E., and Pagni, C. A. Surgical treatment of dystonia and choreoathetosis in infantile cerebral palsy by pedunculotomy. Pathophysiological observations and therapeutic results. *Journal of Neurosurgery*, 1964, **21**, 1076–1086.[97]

Matthews, B. H. C. A special purpose amplifier. *Journal of Physiology (London)*, 1934, **57**, 28P–29P. [231]

Matzke, H. A. The course of fibers arising from the nucleus gracilis and cuneatus of the cat. *Journal of Comparative Neurology*, 1951, **94**, 439–452. [171]

McBride, R. L., and Klemm, W. R. Mechanisms of the immobility reflex ("animal hypnosis") I. Influences of repetition of induction, restriction of auditory-visual input, and destruction of brain areas. *Communications in Behavioral Biology,* 1969, **3**, 33–41. [250]

McCleary, R. A. Response specificity in the behavioral effects of limbic system lesions in the cat. *Journal of Comparative and Physiological Psychology,* 1961, **54**, 605–613. [14, 131, 206]

McCleary, R. A. Response-modulating functions of the limbic system–initiation and suppression. In E. Stellar and J. Sprague (Eds.), *Progress in Physiological Psychology.* Vol. 1. New York: Academic Press, 1966. [14, 16, 131, 206]

McLardy, T. Hippocampal formation of brain as detector-coder of temporal patterns of information. *Perspectives in Biology and Medicine,* 1959, **2**, 443–452. [132]

McLardy. T. Some cell and fibre peculiarities of uncal hippocampus. In W. Bargmann and J. P. Schade (Eds.), *Progress in Brain Research.* Vol. 3. The rhinencephalon and related structures. New York: Elsevier, 1963. [132]

Mehler, W. R. Further notes on the center median nucleus of Luys. In D. P. Purpura and M. D. Yahr (Eds.), *The Thalamus.* New York: Columbia University Press, 1966. [169, 171]

Mehler, W. R., Feferman, M. E., and Nauta, W. J. H. Ascending axon degeneration following anterolateral cordotomy. An experimental study in the monkey. *Brain,* 1960, **83**, 718–750. [171]

Mehler, W. R., Vernier, V. G., and Nauta, W. J. H. Efferent projections from the dentate and interpositus nuclei in primates. *Anatomical Record,* 1958, **130**, 430–431. [171]

Merzabacher, L., and Spielmeyer, W. Beiträge zur Kenntnis des Fledermausgehirns besonders der corticomotorischen Bahnen. *Neurologisches Zentralblatt,* 1903, **22**, 1050–1053. [73, 76]

Mettler, F. A. Extensive unilateral cerebral removals in the primate. Physiologic effects and resultant degeneration. *Journal of Comparative Neurology,* 1943, **79**, 185–243. [155]

Mettler, F. A. On the origin of the fibers in the pyramid of the primate brain. *Proceeding of the Society for Experimental Biology, New York,* 1944, **57**, 111–113. [74]

Mettler, F. A. Extracortical connections of the primate frontal cerebral cortex. I. Thalamo-cortical connections. *Journal of Comparative Neurology,* 1947, **86**, 95–117. [165, 166]

Mettler, F. A. The nonpyramidal projections from the frontal cerebral cortex. *Research Publications of the Association for Research in Nervous and Mental Diseases Monograph,* 1948, **27**, 162–199. [103]

Mettler, F. A. Muscular tone and movement: Their cerebral control in primates. In S. Ehrenpreis and O. C. Solnitzky (Eds.), *Neurosciences Research.* Vol. 1. New York: Academic Press, 1968. [7]

Mettler, F. A. Nigrofugal connections in the primate brain. *Journal of Comparative Neurology,* 1970, **138**, 291–319. [155]

Mettler, F. A., Mettler, G. C., and Culler, E. A. The effects of total removal of the cerebral cortex. *American Medical Association Archives of Neurology and Psychiatry,* 1935, **34**, 1238–1249. [104, 106]

Meyer, M. Study of efferent connections of the frontal lobe in the human brain after leucotomy. *Brain,* 1949, **72**, 265–296. [172]

Micco, D. J., and Schwartz, M. Effects of hippocampal lesions upon the development of Pavlovian internal inhibition in rats. *Journal of Comparative and Physiological Psychology,* 1971, **76**, 371–377. [16]

Miles, P. R., and Gladfelter, W. E. Lateral hypothalamus and reflex discharges over ventral roots of rat spinal nerves. *Physiology and Behavior,* 1969, **4**, 671–675. [9]

Miller, N. E. Motivational effect of brain stimulation and drugs. *Federation Proceedings,* 1960, **19**, 846–854. [205, 220]

Miller, N. E. Learning of visceral and glandular responses. *Science,* 1969, **163**, 434–445. [5, 56]

Millhouse, O. E. A Golgi study of the descending medial forebrain bundle. *Brain Research,* 1969, **15**, 341–363. [209, 288]

Milner, B. Psychological defects produced by temporal lobe excision. *Research Publication of the Association for Research in Nervous and Mental Diseases,* 1958, **36**, 244–257. [132]

Milner, B., and Teuber, H.-L. Alteration of perception and memory in man: Reflection on methods. In L. Weiskrantz (Ed.), *Analysis of Behavioral Change.* New York: Harper and Row, 1968. [132]

Milner, P. M. *Physiological Psychology.* New York: Holt, Rinehart, and Winston, 1970. [17]

Minckler, J., Klemme, R. M., and Minckler, D. The course of efferent fibers from the human premotor cortex. *Journal of Comparative Neurology,* 1944, **81**, 259–277. [74]

Mishkin, M. Effects of small frontal lesions on delayed alternation in monkeys. *Journal of Neurophysiology,* 1957, **20**, 615–622. [191, 196]

Mishkin, M. Perseveration of central sets after frontal lesions in monkeys. In J. M. Warren and K. Akert (Eds.), *The frontal granular cortex and behavior.* New York: McGraw-Hill, 1964. Pp. 219–241. [130, 195, 196]

Mishkin, M., Vest, B., Waxler, M., and Rosvold, H. E. A re-examination of the effects of frontal lesions on object alternation. *Neuropsychologia,* 1969, **7**, 357–363. [194, 197]

Mizuno, N. Projection fibers from the main sensory trigeminal nucleus and the supratrigeminal region. *Journal of Comparative Neurology,* 1970, **139**, 457–471. [171]

Moersch, F. P., and Kernohan, J. W. Hemiballismus, a clinicopathologic study. *Archives of Neurology and Psychiatry,* 1939, **41**, 365–372. [165]

Mogenson, G. J. Effects of sodium pentobarbital on brain self-stimulation. *Journal of Comparative and Physiological Psychology,* 1964, **58**, 461–462. [266]

Mogenson, G. J. General and specific reinforcement systems for drinking behavior. *Annals of the New York Academy of Sciences,* 1969, **157**, 779–797. [251]

von Monakow, C. Experimentelle und pathologisch-anatomische Untersuchungen über die Haubenregion, den Sehhugel und die Regio subthalamica. *Archiv für Psychiatrie und Nervenkrankheiten,* 1895, **27**, 1–219. [154]

Monnier, M. *Functions of the nervous system.* Vol. 2. Motor and psychomotor functions. Amsterdam: Elsevier, 1970. [7, 10]

Morgan, C. T. Physiological mechanisms of motivation. *Nebraska Symposium on Motivation,* 1957, **5**, 1–35. [17]

Mori, S. Some observations on the fine structure of the corpus striatum of the rat brain. *Zeitschrift für Zellforschung und mikroskopische Anatomie,* 1966, **70**, 461–488. [155]

Morris, H., Walker, R., and Margules, D. L. A cannula of variable depth for chemical stimulation of the brain. *Electroencephalography and Clinical Neurophysiology,* 1970, **29**, 521–523. [209]

Morrison, L. R. *Anatomical studies of the central nervous systems of dogs without forebrain or cerebellum.* Haarlem: De Erven F. Bohn, 1929. (Reviewed in *Archives of Neurology and Psychiatry,* 1930, **24**, 218–220.) [155]

Moruzzi, G., and Magoun, H. W. Brain stem reticular formation and activation of the EEG. *Electroencephalography and Clinical Neurophysiology,* 1949, **1**, 455–473. [236, 271, 301]

Munzer, E., and Wiener, H. Das zwischen- und Mittelhirn des Kanincheus und die Beziehungen dieser Teil zum übrigen Centralnervensystem, mit besonderer Berücksichtigung der Pyramidenbahn und Schleife. *Monatsschrift für Psychiatrie Neurologie,* 1902, **12**, 241–279. [75]

Murphy, J. P., and Gellhorn, E. The influence of hypothalamic stimulation on cortically induced movement and on action potentials of the cortex. *Journal of Neurophysiology,* 1945, **8**, 341–364. [261]

Myer, J. S., and Baenninger, R. Some effects of punishment and stress on mouse killing by rats. *Journal of Comparative and Physiological Psychology*, 1966, **62**, 292–297. [8]

Naito, H., Nakamura, K., Kurosaki, T., and Tamura, Y. Transcallosal excitatory postsynaptic potentials of fast and slow pyramidal tract cells in cat sensorimotor cortex. *Brain Research*, 1970, **19**, 299–301. [88]

Nauta, W. J. H. Silver impregnation of degenerating axons. In W. F. Windle (Ed.), *New research techniques in neuroanatomy*. Springfield, Illinois: Thomas, 1957. [273]

Nauta, W. J. H. Hippocampal projections and related neural pathways to the midbrain of the cat. *Brain*, 1958, **81**, 340–391. [132]

Nauta, W. J. H. Some efferent connections of the prefrontal cortex in the monkey. In J. M. Warren and K. Akert (Eds.), *The frontal granular cortex and behavior*. New York: McGraw-Hill, 1964. [130]

Nauta, W. J. H., and Gygax, P. Silver impregnation of degenerating axons in the central nervous system: A modified technique. *Stain Technology*, 1954, **29**, 91–93. [138, 152]

Nauta, W. J. H., and Mehler, W. R. Projections of the lentiform nucleus in the monkey. *Brain Research*, 1966, **1**, 3–42. [139, 145, 149, 150, 159, 166, 169, 172]

Nauta, W. J. H., and Whitlock, D. G. An anatomical analysis of the non-specific thalamic projection system. In J. F. Delafresnaye (Ed.), *Brain Mechanisms and Consciousness*. Springfield, Illinois: Thomas, 1954. [166]

Nehlil, J. La voie pyramidale dans la capsule interne. Rôle de la lésion dans le traitement des mouvements involontaires. Utilité de son repérage. *Neuro-Chirurgie*, 1964, **10**, 443–446. [97]

Newman, B. I., and Feldman, S. M. Electrophysiological activity accompanying intracranial self-stimulation. *Journal of Comparative and Physiological Psychology*, 1964, **57**, 244–247. [266]

Nicolesco, J., and Hornet, T. Contributions à l'étude du faisceau pyramidal direct de Türck. *L'encéphalé*, 1933, **28**, 10-33. [74]

Niimi, K., Katayama, K., Kanaseki, T., and Morimoto, K. Studies on the derivation of the centre median nucleus of Luys. *Tokushima Journal of Experimental Medicine*, 1960, **6**, 261–268. [169]

Niimi, K., Kishi, S., Miki, M., and Fujita, S. An experimental study of the course and termination of the projection fibers from cortical areas 4 and 6 in the cat. *Folia Psychiatrica et Neurologica Japonica*, 1963, **17**, 167–216. [72, 75, 83]

Novick, I., and Phil, R. Effect of amphetamine on the septal syndrome in rats. *Journal of Comparative and Physiological Psychology*, 1969, **68**, 220–225. [15]

Nyberg-Hansen, R. Further studies on the origin of corticospinal fibers in the cat. An experimental study with the Nauta method. *Brain Research*, 1969, **16**, 39–54.

Nyberg-Hansen, R., and Brodal, A. Sites of termination of corticospinal fibers in the cat. An experimental study in silver impregnation methods. *Journal of Comparative Neurology*, 1963, **120**, 369–391. [74, 75, 83, 84]

Nyberg-Hansen, R., and Rinvik, E. Some comments on the pyramidal tract, with special reference to its individual variations in man. *Acta Neurologica Scandinavica*, 1963, **39**, 1–30. [74]

Obersteiner, H. *Anleitung beim Studium des Baues der nervösen Centralorgane*. Leipzig: Deutike, 1896. [74, 75, 85]

O'Keefe, J., and Bouma, H. Complex sensory properties of certain amygdala units in the freely moving cat. *Experimental Neurology*, 1969, **23**, 384–398. [132]

Olds, J. A preliminary mapping of electrical reinforcing effects in the rat brain. *Journal of Comparative and Physiological Psychology*, 1956, **49**, 281–285. [266]

Olds, J. Mechanisms of instrumental conditioning. *Electroencephalography and Clinical Neurophysiology*, 1963, *Supplement 24*, 219–234. [7]

Olds, J. The limbic system and behavioral reinforcement. In W. R. Adey and T. Tokizane (Eds.), *Progress in Brain Research.* Vol. 27. Amsterdam: Elsevier, 1967. [267]

Olds, J. The central nervous system and the reinforcement of behavior. *American Psychologist,* 1969, **24,** 112–132.[226, 267]

Olds, J., and Hirano, T. Conditioned response of hippocampal and other neurons. *Electroencephalography and Clinical Neurophysiology,* 1969, **26,** 159–166. [132]

Olds, J., and Milner, P. Positive reinforcement produced by electrical stimulation of septal area and other regions of rat brain. *Journal of Comparative and Physiological Psychology,* 1954, **47,** 419–427. [206, 264, 265]

Olds, J., and Peretz, B. A motivational analysis of the reticular activating system. *Electroencephalography and Clinical Neurophysiology,* 1960, **12,** 445–454. [271, 292]

Olds, M. E., and Olds, J. Approach-escape interactions in rat brain. *American Journal of Physiology,* 1962, **203,** 803–810. [296]

Olds, M. E., and Olds, J. Approach-avoidance analysis of rat diencephalon. *Journal of Comparative Neurology,* 1963, **120,** 259–295. [266]

Olds, J., and Olds, M. E. The mechanisms of voluntary behavior. In R. Heath (Ed.), *The Role of Pleasure in Behavior.* New York: Harper and Row, 1964. [267, 275]

Olszewski, J. *The Thalamus of the Macaca mulatta. An Atlas for Use with the Stereotaxic Instrument.* New York: Karger, 1952. [138, 149, 163, 165]

Olszewski, J., and Baxter, D. *Cytoarchitecture of the Human Brain Stem.* Philadelphia, Pennsylvania: Lippincott, 1954. [150]

Overton, D. A. State-dependent learning produced by depressant and atropine-like drugs. *Psychopharmacologia,* 1966, **10,** 6–31.[259]

Paillard, J. The patterning of skilled movements. In J. Field (Ed.), *Handbook of Physiology.* Section 1, Neurophysiology. Vol. 3. Washington, D.C.: American Physiological Society, 1960. Pp. 1679–1708.[7, 10]

Papez, J. W. A summary of fiber connections of the basal ganglia with each other and with other portions of the brain. *Association for Research in Nervous and Mental Disease,* 1942, **21,** 21–68.[166]

Papez, J. W., Bennett, A. E., and Cash, P. T. Hemichorea (Hemiballismus), associated with a pallidal lesion involving afferent and efferent connections of the subthalamic nucleus: curare therapy. *Archives of Neurology and Psychiatry,* 1942, **47,** 667–676. [139, 165]

Pappas, B. A., DiCara, L. V., and Miller, N. E. Learning of blood pressure responses in the noncurarized rat: Transfer to the curarized state. *Physiology and Behavior,* 1970, **5,** 1029–1032.[5]

Parmeggiani, P. L., and Rapisarda, C. Hippocampal output and sensory mechanisms. *Brain Research,* 1969, **14,** 387–400.[133]

Patton, H. D., and Amassian, V. E. Single- and multiple-unit analysis of cortical stage of pyramidal tract activation. *Journal of Neurophysiology,* 1954, **17,** 345–363.[69, 91]

Patton, H. D., and Amassian, V. E. The pyramidal tract: its excitation and function. In J. Field (Ed.), *Handbook of Physiology.* Section 1, Vol. 2, Neurophysiology. Washington, D.C.: American Physiological Society, 1960. Pp. 837–861. [69, 91]

Pavlov, I. P. *Conditioned reflexes.* New York: 1927; Dover edition, 1960. [4, 16, 56, 61, 104]

Paxinos, G., and Bindra, D. Rewarding intracranial stimulation, movement and the hippocampal theta rhythm. *Physiology and Behavior,* 1970, **5,** 227–232. [307]

Peacock, S. M., Jr., and Hodes, R. Influence of the forebrain on somato-motor activity. II. Facilitation. *Journal of Comparative Neurology,* 1951, **94,** 409–426.[261]

Peele, T. J. Acute and chronic parietal lobe ablations in monkey. *Journal of Neurophysiology,* 1944, **7,** 269–286.[74]

Pelligrino, L. J., and Cushman, A. J. *A Stereotaxic Atlas of the Rat Brain.* New York: Appleton-Century-Crofts, 1967.[279]

Penfield, W. F., and Milner, B. Memory deficit produced by bilateral lesions in the hippocampal zone. *American Medical Association Archives of Neurology and Psychiatry,* 1958, 79, 475–497. [132]

Penfield, W., and Rasmussen, T. *The Cerebral Cortex.* New York: Macmillan, 1952. [69]

Penfield, W., and Welch, K. The supplementary motor area of the cerebral cortex. A clinical and experimental study. *Archives of Neurology and Psychiatry (Chicago),* 1951, 66, 289–317. [69]

Pennington, L. A. The function of the brain in auditory localization. III. Post-operative solution of an auditory spatial problem. *Journal of Comparative Neurology,* 1937, 67, 33–48. [103]

Peters, R. H., Rosvold, H. E., and Mirsky, A. F. The effect of thalamic lesions upon delayed response-type test in the rhesus monkey. *Journal of Comparative and Physiological Psychology,* 1956, 49, 111–116. [131]

Petras, J. M. Some fiber connections of the precentral cortex (areas 4 and 6) with the diencephalon in the monkey *(Macaca mulatta). Anatomical Record,* 1964, 148, 322. [169]

Petras, J. M. Some fiber connections of the precentral and postcentral cortex with the basal ganglia, thalamus, and subthalamus. *Transactions of the American Neurological Association,* 1965, 90, 274–275. [169, 172]

Petras, J. M. Fiber degeneration in the basal ganglia and diencephalon following lesions in the precentral and postcentral cortex of the monkey *(Macaca mulatta);* with additional observations in the chimpanzee. *International Congress of Anatomy, Wiesbaden.* Vol. 8, 1966. [169]

Petras, J. M. Some efferent connections of the motor and somatosensory cortex of simian primates and Felid, Canid and Procyonid carnivores. *Annals of the New York Academy of Sciences,* 1969, 167, 469–505. [83, 169, 172]

Petras, J. M., and Lehman, R. A. W. Corticospinal fibers in the raccoon. *Brain Research,* 1966, 3, 195–197. [83]

Petsche, H., Stumpf, Ch., and Gogolak, G. The significance of the rabbit's septum as a relay station between the midbrain and the hippocampus. I. The control of hippocampus arousal activity by the septum cells. *Electroencephalography and Clinical Neurophysiology,* 1962, 14, 202–211. [17, 297]

Pfaffman, C. Taste preference and reinforcement. In J. T. Tapp(Ed.), *Reinforcement and Behavior.* New York: Academic Press, 1969. Pp. 215–241. [221]

Phillips, C. G., and Porter, R. The pyramidal projection to motoneurons of some muscle groups of the baboon's forelimb. In J. C. Eccles and J. P. Schade (Eds.), *Progress in brain research.* Vol. 12. Physiology of spinal neurons. Amsterdam: Elsevier, 1964. Pp. 222–245. [90, 91, 92, 93]

Piaget, J. *The origins of intelligence in children.* (Translated by M. Cook.) New York: International University Press, 1952. [100]

Pickenhain, L., and Klingberg, F. Hippocampal slow activity as a correlate of basic behavioral mechanisms in the rat. In W. R. Adey and T. Tokizane (Eds.), *Progress in brain research.* Vol. 27. Amsterdam: Elsevier, 1967. Pp. 218–227. [307]

Pinto, T., and Bromiley, R. G. A search for "spinal conditioning" and for evidence that it can become a reflex. *Journal of Experimental Psychology,* 1950, 40, 121–130. [113, 117]

Pliskoff, S. S., Wright, J. E., and Hawkins, D. T. Brain stimulation as a reinforcer: intermittent schedules. *Journal of the Experimental Analysis of Behavior,* 1965, 8, 75–88. [266]

Poirier, L. J., and Sourkes, T. L. Influence of the substantia nigra on the catecholamine content of the striatum. *Brain,* 1965, 88, 181–192. [137, 155, 168]

Poltyrev, S. S., and Zeliony, G. P. Der Hund ohne Grosshirn. *American Journal of Physiology,* 1929, **90,** 475–476. [104]

Poltyrev, S. S., and Zeliony, G. P. Grosshirnrinde und Associations-funktion. *Zeitschrift für Biologie,* 1930, **90,** 157–160. [104]

Pompeiano, O. The neurophysiological mechanisms of the postural and motor events during desynchronized sleep. *Research Publications of the Association for Research in Nervous and Mental Disease,* 1967, **45,** 351–423. [250]

Pond, F. J., and Schwartzbaum, J. S. Hippocampal electrical activity evoked by rewarding and aversive brain stimulation in rats. *Communications in Behavioral Biology,* 1970, **5,** 89–103. [250]

Porter, R. Early facilitation at corticomotoneuronal synapses. *Journal of Physiology, London,* 1970, **207,** 733–745. [91, 93]

Porter, R., and Hore, J. Time course of minimal corticomotoneuronal excitatory postsynaptic potentials in lumbar motoneurons of the monkey. *Journal of Neurophysiology,* 1969, **32,** 443–451. [90, 91]

Posluns, D. An analysis of chlorpromazine-induced suppression of the avoidance response. *Psychopharmacologia,* 1962, **3,** 361–373. [258]

Powell, T. P. S. The organization and connexions of the hippocampal and intralaminar systems. *Recent Progress in Psychiatry,* 1958, **3,** 54–74. [166]

Powell, T. P. S., and Cowan, W. M. A study of thalamo-striate relations in the monkey. *Brain,* 1956, **79,** 364–390. [139, 166]

Preston, J. B., and Whitlock, D. G. Intracellular potentials recorded from motoneurons following precentral gyrus stimulation in primate. *Journal of Neurophysiology,* 1961, **24,** 91–100. [90]

Pribram, K. H. A review of theory in physiological psychology. *Annual Review of Psychology,* 1960, **11,** 1–40. [15]

Pribram, K. H. The limbic systems, efferent control of neural inhibition and behavior. In W. R. Adey and T. Tokizane (Eds.), *Progress in brain research.* Vol. 27, Structure and function of the limbic system. New York: Elsevier, 1967. [133]

Pribram, K. H. *Brain and behavior 2: perception and action.* Baltimore, Maryland: Penguin Books, 1969. [9]

Probst, M. Zur Kenntnis der Pyramidenbahn. (Normale und abnormale Pyramidenbündel und Reizversuche der Kleinhirnrinde.) *Monatsschrift für Psychiatrie Neurologie,* 1899, **6,** 91–113. [74, 77]

Probst, M. Ueber die anatomischen und physiologischen Folgen der Halbseitendurch-schneidung des Mittelhirns. *Jahrbuch für Psychiatrie, Leipzig und Wien,* 1903, **24,** 219–325. [83]

Purpura, D. P., Frigyesi, T. L., McMurtry, J. G., and Scarf, T. Synaptic mechanisms in thalamic regulation of cerebellocortical projection activity. In D. P. Purpura and M. D. Yahr (Eds.), *Thalamic Integration of Sensory and Motor Activities.* New York: Columbia University Press, 1966. [165]

Rall, W., and Shepherd, G. M. Theoretical reconstruction of field potentials and dendrodendritic synaptic interactions in olfactory bulb. *Journal of Neurophysiology,* 1968, **31,** 884–915. [209]

Ramon-Moliner, E., and Nauta, W. J. H. The isodendritic core of the brain stem. *Journal of Comparative Neurology,* 1966, **126,** 311–336. [209]

Ramon Y Cajal, S. *Recollections of my life.* Philadelphia, Pennsylvania: American Philosophical Society, 1937. [313]

Ranson, S. W. The fasciculus cerebro-spinalis in the albino rat. *American Journal of Anatomy,* 1913, **14,** 411–424. [76]

Ranson, S. W. Rigidity caused by pyramidal lesions in the cat. *Journal of Comparative Neurology,* 1932, **55,** 91–97. [89]

Rasmussen, A. T., and Peyton, W. T. The course and termination of the medial lemniscus in man. *Journal of Comparative Neurology,* 1948, **88,** 411–424. [171]

Redding, F. K. Modification of sensory cortical evoked potentials by hippocampal stimulation. *Electroencephalography and Clinical Neurophysiology,* 1967, **22,** 74–83. [133]

Rescorla, R. A. Pavlovian conditioning and its proper control procedures. *Psychological Review,* 1967, **74,** 71–80. [4]

Rescorla, R. A., and LoLordo, V. M. Inhibition of avoidance behavior. *Journal of Comparative and Physiological Psychology,* 1965, **59,** 406–412. [4]

Reveley, I. L. The pyramidal tract in the guinea-pig (*Cavia aperea*). *Anatomical Record,* 1915, **9,** 297–305. [76]

Revzin, A. M. A specific visual projection area in the hyperstriatum of the pigeon (*Columba livia*). *Brain Research,* 1969, **15,** 246–249. [86]

Revzin, A. M. Some characteristics of wide-field units in the brain of the pigeon. *Brain, Behavior and Evolution,* 1970, **3,** 195–204. [86]

Revzin, A. M., and Karten, H. J. Rostral projections of the optic tectum and nucleus rotundus in the pigeon. *Brain Research,* 1966, **3,** 264–276. [86]

Rinvik, E. The cortico-nigral projection in the cat. An experimental study with silver impregnation methods. *Journal of Comparative Neurology,* 1966, **126,** 241–254. [172]

Rinvik, E. The corticothalamic projection from the pericruciate and coronal gyri in the cat. An experimental study with silver impregnation methods. *Brain Research,* 1968, **10,** 79–119. [169, 170]

Rinvik, E. The corticothalamic projection from the gyrus proreus and the medial wall of the rostral hemisphere in the cat. An experimental study with silver impregnation methods. *Experimental Brain Research,* 1968, **5,** 129–152. (a) [170]

Rinvik, E., and Walberg, F. Demonstration of a somatotopically arranged cortico-rubral projection in the cat. An experimental study with silver methods. *Journal of Comparative Neurology,* 1963, **120,** 393–407. [8]

Rinvik, E., and Walberg, F. Is there a cortico-nigral tract? A comment based on experimental electron microscopic observations in the cat. *Brain Research,* 1969, **14,** 742–744. [172]

Rioch, D. M. Certain aspects of the behavior of decorticate cats. *Psychiatry,* 1938, **1,** 339–345. [106, 107]

Rioch, D. M., and Brenner, C. Experiments on the corpus striatum and rhinencephalon. *Journal of Comparative Neurology,* 1938, **68,** 491–507. [105, 106, 107, 111]

Roberts, T. D. M. *Neurophysiology of postural mechanisms.* New York: Plenum Press, 1967. [7, 10]

Robichaud, R. C., and Sledge, K. L. The effects of p-chlorophenylalanine on experimentally induced conflict in the rat. *Life Sciences.* 1969, **8,** 965–969. [224]

Roeder, F., and Ortheer, H. Erfahrungen mit stereotaktischen Eingriffen. I. Mitteilung: Zur Pathogenese und Therapie extrapyramidalmotorischer Bewegungsstörungen. Erfolgreiche Behandlung eines Falles schwerem Hemiballismus mit gezielter Elektrokoagulation des Globus pallidus. *Deutsche Zeitschrift für Nervenheilkunde,* 1956, **175,** 419–434. [165]

Robinson, B. W. Forebrain alimentary responses: Some organizational principles. In M. J. Wayner (Ed.), *Thirst in the regulation of body water.* New York: Pergamon, 1964. [269]

Rosvold, G. E., and Delgado, J. M. R. The effect on delayed-alternation test performance of stimulating or destroying electrically structures within the frontal lobes of the monkey's brain. *Journal of Comparative and Physiological Psychology,* 1956, **49,** 365–372. [130]

Roth, S. R., Sterman, M. B., and Clemente, C. D. Comparison of the EEG correlates of reinforcement, internal inhibition, and sleep. *Electroencephalography and Clinical Neurophysiology,* 1967, **23**, 509–520.[236]

Rothman, H. Zusammenfassender Bericht über den Rothmannschen grosshirnlosen Hund nach klinischer und anatomischer Untersuchung. *Zeitschrift für die gesamte Neurologie und Psychiatrie,* 1923, **87**, 247–313. [102]

Rothmann, M. Ueber die Pyramidenkreuzung. *Archiv für Psychiatrie und Nervenkrankheiten,* 1900, **33**, 292–310.[74, 75]

Routtenberg, A. Neural mechanisms of sleep: changing view of reticular formation function. *Psychological Review,* 1966, **73**, 481–499.[307]

Routtenberg, A. The two-arousal hypothesis: Reticular formation and limbic system. *Psychological Review,* 1968, **75**, 51–80. (a) [265, 270, 292, 296, 307]

Routtenberg, A. Hippocampal correlates of consummatory and observed behavior. *Physiology and Behavior,* 1968, **3**, 533–535. (b)[302, 306]

Routtenberg, A. Hippocampal activity and brainstem reward-aversion loci. *Journal of Comparative and Physiological Psychology,* 1970, **72**, 161–170. [251. 309, 317]

Routtenberg, A. Forebrain pathways of reward in *Rattus norvegicus. Journal of Comparative and Physiological Psychology,* 1971, **75**, 269–276. (a) [286, 287, 313, 316]

Routtenberg, A. Stimulus processing and response execution: A neurobehavioral theory. *Physiology and Behavior,* 1971, **6**, 589–596. (b) [10, 307, 308, 315]

Routtenberg, A., Gardner, E. L., and Huang, Y. H. Self-stimulation pathways in the monkey, *Macaca mulatta. Experimental Neurology,* 1971, **33**, 213–224.[289]

Routtenberg, A., and Huang, Y. H. Reticular formation and brainstem unitary activity: Effects of posterior hypothalamic and septal-limbic stimulation at reward loci. *Physiology and Behavior,* 1968, **3**, 611–617. [277, 282, 292, 296, 297, 300]

Routtenberg, A., and Kane, R. S. Weight loss following lesions at the self-stimulation point: Ventral midbrain tegmentum. *Canadian Journal of Psychology,* 1966, **20**, 343–351. [271, 272, 310]

Routtenberg, A., and Kramis, R. C. "Foot-stomping" in the gerbil: Rewarding brain stimulation, sexual behavior and foot shock. *Nature,* 1967, **214**, 173–174. [305, 306]

Routtenberg, A., and Kramis, R. C. Hippocampal correlates of aversive midbrain stimulation. *Science,* 1968, **160**, 1363–1365.[250, 251, 303, 309]

Routtenberg, A., and Lindy, J. Effects of the availability of rewarding septal and hypothalamic stimulation on bar pressing for food under conditions of deprivation. *Journal of Comparative and Physiological Psychology,* 1965, **60**, 158–161.[267]

Routtenberg, A., and Malsbury, C. Brainstem pathways of reward. *Journal of Comparative and Physiological Psychology,* 1969, **68**, 22–30. [264, 272, 274, 275, 278, 279, 282, 283, 296, 310, 312, 314]

Routtenberg, A., and Sugar, R. Runway performance following lesions at the self-stimulation point in midbrain tegmentum. Unpublished manuscript, Northwestern University, 1966. [272]

Routtenberg, A., and Vern, B. Septal-limbic response to stimulation at hypothalamic reward sites: microelectrode study. Unpublished manuscript, Northwestern University, 1968. [293, 297]

Routtenberg, A., Zechmeister, E. B., and Benton, C. Hippocampal activity during memory disruption of passive avoidance by electroconvulsive shock. *Life Sciences,* 1970, **9**, 909–918. [307, 312]

Rozkowska, E., and Fonberg, E. The effects of lateral hypothalamic lesions on food intake and instrumental alimentary reflex in dogs. *Acta Neurobiologiae Experimentalis,* 1970, **30**, 59–68. [179]

Rożkowska, E., and Fonberg, E. Effect of ventromedial hypothalamic lesions on food intake and alimentary instrumental conditioned reflexes in dogs. *Acta Neurobiologiae Experimentalis,* 1971, **31,** 351–364. [183]

Ruch, T. C., Chang, H. T., and Ward, A. A., Jr. The pattern of muscular response to evoked cortical discharge. *Proceedings of the Association for Research in Nervous and Mental Disease,* 1946, **26,** 61–83. [95]

Runnels, P., and Thompson, R. Hypothalamic structures critical for the performance of a locomotor escape response in the rat. *Brain Research,* 1969, **13,** 328–337. [11]

Russell, J. R., and DeMyer, W. The quantitative cortical origin of pyramidal axons of *Macaca rhesus. Neurology,* 1961, **11,** 96–109. [72, 74]

Sacher, G. A. Allometric and factorial analysis of brain structure in insectivores and primates. In C. R. Noback and M. Montagna (Eds.), *Advances in primatology.* Vol. 1, The primate brain. New York: Appleton-Century-Crofts, 1970. Pp. 245–287. [81]

Sachs, E., Jr. and Brendler, S. J. Some effects of stimulation of the orbital surface of the frontal lobe in the dog and monkey. *Federation Proceedings,* 1948, **7,** 107. [13]

Sainsbury, R. S. Hippocampal activity during natural behavior in the guinea pig. *Physiology and Behavior,* 1970, **5,** 317–324. [230]

Sawa, M., and Delgado, J. Amygdala unitary activity in the unrestrained cat. *Electroencephalography and Clinical Neurophysiology,* 1963, **15,** 637–650. [132]

Schäfer, E. A. Experiments on the paths taken by volitional impulses passing from the cerebral cortex to the cord: The pyramids and the ventro-lateral descending paths. *Quarterly Journal of Experimental Physiology,* 1910, **3,** 355–373. [71, 89]

Schaltenbrand, G., and Cobb, S. Clinical and anatomical studies on two cats without neocortex. *Brain,* 1931, **53,** 449–488. [105, 106]

Scheibel, M. E., and Scheibel, A. B. Terminal axonal patterns in cat spinal cord. I. The lateral corticospinal tract. *Brain Research,* 1966, **2,** 333–350. [83, 84]

Schoen, J. H. R. Corticospinal projections in some primates. *Acta Morphologica Neerlando-Scandinavica,* 1966, **6,** 408–409. [75]

Schreiner, L. H., Rioch, D. McK., Pechtel, C., and Masserman, J. H. Behavioral changes following thalamic injury in cat. *Journal of Neurophysiology,* 1953, **16,** 234–246. [131]

Schwartzbaum, J. S., Kellicutt, M. H., Spieth, T. M., and Thompson, J. B. Effect of septal lesions in rats on response inhibition associated with food-reinforced behavior. *Journal of Comparative and Physiological Psychology,* 1964, **58,** 217–224. [14]

Sclafani, A., and Grossman, S. P. Reactivity of hyperphagic and normal rats to quinine and electric shock. *Journal of Comparative and Physiological Psychology,* 1971, **74,** 157–166. [211]

Scott, J. W. Brain stimulation reinforcement with distributed practice: Effects of electrode locus, previous experience and stimulus intensity. *Journal of Comparative and Physiological Psychology,* 1967, **63,** 175–183. [266]

Scoville, W. B., and Milner, B. Loss of recent memory after bilateral hippocampal lesions. *Journal of Neurology, Neurosurgery, and Psychiatry,* 1947, **20,** 11–21. [132]

Semmes, J., Mishkin, J., and Cole, M. Effects of isolating sensorimotor cortex in monkeys. *Cortex,* 1968, **4,** 301–327. [96]

Sepinwall, J., and Grodsky, F. S. Effects of cholinergic stimulation or blockade of the rat hypothalamus on discrete-trial conflict behaviour. *Life Sciences,* 1969, 8, 45–52. [212, 214]

Sharpless, S. Designated discussion. In H. H. Jasper (Ed.), *Reticular formation of the brain.* Boston, Massachusetts: Little, Brown, 1958. [271, 292]

Shibasaki, H. Fiber-analytical studies on the pyramidal tracts in cerebrovascular and motor neuron diseases. *Folia Psychiatrica et Neurologica Japonica,* 1968, **22,** 205–226. [78]

Shibasaki, H., and Wasano, T. Fiber-analytical studies of the pyramidal tracts following unilateral motor cortex ablation in monkeys. *Okajimas Folia Anatomica Japonica,* 1969, **45**, 227–240. [78]

Shriver, J. E., and Matzke, H. A. Corticobulbar and corticospinal tracts in the marmoset monkey (*Oedipomidas oedipus*). *Anatomical Record,* 1965, **151**, 416. [75]

Shurrager, P. S., and Culler, E. A. Phenomena allied to conditioning in the spinal dog. *American Journal of Physiology,* 1938, **123**, 186–187. [112, 113]

Shurrager, P. S., and Culler, E. A. Conditioning in the spinal dog. *Journal of Experimental Psychology,* 1940, **26**, 133–159. [112, 113]

Shurrager, P. S., and Culler, E. A. Conditioned extinction of a reflex in the spinal dog. *Journal of Experimental Psychology,* 1941, **28**, 287–303. [112, 113]

Shute, C. C. D., and Lewis, P. R. The ascending cholinergic reticular system: Neocortical, olfactory and subcortical projections. *Brain,* 1967, **90**, 497–518. [209, 219]

Simpson, S. The motor cortex and pyramidal tract in the raccoon (*Procyon lotor,* Linn.). *Proceedings of the Society for Experimental Biology and Medicine, New York,* 1912, **10**, 46–47. [75]

Simpson, S. The pyramid tract in the red squirrel (*Sciurus hudsonius loquax*) and chipmunk (*Tamias striatus lysteri*). *Journal of Comparative Neurology,* 1914, **24**, 137–160. [76]

Simpson, S. The motor areas and pyramid tract in the Canadian porcupine (*Erethizon dorsatus,* Linn.). *Quarterly Journal of Experimental Physiology,* 1915, **8**, 79–102. (a) [76]

Simpson, S. The pyramid tract in the striped gopher (*Spermophilus tridecemlineatus* [Mitchell]). *Quarterly Journal of Experimental Physiology,* 1915, **8**, 383–390. (b) [76]

Simpson, S., and King, J. L. Localisation of the motor area in the sheep. *Quarterly Journal of Experimental Physiology,* 1911, **4**, 53–65. [95]

Skinner, B. F. *The behavior of organisms.* New York: Appleton-Century-Crofts, 1938. [4]

Skinner, B. F. Operant behavior. In W. K. Honig (Ed.), *Operant behavior: Areas of research and application.* New York: Appleton-Century-Crofts, 1966. [3]

Slotnick, B. M. Disturbances of maternal behaviour in the rat following lesions of the cingulate cortex. *Behaviour,* 1967, **29**, 204–236. [260]

Smith, A. M. The effects of rubral lesions and stimulation on conditioned forelimb flexion responses in the cat. *Physiology and Behavior,* 1970, **5**, 1121–1126. [9]

Smith, K. U., and Ansell, S. Closed-loop digital computer system for study of sensory feedback effects of brain rhythms. *American Journal of Physical Medicine,* 1965, **44**, 125–137. [59]

Smith, K. U., and Henry, J. P. Cybernetic foundations for rehabilitation. *American Journal of Physical Medicine,* 1967, **46**, 379–467. [46]

Smith, K. U., and Luetke, A. F. Experimental feedback analysis of external respiration and behavior. Madison, Wisconsin: University of Wisconsin Behavioral Cybernetics Laboratory, 1969. [52]

Smith, K. U., and Putz, V. Feedback analysis of learning and performance in steering and tracking behavior. *Journal of Applied Psychology,* 1970, **54**, 239–247. [46]

Smith, K. U., and Sussman, H. Cybernetic theory and analysis of motor learning and memory. In E. Bilodeau (Ed.), *Principles of skill acquisition.* New York: Academic Press, 1969. [46]

Smith, N. S., and Coons, E. E. Temporal summation and refractoriness in hypothalamic reward neurons as measured by self-stimulation behavior. *Science,* 1970, **169**, 782–785. [299]

Smythies, J. R., Gibson, W. C., Purkis, V. A., and Lowes, I. A. Some efferent connexions of the frontal lobe with a critique of the method of terminal degeneration. *Journal of Comparative Neurology,* 1957, **107**, 57–107. [172]

Sokolov, E. N. Higher nervous functions: the orienting reflex. *Annual Review of Physiology,* 1963, **25**, 545–580. [133]

Soltysik, S., and Jaworska, K. Prefrontal cortex and fear-motivated behaviour. *Acta Biologiae Experimentalis,* 1967, **27**, 429–448. [183]

Sperry, R. W., and Miner, N. Pattern perception following insertion of mica plates into visual cortex. *Journal of Comparative and Physiological Psychology,* 1955, **48**, 463-469. [103]

Spies, G. Food versus intracranial self-stimulation reinforcement in food-deprived rats. *Journal of Comparative and Physiological Psychology,* 1965, **60**, 153–157. [273]

Stanley, W. C., and Jaynes, J. The function of the frontal cortex. *Psychological Review,* 1949, **56**, 18–32. [13]

Stark, P., and Totty, C. W. Effects of amphetamines on eating elicited by hypothalamic stimulation. *Journal of Pharmacology and Experimental Therapy,* 1967, **158**, 272–278. [220]

Stark, P., Totty, C. W., Turk, J. A., and Henderson, J. K. A possible role of a cholinergic system affecting hypothalamic-elicited eating. *American Journal of Physiology,* 1968, **214**, 463–468. [205, 221]

Stavraky, G. W. *Supersensitivity following lesions of the nervous system.* Toronto, Canada: University of Toronto Press, 1961. [115]

Stein, L. Facilitation of avoidance behavior by positive brain stimulation. *Journal of Comparative and Physiological Psychology,* 1965, **60**, 9–19. [296]

Stein, L. Chemistry of purposive behavior. In J. T. Tapp (Ed.), *Reinforcement and behavior.* New York: Academic Press, 1969. [204, 207, 224]

Stein, L., and Wise, C. D. Release of norepinephrine from hypothalamus and amygdala by rewarding medial forebrain bundle stimulation and amphetamine. *Journal of Comparative and Physiological Psychology,* 1969, **67**, 189–198. [220]

Stępień, I., and Stamm, J. S. Locomotor delayed response in frontally ablated monkeys. *Acta Neurobiologiae Experimentalis,* 1970, **30**, 13–18.   (a) [189]

Stępień, I., and Stamm, J. Impairments on locomotor task involving spatial opposition between cue and reward in frontally ablated monkeys. *Acta Neurobiologiae Experimentalis,* 1970, **30**, 1–12.   (b) [197]

Stepien, I., and Stępień, L. The effects of bilateral lesions in precruciate cortex on simple locomotor conditioned response in dogs. *Acta Biologiae Experimentalis,* 1965, **25**, 387–394. [179]

Stępień, I., Stępień, L., and Konorski, J. The effects of bilateral lesions in the premotor cortex on type II conditioned reflexes in dogs. *Acta Biologiae Experimentalis,* 1960, **20**, 225–242. [179]

Stępień, I., Stępień, L., and Kreiner, J. The effects of total and partial ablations of the premotor cortex on the instrumental conditioned reflexes in dogs. *Acta Biologiae Experimentalis,* 1963, **23**, 45–60. [179]

Stępień, I., Stępień, L., and Sychowa, B. Disturbance of motor conditioned behaviour following bilateral ablations of the precruciate area in dogs and cats. *Acta Biologiae Experimentalis,* 1966, **26**, 323–340. [179]

Stetsen, R. H. *Motor phonetics.* Amsterdam: North–Holland Publ., 1951. [55]

Stewart, D. H., Jr., and Preston, J. B. Functional coupling between the pyramidal tract and segmental motoneurons in cat and primate. *Journal of Neurophysiology,* 1967, **30**, 453–465. [89]

Stewart, W. A., and King, R. B. Fiber projections from the nucleus caudalis of the spinal trigeminal nucleus. *Journal of Comparative Neurology,* 1963, **121**, 271–286. [171]

Stolerman, I. P. Factors determining the effect of chlorpromazine on the food intake of rats. *Nature,* 1967, **215**, 1518–1519. [221]

Strominger, N. L. A comparison of the pyramidal tracts in two species of edentate. *Brain Research,* 1969, **15,** 259–262. [77]

Stumpf, Ch. The fast component in the electrical activity of the rabbits' hippocampus. *Electroencephalography and Clinical Neurophysiology,* 1965, **18,** 477–486.   (a) [230]

Stumpf, Ch. Drug action on the electrical activity of the hippocampus. *International Review of Neurobiology,* 1965, **8,** 77–138.   (b) [246, 253, 254]

Stumpf, Ch., Petsche, H., and Gogolak, G. The significance of the rabbit's septum as a relay station between the midbrain and the hippocampus. II. The differential influence of drugs upon both septal cell firing pattern and the hippocampus theta activity. *Electroencephalography and Clinical Neurophysiology,* 1962, **14,** 212–219. [17]

Sugar, O., Chusid, J. G., and French, J. D. A second motor cortex in the monkey (*Macaca mulatta*). *Journal of Neuropathology and Experimental Neurology,* 1948, 7, 182–189. [69]

Szabo, J. Topical distribution of the striatal efferents in the monkey. *Experimental Neurology,* 1962, **5,** 21–36. [139, 168, 172, 173]

Szabo, J. The efferent projections of the putamen in the monkey. *Experimental Neurology,* 1967, **19,** 463–476. [139, 168, 172, 173]

Szabo, J. Projections from the body of the caudate nucleus in the rhesus monkey. *Experimental Neurology,* 1970, **27,** 1–15. [139, 172, 173]

Szentágothai-Schimert, J. Die Endigungweise der absteigenden Rückenmarksbahnen. *Zeitschrift für Anatomie und Entwicklungsgeschichte,* 1941, **111,** 322–330. [83]

Szwejkowska, G. Further properties of the alternation conditioned reflexes in dogs. *Acta Biologiae Experimentalis,* 1965, **25,** 3–11.   (a) [198]

Szwejkowska, G. The effect of prefrontal lesions on instrumental conditioned alternation reflexes in dogs. *Acta Biologiae Experimentalis,* 1965, **25,** 379–386.   (b) [198, 199]

Szwejkowska, G., Kreiner, J., and Sychowa, B. The effect of partial lesions of the prefrontal area on alimentary conditioned reflexes in dogs. *Acta Biologiae Experimentalis,* 1963, **23,** 181–192. [182]

Szwejkowska, G., Ławicka, W., and Konorski, J. The properties of alternation of conditioned reflexes in dogs. *Acta Biologiae Experimentalis,* 1964, **24,** 135–144. [198]

Szwejkowska, G., Stępień, L., and Kreiner, J. The effect of subproreal lesions of the prefrontal area on alimentary conditioned reflexes in dogs. *Acta Biologiae Experimentalis,* 1965, **25,** 373–378. [182]

Szwejkowska, G., and Sychowa, B. The effect of lesions of auditory cortex on discrimination of sound localization in dogs. *Acta Neurobiologiae Experimentalis,* 1971, **31,** 237–250. [182]

Taeschler, M., and Cerletti, A. Differential analysis of the effects of phenothiazine tranquilizers on emotional and motor behavior in experimental animals. *Nature,* 1959, **184,** 823–824. [258]

Talairach, J., Paillas, J. E., and David, M. Dyskinésie de type hémiballique traitée par cortectomie frontale limitée puis par coagulation de l'anse lenticulaire et de la portion interne du globus pallidus. *Revue Neurologique,* 1950, **83,** 440–451. [165]

Teitelbaum, H., and Milner, P. Activity changes following hippocampal lesions in rats. *Journal of Comparative and Physiological Psychology,* 1963, **56,** 284–289. [260]

ten Cate, J. Können die bedingten Realisationen sich auch ausserhalb der Grosshirnrinde bilden? *Archives Néerlandaises de Physiologie,* 1934, **19,** 469–481. [102]

Takahashi, K. Slow and fast groups of pyramidal tract cells and their respective membrane properties. *Journal of Neurophysiology,* 1965, **28,** 908–924. [88]

Takahashi, K., Kubota, K., and Uno, M. Recurrent facilitation in cat pyramidal tract cells. *Journal of Neurophysiology,* 1967, **30,** 22–34. [88]

Thomas, G. J., Hostetter, G., and Barker, D. J. Behavioral functions of the limbic system. In E. Stellar and J. M. Sprague (Eds.), *Progress in Physiological Psychology.* Vol. 2. New York: Academic Press, 1968. [15]

Thomas, G. J., and Otis, L. S. Effects of rhinencephalic lesions on maze learning in rats. *Journal of Comparative and Physiological Psychology,* 1958, **51**, 161–166. [260]

Thompson, R., and Massopust, L. C., Jr. The effect of subcortical lesions on retention of a brightness discrimination in rats. *Journal of Comparative and Physiological Psychology,* 1960, **53**, 488–496. [131]

Thorndike, E. L. *The fundamentals of learning.* New York: Teachers College, Columbia University, 1932. [61]

Thorpe, W. H. *Learning and instinct in animals.* London: Methuen, 1963. [101]

Tilney, F. The brain stem of *Tarsius.* A critical comparison with other primates. *Journal of Comparative Neurology,* 1927, **43**, 342–371. [75]

Torii, S. Two types of pattern of hippocampal electrical activity induced by stimulation of hypothalamus and surrounding parts of rabbit's brain. *Japanese Journal of Physiology,* 1961, **11**, 147–157. [311, 312]

Towe, A. L. Sensory-motor organization and movement. In E. V. Evarts, E. Bizzi, R. E. Burke, M. DeLong, and W. T. Thach, Jr. (Eds.), *Neurosciences Research Program Bulletin,* 1971, **9** (1), 40–48. [206]

Towe, A. L. Relative numbers of pyramidal tract neurons in mammals of different sizes. *Brain, Behavior, and Evolution,* 1972, in press. [81]

Towe, A. L., and Biedenbach, M. A. Observations on the primitive pyramidal system of the American opossum. *Brain, Behavior and Evolution,* 1969, **2**, 498–529. [71, 74, 76, 96]

Towe, A. L., and Harding, G. W. Extracellular microelectrode sampling bias. *Experimental Neurology,* 1970, **29**, 366–381. [78, 88]

Towe, A. L., Whitehorn, D., and Nyquist, J. K. Differential activity among wide-field neurons of the cat postcruciate cerebral cortex. *Experimental Neurology,* 1968, **20**, 497–521. [87]

Tower, S. S. The dissociation of cortical excitation from cortical inhibition by pyramid section, and the syndrome of that lesion in the cat. *Brain,* 1935, **58**, 238–255. [89]

Toyama, K., Tsukahara, N., Kosaka, K., and Matsunami, K. Synaptic excitation of red nucleus neurones by fibres from interpositus nucleus. *Experimental Brain Research,* 1970, **11**, 187–198. [285]

Travis, A. M., and Woolsey, C. N. Motor performance of monkeys after bilateral partial and total cerebral decortications. *American Journal of Physical Medicine,* 1956, **35**, 273–310. [69, 89, 95]

Trowill, J. A., Panksepp, J., and Gandelman, R. An incentive model of rewarding brain stimulation. *Psychological Review,* 1969, **76**, 264–281. [266]

Tsukahara, N., and Fuller, D. R. G. Conductance changes during pyramidally induced postsynaptic potentials in red nucleus neurons. *Journal of Neurophysiology,* 1969, **32**, 35–42. [72, 83, 88]

Tsukahara, N., Fuller, D. R. G., and Brooks, V. B. Collateral pyramidal influences on the corticorubrospinal system. *Journal of Neurophysiology,* 1968, **31**, 467–484. [72, 83, 88]

Tunturi, A. R. Effects of lesions of the auditory and adjacent cortex on conditioned reflexes. *American Journal of Physiology,* 1955, **181**, 225–227. [103]

Turner, E. Hippocampus and memory. *Lancet,* 1969, **2**, 1123–1126. [132]

Uesugi, M. Über die corticalen extrapyramidalen Faser aus den sog. sensiblen Rindenfeldern (Areae 1 und 2) beim Affen. *Anatomischer Anzeiger,* 1937, **83**, 179–197. [74]

Ursin, H., Linck, P., and McCleary, R. A. Spatial differentiation of avoidance deficit following septal and cingulate lesions. *Journal of Comparative and Physiological Psychology,* 1969, **68**, 74–79. [2]

Valenstein, E. S. Problems of measurement and interpretation with reinforcing brain stimulation. *Psychological Review,* 1964, 71, 415–437. [270]

Valenstein, E. S. The anatomical locus of reinforcement. In E. Steller (Ed.), *Progress in physiological psychology.* Vol. 1. New York: Academic Press, 1966. [267]

Valenstein, E. S. Behavior elicited by hypothalamic stimulation: A prepotency hypothesis. *Brain, Behavior and Evolution,* 1969, 2, 295–316. [11]

Valenstein, E. S. Stability and plasticity of motivation systems. In F. O. Schmitt (Ed.), *The neurosciences: Second study program.* New York: Rockefeller University Press, 1970. [11, 12]

Valenstein, E. S., and Campbell, J. F. Medial forebrain bundle-lateral hypothalamic area and reinforcing brain stimulation. *American Journal of Physiology,* 1964, 210, 270–274. [267]

Valenstein, E. S., Cox, V. C., and Kakolewski, J. W. The Hypothalamus and motivated behavior. In J. Tapp (Ed.), *Reinforcement and behavior.* New York: Academic Press, 1969. [6, 11]

Valenstein, E. S., Cox, V. C., and Kakolewski, J. W. Reexamination of the role of the hypothalamus in motivation. *Psychological Review,* 1970, 77, 16–31. [11]

Valverde, F. The pyramidal tract in rodents. A study of its relations with the posterior column nuclei, dorsolateral reticular formation of the medulla oblongata, and cervical spinal cord. *Zeitschrift für Zellforschung und mikroskopische Anatomie,* 1966, 71, 297–363. [73, 76, 83, 84]

van Crevel, H., and Verhaart, W. J. C. The rate of secondary degeneration in the central nervous system. I. The pyramidal tract of the cat. *Journal of Anatomy (London),* 1963, 97, 429–449. (a) [72]

van Crevel, H., and Verhaart, W. J. C. The "exact" origin of the pyramidal tract. A quantitative study in the cat. *Journal of Anatomy (London),* 1963, 97, 495–515. (b) [74, 79, 80]

Vanderwolf, C. H. Medial thalamic functions in voluntary behavior. *Canadian Journal of Psychology,* 1962, 16, 318–330. [246]

Vanderwolf, C. H. Hippocampal electrical activity and voluntary movement in the rat. *Electroencephalography and Clinical Neurophysiology,* 1969, 26, 407–418. [230, 248, 306]

Vanderwolf, C. H. Limbic-diencephalic mechanisms of voluntary movement. *Psychological Review,* 1971, 78, 83–113. [230, 246, 261]

van der Vloet, A. Ueber den Verlauf der Pyramidenbahn bei neideren Säugetieren. *Anatomischer Anzeiger (Jena),* 1906, 29, 113–132. [73, 75, 76]

van Lenhossék, M. Über die Pyramidenbahnen in Rückenmarke einiger Säugetiere. *Anatomischer Anzeiger,* 1889, 4, 208–219. [74, 75, 76]

Verhaart, W. J. C. The pes pedunculi and pyramid. *Journal of Comparative Neurology,* 1948, 88, 139–155. [78]

Verhaart, W. J. C. Fiber tracts and fiber patterns in the anterior and the lateral funiculus of the cord in *Macaca ira. Acta Anatomica (London),* 1954, 20, 330–373. [75]

Verhaart, W. J. C. Pyramidal tract in the cord of the elephant. *Journal of Comparative Neurology,* 1963, 121, 45–49. [76]

Verhaart, W. J. C. The pyramidal tract of *Tupaia,* compared to that in other primates. *Journal of Comparative Neurology,* 1966, 126, 43–50. [75]

Verhaart, W. J. C. The non-crossing of the pyramidal tract in *Procavia capensis* (Storr) and other instances of absence of the pyramidal crossing. *Journal of Comparative Neurology,* 1967, 137, 387–392. [73, 76]

Verhaart, W. J. C. The pyramidal tract in the primates. In C. R. Noback and W. Montagna (Eds.), *Advances in primatology.* Vol. 1, The primate brain. New York: Appleton-Century-Crofts, 1970. Pp. 83–108. [75, 77, 78, 79]

Verhaart, W. J. C., and Kramer, W. The uncrossed pyramidal tract. *Acta Psychiatrica et Neurologica Scandinavica*, 1952, **27**, 181–200. [75]

Verhaart, W. J. C., and Kramer, W. The pyramid in the medulla and the cord of the elephant. *Acta Morphologica Neerlando-Scandinavica*, 1959, **2**, 174–181. [76]

Verhaart, W. J. C., and Noorduyn, N. J. A. The cerebral peduncle and the pyramid. *Acta Anatomica*, 1961, **45**, 315–343. [74, 77, 79, 80, 84, 85]

Villablanca, J. Personal communication, 1971. [109, 110, 111]

Vinogradova, O. S. Dynamic classification of the reactions of hippocampal neurons to sensory stimuli. *Federation Proceedings, Translation Supplement*, 1966, **25**, T397–T403. [132]

Vogt, C., and Vogt, O. Allgemeinere Ergebnisse unserer Hirnforschung. *Journal für Psychologie und Neurologie (Leipzig)*, 1919, **25**, 277–462. [69]

Voneida, T. J. An experimental study of the course and destination of fibers arising from the head of the caudate nucleus in the cat and monkey. *Journal of Comparative Neurology*, 1960, **115**, 75–87. [139, 168, 172]

Walberg, F., and Brodal, A. Pyramidal tract fibers from temporal and occipital lobes. An experimental study in the cat. *Brain*, 1953, **76**, 491–508. [74]

Walker, A. E. *The primate thalamus*. Chicago, Illinois: University of Chicago Press, 1938. [165, 171]

Walker, A. E. Afferent connections. In P. C. Bucy (Ed.), *The precentral motor cortex*, 2nd ed., Chapter 4. Urbana, Illinois: University of Illinois, 1949. Pp. 112–132. [165]

Walters, G. C., and Glazer, R. D. Punishment of instinctive behavior in the Mongolian gerbil. *Journal of Comparative and Physiological Psychology*, 1971, **75**, 331–340. [8]

Wang, G. H., and Akert, K. Behavior and reflexes of chronic striatal cats. *Archives Italiennes Biologie*, 1962, **100**, 48–85. [105, 106, 261]

Warren, J. M., and Akert, K. Impaired problem solving by cats with thalamic lesions. *Journal of Comparative and Physiological Psychology*, 1960, **53**, 207–211. [131]

Weber, D., and Buchwald, J. S. A technique for recording and integrating multiple unit activity simultaneously with the EEG in chronic cats. *Electroencephalography and Clinical Neurophysiology*, 1965, **19**, 190–192. [118]

Weed, L. H. The reactions of kittens after decerebration. *American Journal of Physiology*, 1917, **43**, 131–157. [109]

Webster, K. E. Cortico-striate interrelations in the albino rat. *Journal of Anatomy*, 1961, **95**, 532–544. [139, 172]

Webster, K. E. The cortico-striatal projection in the cat. *Journal of Anatomy*, 1965, **99**, 329–337. [172]

Weil, A. A rapid method of staining myelin sheaths. *Archives of Neurology and Psychiatry*, 1928, **20**, 392–393. [289]

Weil, A., and Lassek, A. M. The quantitative distribution of the pyramidal tract in man. *Archives of Neurology and Psychiatry*, 1929, **22**, 495–510. [75, 82]

Weiskrantz, L. Behavioral changes associated with ablation of the amygdaloid complex in monkeys. *Journal of Comparative and Physiological Psychology*, 1956, **49**, 381–391. [132]

Weiskrantz, L., and Mishkin, M. Effects of temporal and frontal cortical lesions on auditory discrimination in monkeys. *Brain*, 1958, **81**, 406–414. [186]

Weissman, A. Licking behavior of rats on a schedule of food reinforcement. *Science*, 1962, **135**, 99–101. [220]

Welker, W. I., Benjamin, R. M., Miles, R. C., and Woolsey, C. N. Motor effects of cortical stimulation in squirrel monkey (*Saimiri sciureus*). *Journal of Neurophysiology*, 1957, **20**, 347–364. [69, 96]

Werman, R., Davidoff, R. A., and Aprison, M. H. Inhibitory action of glycine on spinal neurons in the cat. *Journal of Neurophysiology*, 1968, **31**, 81–95. [214, 215]

Wetzel, M. C. Self-stimulation's anatomy: data needs. *Brain Research,* 1968, **10**, 287–296. [268]

Whishaw, I. Q. *Comparative studies of the relation of hippocampal electrical activity to behavior.* Unpublished Ph.D. thesis, University of Western Ontario, 1971. [230, 240, 241, 242, 243, 244, 245, 248, 249, 253]

Whishaw, I. Q., and Vanderwolf, C. H. Hippocampal EEG and behavior: Effects of variation in body temperature and relation of EEG to vibrissae movement, swimming and shivering. *Physiology and Behavior,* 1971, **6**, 391–397. [230, 261]

Whishaw, I. Q., Bland, B. H., and Vanderwolf, C. H. Hippocampal activity, behavior, self-stimulation and heart rate during electrical stimulation of the lateral hypothalamus. *Journal of Comparative and Physiological Psychology,* 1972, **79**, 115–127. [251, 252, 253]

White, A., Handler, P., and Smith, E. L. *Principles of biochemistry.* New York: McGraw-Hill, 1964. [28, 30, 34]

White, R. P., and Rudolph, A. S. Neuropharmacological comparison of subcortical actions of anticholinergic compounds. In P. B. Bradley (Ed.), *Progress in Brain Research. Anticholinergic drugs and brain functions in animals and man.* Vol. 28. Amsterdam: Elsevier, 1968. Pp. 14–26. [236]

Whitlock, D. G., and Nauta, W. J. H. Subcortical projections from the temporal neocortex in *Macaca mulatta. Journal of Comparative Neurology,* 1956, **106**, 183–211. [170]

Whittier, J. R., and Mettler, F. A. Studies on the subthalamus of the rhesus monkey. II. Hyperkinesia and other physiologic effects of subthalamic lesions with special reference to the subthalamic nucleus of Luys. *Journal of Comparative Neurology,* 1949, **90**, 319–372. [165]

Wiesendanger, M. The pyramidal tract. Recent investigations on its morphology and function. *Ergebnisse der Physiologie,* 1969, **61**, 72–136. [87, 89]

Wiesendanger, M., and Tarnecki, R. Die Rolle des pyramidalen Systems bei der sensorimotorischen Integration. *Bulletin der Schweizerischen Akademie der Medizinischen Wissenschaften,* 1966, **22**, 306–328. [89]

Wiitanen, J. T. Selective silver impregnation of degenerating axons and axon terminals in the central nervous system of the monkey (*Macaca mulatta*). *Brain Research,* 1969, **14**, 546–548. [138, 155]

Winer, B. J. *Statistical principles in experimental design.* New York: McGraw-Hill, 1962. [51]

Woodburne, R. T., Crosby, E. C., and McCotter, R. E. The mammalian midbrain and isthmus regions. II. The fiber connections. A. The relations of the tegmentum of the midbrain with the basal ganglia in *Macaca mulatta. Journal of Comparative Neurology,* 1946, **85**, 67–92. [166]

Woods, J. W. Behavior of chronic decerebrate rats. *Journal of Neurophysiology,* 1964, **27**, 635–644. [109, 259, 261]

Woolsey, C. N. Organization of somatic sensory and motor areas of the cerebral cortex. In H. F. Harlow and C. N. Woolsey (Eds.), *Biological and biochemical bases of behavior.* Madison, Wisconsin: University of Wisconsin Press, 1958. Pp. 63–81. [69, 96]

Woolsey, C. N., Settlage, P. H., Meyer, D. R., Spencer, W., Pinto-Hamuy, T., and Travis, A. M. Patterns of localization in precentral and "supplementary" motor areas and their relation to the concept of a premotor area. *Research Publication of the Association for Research in Nervous and Mental Disease,* 1951, **30**, 238–264. [69]

Woolsey, C. N., Travis, A. M., Barnard, J. W., and Ostenso, R. S. Motor representation in the postcentral gyrus after chronic ablation of precentral and supplementary motor areas. *Federation Proceedings,* 1953, **12**, 160. [69, 96]

Wyrwicka, W. Studies on motor conditioned reflexes. 5. On the mechanism of the motor conditioned reaction. *Acta Biologiae Experimentalis,* 1952, **16**, 131–137. [179]

Yahr, M. D., and Purpura, D. P. (Eds.), *Neurophysiological basis of normal and abnormal motor activities.* New York: Raven Press, 1967.[264]

Zecha, A. The "pyramidal tract" and other telencephalic efferent in birds. *Acta Morphologica Neerlando-Scandinavica,* 1961, **5,** 194–195.[86]

Zeliony, G. *Transactions of the Society of Russian Physicians* (in Russian), 1911. Pp. 50, 147. Cited by Culler and Mettler, 1934.[104]

Zeliony, G. P. Effets de l'ablation des hémisphères cérébraux. *Revue Médicale, Paris,* 1929, **46,** 191–214. Cited by Girden *et al.,* 1936.[103]

Zeliony, G. P. Observations sur des chiens ausquels on a enlevé les hémisphères cérébraux. *Comptes Rendus de la Société de Biologie,* 1913, **74,** 707–708. [104]

Żernicki, B., Doty, R. W., and Santibanez-H. G. Isolated midbrain in cats. *Electroencephalography and Clinical Neurophysiology,* 1970, **28,** 221–235.[110]

Ziehen, T. Der Aufbau des Cervicalmarks und der Oblongata bei Marsupialiern und Monotremen. *Anatomischer Anzeiger,* 1897, **13,** 171–174.[76]

Ziehen, T. Das Centralnervensystem der Monotremen und Marsupialier. II. Teil. Zweiter Abschnitt. Der Faserverlauf im Gehirn von Echidna und Ornithorhynchus nebst vergleichenden Angaben über den Faserverlauf des Gehirns von Perameles und Macropus. Jena: Fischer, 1908. Pp. 789–921.[76]

Zimmerman, E. A., Chambers, W. W., and Liu, C. N. An experimental study of the anatomical organization of the cortico-bulbar system in the albino rat. *Journal of Comparative Neurology,* 1964, **123,** 301–324. [83, 84, 86]

Zucker, I., and McCleary, R. A. Perseveration in septal cats. *Psychonomic Science,* 1964, **1,** 387–388. [14]

Subject Index